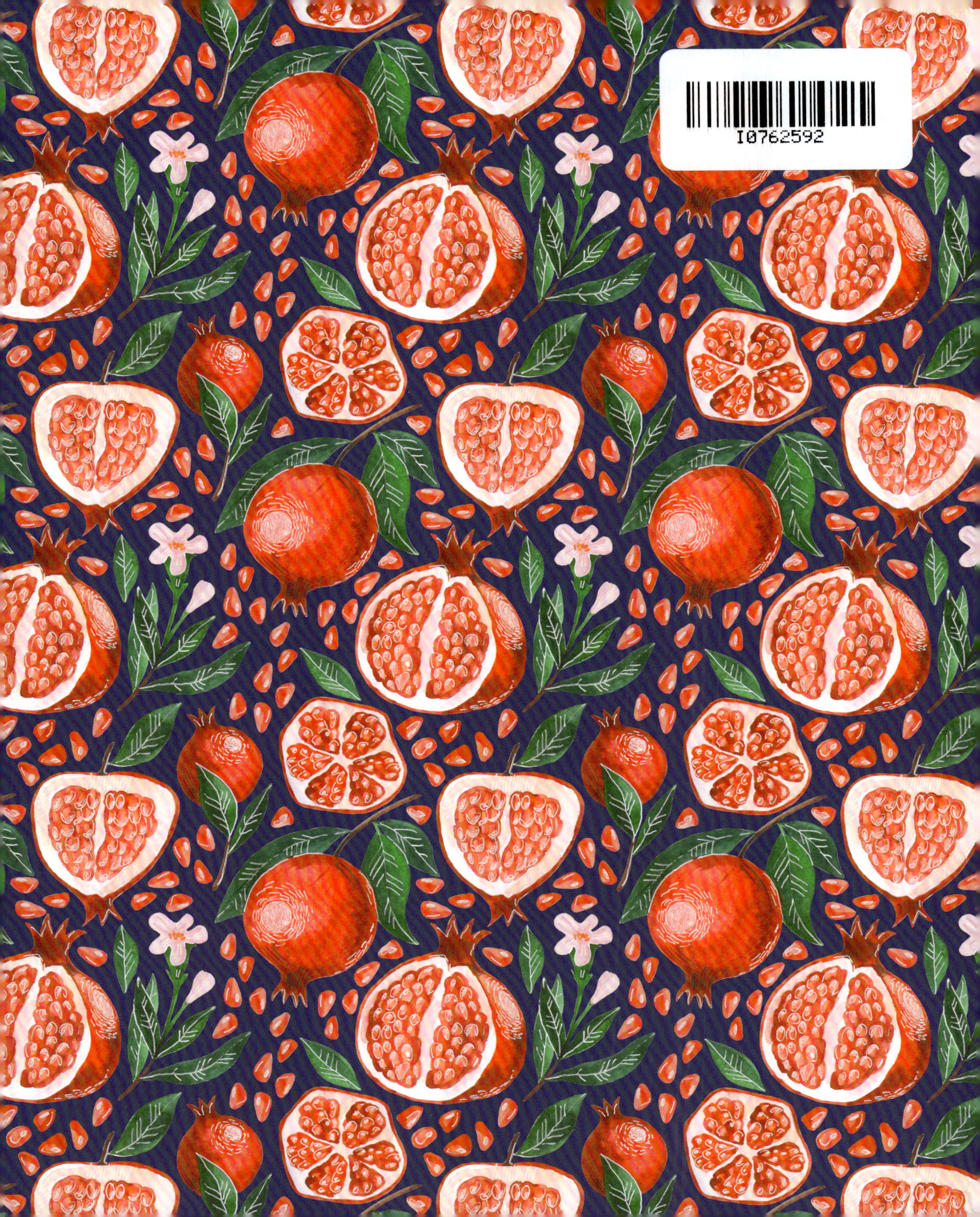

"*The Food Doula Cookbook* should be required reading (and cooking) for all mothers-to-be. It is, hands down, the best pre- and post-natal culinary nutrition-infused cookbook out there. The evidence-based insights, nutrition guidance, menu inspiration, and nutrient-dense, easy-to-make, delicious and beautiful recipes make it an incredible guide for optimal nourishment for expectant mothers. And I have no doubt the recipes will become family staples and favourites long after baby arrives. *The Food Doula Cookbook* is now my go-to recommendation for all expectant moms."

— MEGHAN TELPNER,
BESTSELLING AUTHOR, *THE UNDIET COOKBOOK*, AND
FOUNDER OF THE ACADEMY OF CULINARY NUTRITION

"I was initially drawn to *The Food Doula Cookbook* for the recipes, but Lindsay's comforting words and sage advice stayed with me long after I was hungry. Following the birth of my second child, I was often so exhausted and sleep-deprived that opening the first bag of chips in sight seemed like a good idea. Wrong! That's when I took Lindsay's words to heart and started eating nourishing food. The recipes are beautifully laid out and organized, making it easy for my husband and me to plan meals and snacks that helped me keep my health and well-being a priority. I will continue to revisit this cookbook long after my babies are grown."

— EVANKA OSMAK,
SPORTS ANCHOR, SPORTSNET, AND CO-HOST,
MOMS IN THE MIDDLE PODCAST

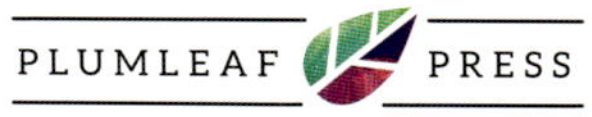

www.plumleafpress.com

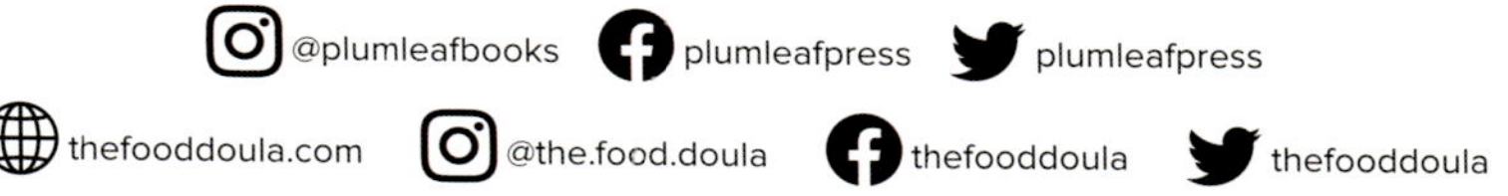

Photography and food styling on recipe pages by Lindsay Taylor
Author photos by Kelly Wilk Photography

Associate Publisher: Kim Koh
Copyeditor: Christine Pillman
Creative Director: Jennifer Drew
Assistant Designer: Robin Forsyth

25 26 27 28 29 8 7 6 5 4

ISBN 978-1-894915-98-4

Printed in China

The FOOD DOULA COOKBOOK

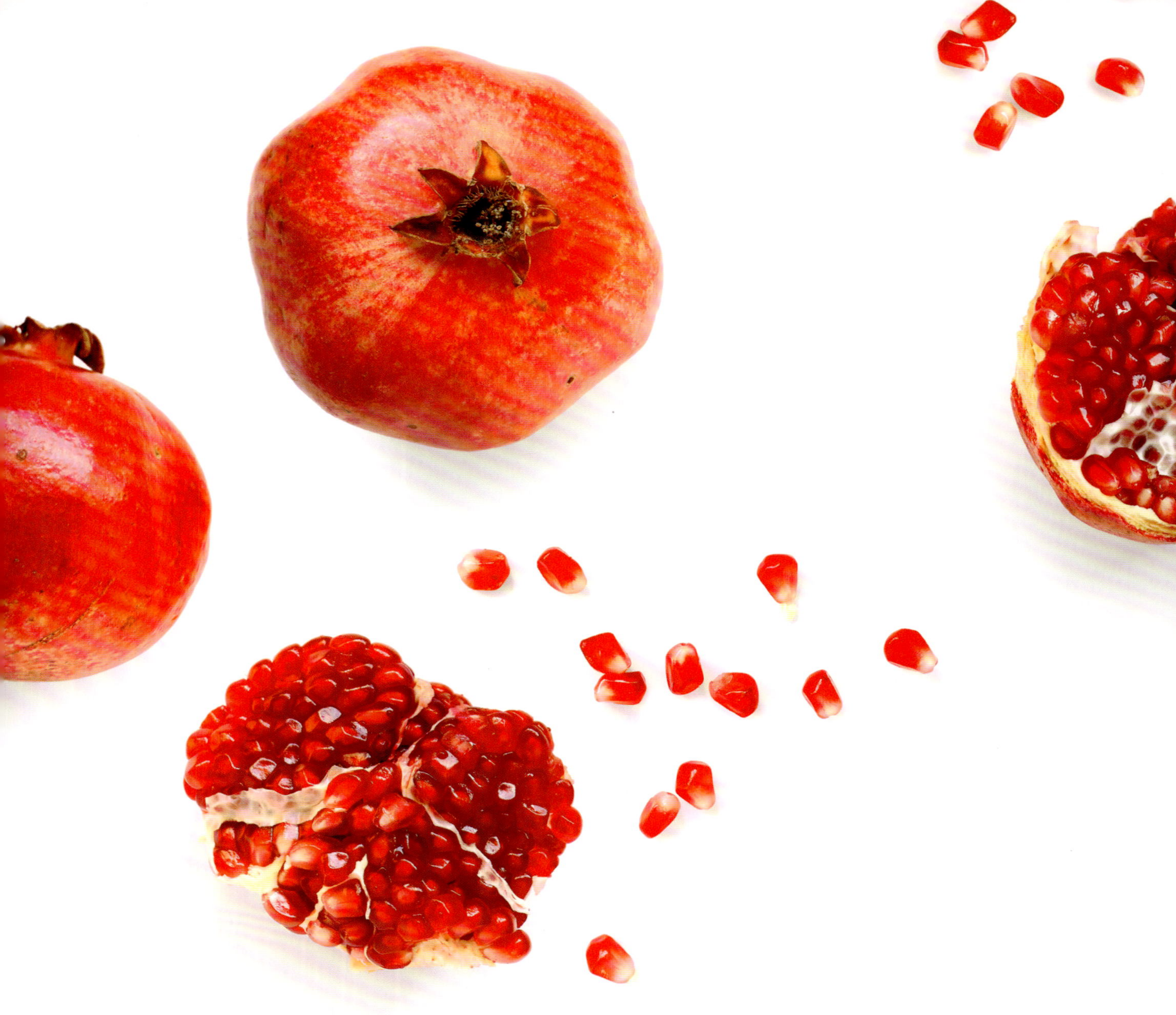

dedication

To Charlotte and Penny, may you bravely
follow that voice inside that wants to be heard.

To Mike, in you I've found the true meaning of the word partner.

To the women who have supported, inspired, taught,
and stood with me in the waves of motherhood and life,
where would I be without you?

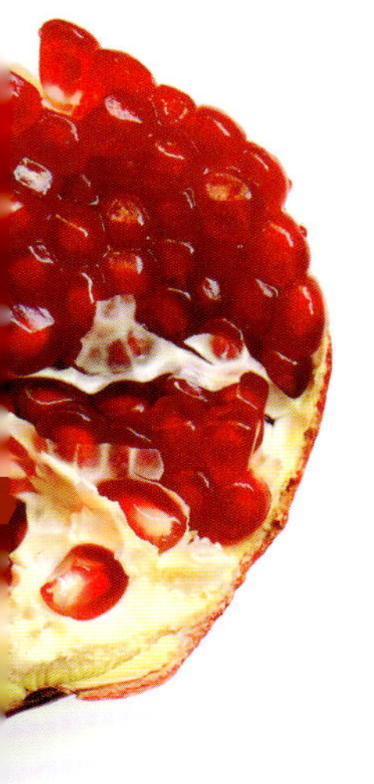

The FOOD DOULA COOKBOOK

A GUIDE TO A HEALTHY PREGNANCY AND A NOURISHED NEW MOM

Lindsay Taylor

CONTENTS

TRIMESTER 3: WEEKS 29–40

TRIMESTER 4: POSTPARTUM

INTRODUCTION

YOU'VE JUST FOUND OUT you're pregnant, and you'd like to eat well for a healthy pregnancy and baby. Questions swirl — *Where do I begin? What can I eat? What should I avoid?*

This feeling of uncertainty and confusion can be overwhelming. I studied nutrition, and yet I was overwhelmed by prenatal nutrition and the application of it in my real life — especially during my first pregnancy. When I looked for information on what to eat, I kept finding prescriptions and charts about the science of nutrition and how much of each macro and micronutrient I should be consuming in one day. None of that helped me at the grocery store when I had to decide what to buy, or in my kitchen when I stared blankly into the fridge wondering what to eat. I came to realize that I didn't need to learn about nutritional science as much as I had to be comfortable choosing, cooking, and eating *real food.*

Knowing what to eat during pregnancy and in the postpartum months can be daunting, and I want to help make it simple and practical, hence this book. As a mom of two, I know you need easy, healthy, and balanced meals, snacks to keep in your purse, and a trusty chocolate treat to keep you going until nap time. I also get that you need a book designed for real life. It is vital to me that this cookbook takes the pressure or guilt off you to do things the "right" way or to always eat the "right" foods. If at times you feel the urge for ice cream, that's okay. I too had a bowl of ice cream on top of the table that was my belly. Sometimes that's just what mama needs. There is no one right way of eating. Just as you are the expert when it comes to your pregnancy and baby, you are also the one who knows best what foods make you feel good.

> Being nourished sufficiently through pregnancy can significantly impact how you feel, how your baby develops, and how your body heals postpartum.

This cookbook focuses on real food for real life, every step of the way. Whether you are feeling good and inspired to prep healthy meals for the week, or you are feeling terrible, have nausea or heartburn, and can't eat much, you'll find a big selection of recipes here to light up your taste buds, satisfy your cravings, and provide essential nutrition for you and baby, plus loads of advice and tips for food prep, meal planning, choosing the most wholesome foods, and cooking up nutritious, delicious meals.

Being nourished sufficiently through pregnancy can significantly impact how you feel, how your baby develops, and how your body heals postpartum. A happy, healthy mother is the most important thing in the world to a baby. As a mom and postpartum doula, I firmly believe that you need care and attention as much as your baby. You deserve to feel good, to receive love and support, to be honoured and appreciated, and to have time to bond with your baby.

Throughout pregnancy and in the first few months postpartum, your nutrition is key to your staying well — mentally, emotionally, and physically.

The Food Doula Cookbook is organized by trimester and offers you real-food solutions to meet your needs as you experience the ebbs and flows that happen in real life from preconception to postpartum.

Do you want chili for breakfast, pancakes for dinner, or soup for an early morning snack? No judgment here. Who needs strict mealtimes when you're feeling nauseated or if you are hungry every hour because you're breastfeeding around the clock? Go ahead and reach for what fuels you and makes you feel your best, no matter the societal norms about what foods suit which time of day.

Good nutrition is key, and what your body needs, what you feel like eating, and what your life looks like will have more to do with what you're going to put on your plate than the time of day.

Wishing you good health and delicious food.

Lindsay

LINDSAY TAYLOR believes in the power of food to help us live our best life, and she believes no one is more deserving of feeling good than mothers and mothers-to-be. With a Master's degree in Public Health, certification as a Postpartum and Infant Care Doula, and an Honours certification as a Culinary Nutrition Expert, Lindsay transforms an academic background in nutritional science into real-food, real-world, and practical solutions to help modern moms feel supported, nourished, and energized as they embrace the challenges and joys of new motherhood.

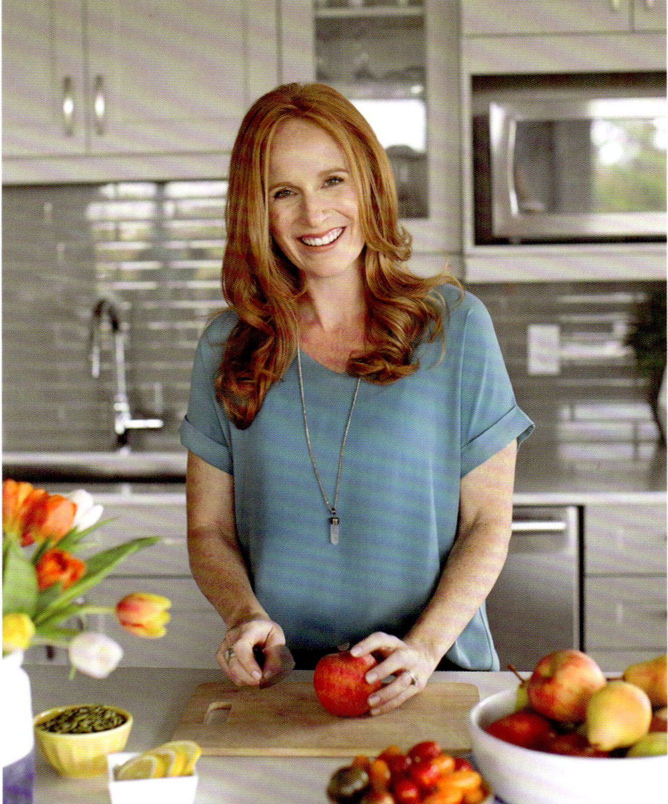

HOW THIS COOKBOOK IS ORGANIZED

This book starts with a look at the benefits of real food for pregnancy, and it includes practical, how-to advice for stocking a prenatal pantry and picking the best foods for mom and baby each step of the way.

The recipes are designed to help you feel your best through each trimester and beyond. They offer healthy and delicious choices to cater to your needs from morning to night. No matter your trimester — feel free to mix and match recipes at any time. The recipes also prioritize plant-based and energizing real-food ingredients, and are perfect additions to your meal rotation for the whole family!

TRIMESTER 1 prioritizes meals that are easy to make, easy to digest, and easy on you if you're feeling tired, terrible, or like you'll be sick forever. You will find recipes for simple comfort foods with ingredients that will pack in the nutrients so that you can eat what you feel like eating and feel confident you're getting in what your baby needs.

TRIMESTER 2 offers recipes that are, hopefully like you at this stage, more colourful and adventurous. The focus is on delicious and satisfying meals you might be craving, including adaptations of typically "off-limits" foods.

TRIMESTER 3 provides lighter, refreshing, and nourishing recipes that won't overstuff your belly, trigger heartburn, or use up all of your energy in the kitchen.

TRIMESTER 4 (POSTPARTUM) presents warming, nutrient-dense, and easily digestible recipes. These are designed to help you heal faster, stabilize your mood, give you energy to get through long nights, and support you in breastfeeding or bottle-feeding around the clock. Even more importantly, these recipes are batch-and-freezer friendly, reducing your time in the kitchen and ensuring you always have nutrient-packed foods at the ready.

All recipes are free of refined sugar, most are dairy and gluten-free, and there're lots to choose from if you're eating fewer grains or animal products. To accommodate a variety of dietary needs, each recipe includes notations to make it quick and easy for you to spot the recipes that will work best for you and your family.

- **Dairy-Free (DF)**: No dairy products used in recipe. Modifications noted for dairy-free option.
- **Gluten-Free (GF)**: No gluten-containing ingredients used in recipe. Some naturally gluten-free ingredients may become cross-contaminated during the manufacturing process — look for products that have gluten-free certification.
- **Grain-Free (GrF)**: No grains used in recipe. Modifications noted for grain-free option.
- **Vegan (V)**: No animal products including meat, egg, dairy, and honey used in recipe. Modifications noted for vegan option.
- **Nut-Free (NF)**: No nuts used in recipe (school safe).
- **Freezer-Friendly (FF)**: Recipe has the seal of approval to be kept in the freezer — make extras and store them.

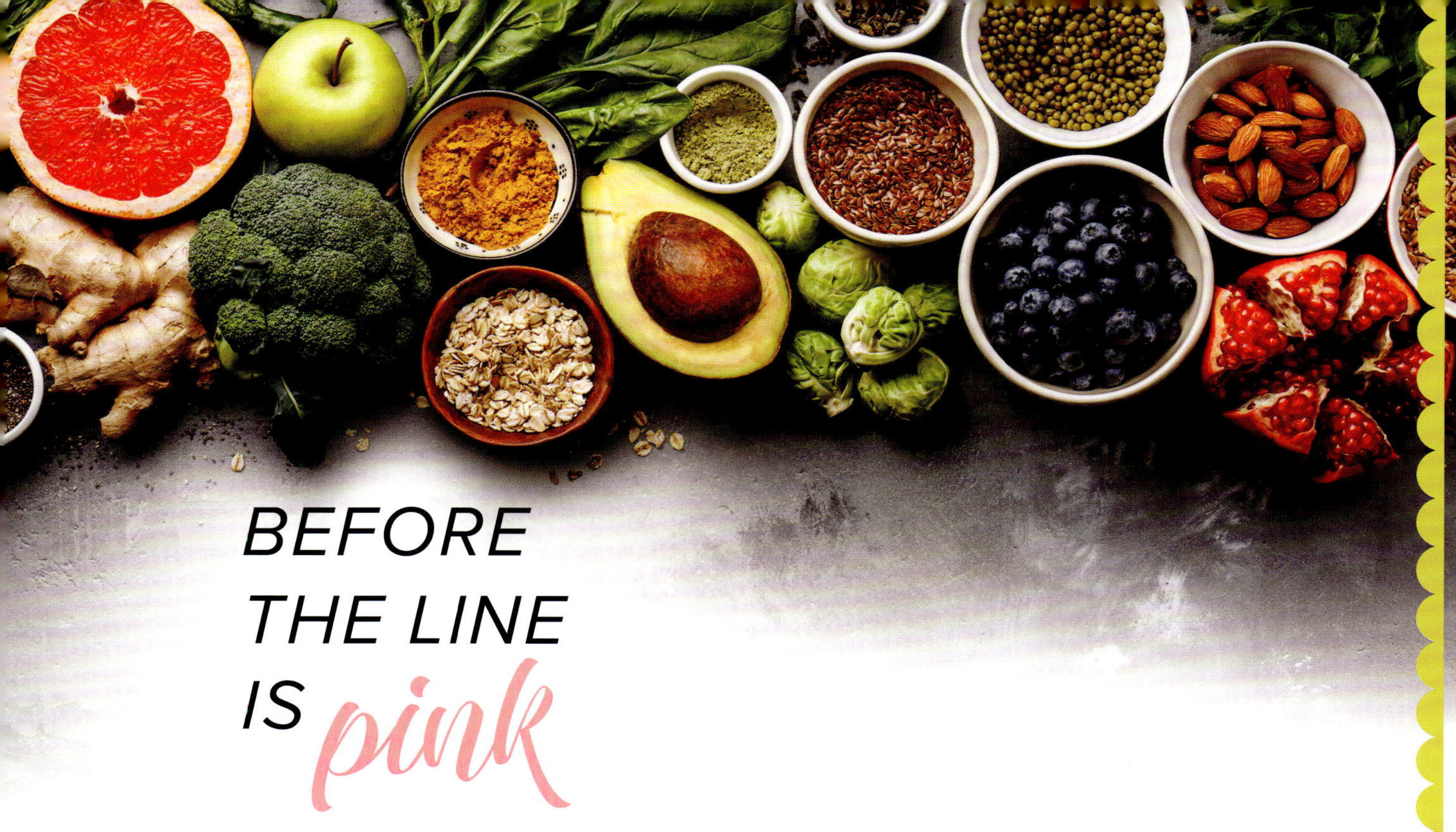

BEFORE THE LINE IS *pink*

THINKING OF HAVING A BABY? Begin by prepping for pregnancy! If you've picked up this book as a preconception resource, you're in the right place! All of the recipes and nutrition tips found throughout this book are just as perfect for preconception as they are for pregnancy. Studies have shown that the health and nutrition of both parents during the preconception stage can influence the well-being of mother and baby.

Consider preconception — at least the three to four months before conception — as a window of opportunity to influence the health and development of the embryo. Prioritizing a diet full of vegetables (leafy greens in particular), fruit, legumes, meat, fish, and nuts and seeds is thought to lower the risk of gestational diabetes, hypertensive disorders of pregnancy such as pre-eclampsia, and preterm birth, while supporting positive delivery and birth outcomes.

Of course, food and nutrition do not stand alone in supporting preconception health. Other important factors come into play — loving and healthy relationships; control of chronic health conditions, environmental toxins, and substance use; as well as access to health care; genetics and mental health; and positive social support from family and friends.

A nutritious diet can contribute to healthy and happy outcomes, especially in improved fertility and a lower risk of miscarriage and neural tube defects.

Real Food — So Good for You

A nutritious diet begins with eating real food. Real food is rich in nutrients, mostly unprocessed, and environmentally friendly. It contains antioxidants, has no chemical additives, and tastes delicious. Real food is a great option for everyone, but especially for mothers-to-be.

REAL FOOD CAN SUPPORT PRECONCEPTION

The link between preconception nutrition and positive pregnancy outcomes is most recognized when it comes to decreasing the risk of neural tube defects (NTDs). NTDs, for example, spina bifida, occur when the neural tube — the place where the baby's brain, spine, and skull will develop — does not close properly in the early weeks of pregnancy.

Several micronutrients appear to play a role in lowering the risk of NTDs, including folate, vitamin B12, and choline. Consuming foods rich in these micronutrients (such as meat and seafood, eggs, leafy greens and cruciferous vegetables, and beans and legumes) and speaking to your healthcare professional about a high-quality folate supplement can significantly reduce your risk of NTDs.

REAL FOOD MAY HELP MANAGE PREGNANCY NAUSEA

The key here is blood sugar control — a major player in the nausea game. Balancing your blood sugar level can make you less likely to experience nausea and vomiting. Starting early is best because it can take some time for your cells to get used to processing blood sugar more efficiently.

When we eat lots of sugar and refined carbohydrates, too much glucose floods our system, triggering the body to push out lots of insulin to get all that glucose out of the bloodstream. The excess insulin makes this process happen at super-speed — so fast that the result is a big drop in the blood sugar levels, which leaves a person feeling nauseous, shaky, anxious, hungry, and craving sugar to get those blood sugar levels back up. It works like one giant roller coaster, and we all know that women do not want to be on roller coasters when pregnant.

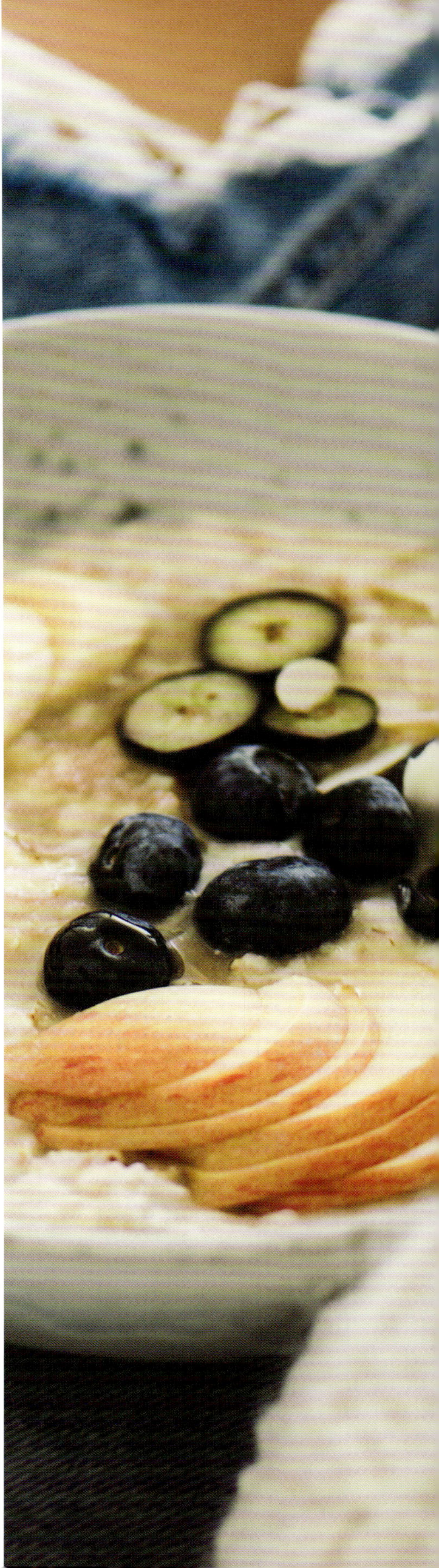

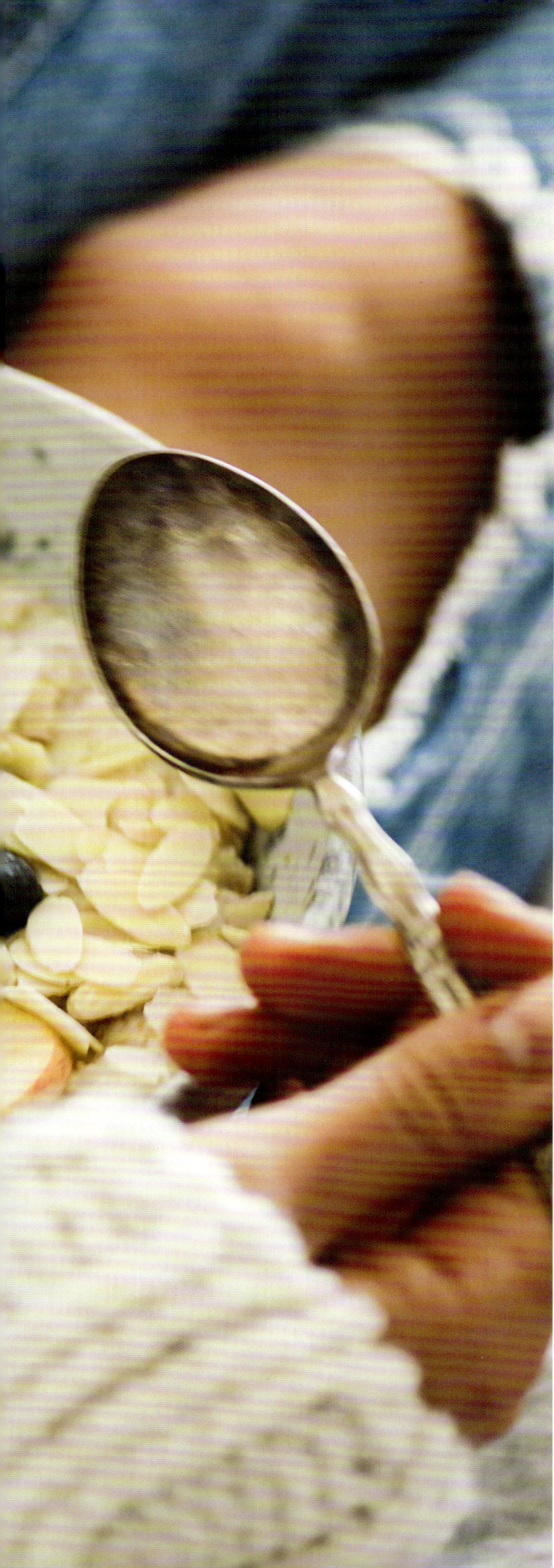

REAL FOOD SUPPORTS BABY AND YOU

We're finding out more all the time about how food and nutrition support pre- and postnatal health. What continues to stand out is this: *It's the overall balance that matter*s. A diet full of vegetables, fruit, legumes, eggs, nuts, seeds, and high-quality fats and proteins means a lower risk of undesirable pregnancy and birth outcomes — from gestational diabetes to pre-eclampsia and pre-term birth to low birth weight.

You may not feel well enough to look at, let alone enjoy, many of the foods in that list some of the time. You're not alone! Just remember that a few weeks here and there of only being able to eat beige foods is simply a blip in the overall picture.

When you're feeling up to it, your efforts in the kitchen will truly pay off! The following are just a few of the benefits of a real-food diet for you and baby.

- A boost to baby's brain, neurological, and behavioural development
- A greater likelihood of happy delivery outcomes such as healthy birth weight and length of gestation
- Healthy function of the placenta
- Support for your immune system (since pregnancy colds seem to last forever!)
- Prevention of nutrient deficiencies and anemia
- A possibly lower risk of perinatal mood disorders such as postpartum depression

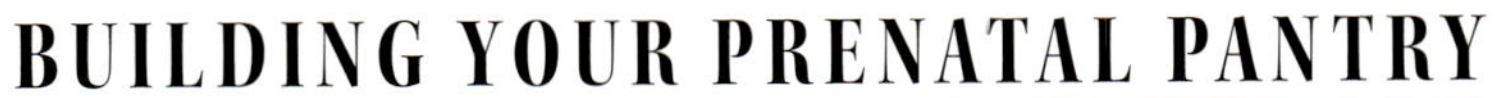

BUILDING YOUR PRENATAL PANTRY

Simple pantry switches can boost the good fats, protein, fibre, vitamins, and minerals in your meals, making healthy eating easier and supporting you to feel good in each trimester.

PANTRY STAPLE	TOP PICKS	WHY SWITCH	RECIPE INSPIRATION
Flour	Oat Flour	Comparable to whole wheat and all-purpose flour but gluten-free and higher in good fats, protein, folate, and calcium	Lemon + Ginger Carrot Muffins (page 51) Sheet Pan Pumpkin Pancakes (page 187) Bedside Granola Clusters (page 45)
	Almond Flour	Big boost of protein and fat, which helps you stay full longer and relieves nausea	Almond Chocolate Oat Bars (page 49) Grain-Free Chicken Fingers (page 106) Preggo Protein Pancakes (page 41)
	Chickpea Flour	Grain-free and nut-free option that's high in protein, folate, zinc, and iron	Summer Veggie Fritters (page 108) Chickpea Flour Ginger Cookies (page 98)
Sweeteners	Unrefined Coconut Sugar	All sweeteners have sugar, but natural and unrefined products don't spike your blood sugar as sharply — less nausea and fewer crashes	Little Lactation Cookies (page 201) Greek Chicken Skewers (page 150) Double Chocolate Lentil Muffins (page 53)
	Pure Maple Syrup	Has a lower effect on blood sugar and contains antioxidants and minerals such as potassium, zinc, calcium, and magnesium	Cinnamon Chocolate Banana Loaf (page 95) Apple Pie Oat Bars (page 196) Seed Strong Chocolate Energy Balls (page 159)
	Raw Honey	Rich in B vitamins, minerals, and is naturally anti-inflammatory, anti-microbial, and anti-viral	Homemade Ginger Ale (page 32) Strawberry Chia Jam (page 42) Heavenly Hot Chocolate (page 119)
Cooking Oils/ Fats	Ghee, Grass-fed Butter, Avocado Oil, and Coconut Oil	Unlike "vegetable" oils, which are refined and prone to damage from heat and light, these fats are stable at high heat	Try mixing melted coconut oil with maple syrup for a pancake topping, or use avocado oil or ghee/butter as your go-to neutral oil for roasting or searing
	Olive Oil	Perfect for low-medium heat cooking — look for unrefined, cold-pressed oils in dark glass bottles	Try it in salad dressings and dips, or use it to sauté food
	Nut and Seed Oils (flax, walnut, etc.)	High in beneficial omega-3 fats, which can be oxidized by heat, so raw use is best (keep in fridge!)	Try adding flax oil to your smoothies for a brain boost

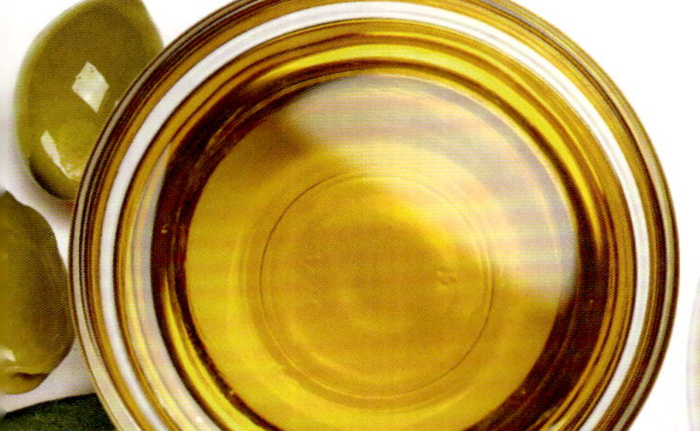

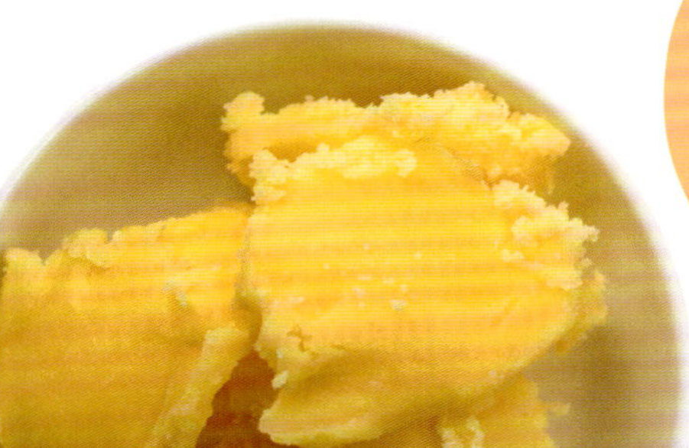

We ♡ fat!

Many vitamins can't be absorbed without fat, and it's essential for a healthy brain and mood — for baby *and* you!

TOP 9 FOODS FOR A HEALTHY NINE MONTHS

PRENATAL SUPERFOOD	GET THE MOST OUT OF IT	RECIPE INSPIRATION
Eggs Back-up: meat or liver	Buy pasture-raised eggs, which have higher vitamin content	7-Minute Ultimate Breakfast Bowl (page 39) Red Pepper Basil Egg Cups (page 185)
Spinach Back-up: kale or romaine	Buy organic and as fresh as possible (try growing in season!)	Chicken + Spinach Enchiladas (page 218) Soothing Mango Green Smoothie (page 35)
Salmon Back-up: sardines or mackerel	Buy wild salmon, which has the best nutrient profile, when available from a sustainable source	Sheet Pan Maple Sesame + Shiitake Salmon (page 67) Simple Salted Lemon Salmon (page 215)
Flaxseeds Back-up: chia seeds or walnuts	Buy whole flaxseeds and grind them yourself for best absorption; keep ground flaxseeds in your refrigerator	Apple Zucchini Oat Bowl (page 37) Overnight Flax + Chia Pudding (page 135)
Raspberries Back-up: blueberries or blackberries	Buy organic, fresh or frozen	Berry Sorbet (page 141) Raspberry Date Labour Prep Smoothie (page 131)
Broccoli Back-up: Brussels sprouts or bok choy	Buy as fresh as possible	Quinoa Fried N'Ice (page 69) Simple Sesame Noodles (page 111)
Lentils Back-up: black beans or chickpeas	Red or green, dry or canned, stock up on this affordable pantry item	Double Chocolate Lentil Muffins (page 53) Slow Cooker Spiced Cauliflower + Sweet Potato Soup (page 65)
Bone Broth Back-up: veggie broth or more water!	Try making it yourself from pastured, organic bones; use in soup or drink like tea	Everyday Bone Broth (page 181) Rosemary Chicken Noodle Soup (page 213)
Chocolate Back-up: *Really?*	Happy hormones and antioxidants; aim for at least 70% cacao and purchase raw cacao for baking	Late-Night Chocolate Avocado Pudding (page 157) Heavenly Hot Chocolate (page 119)

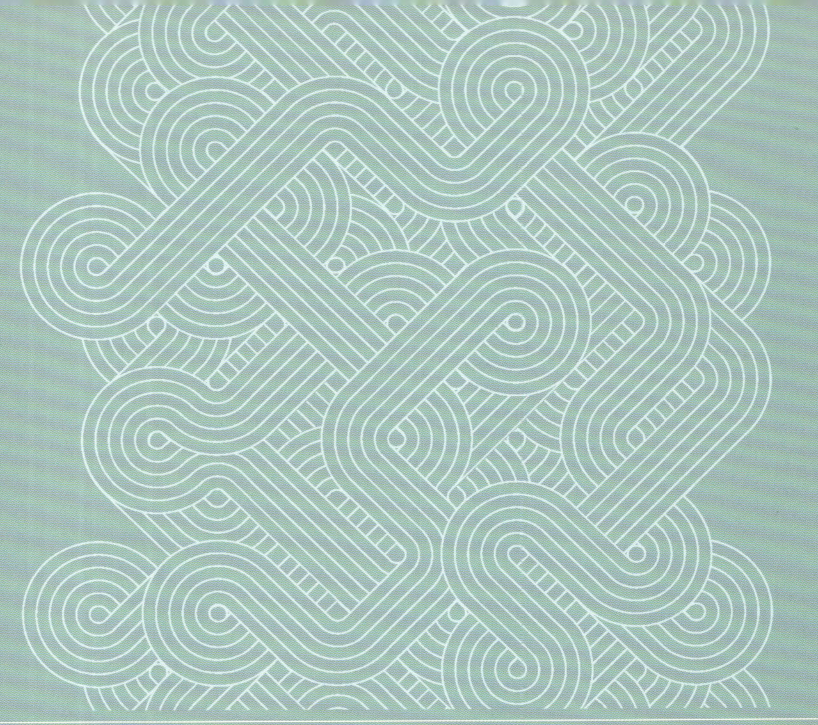

TRIMESTER 1

(WEEKS 1–12)

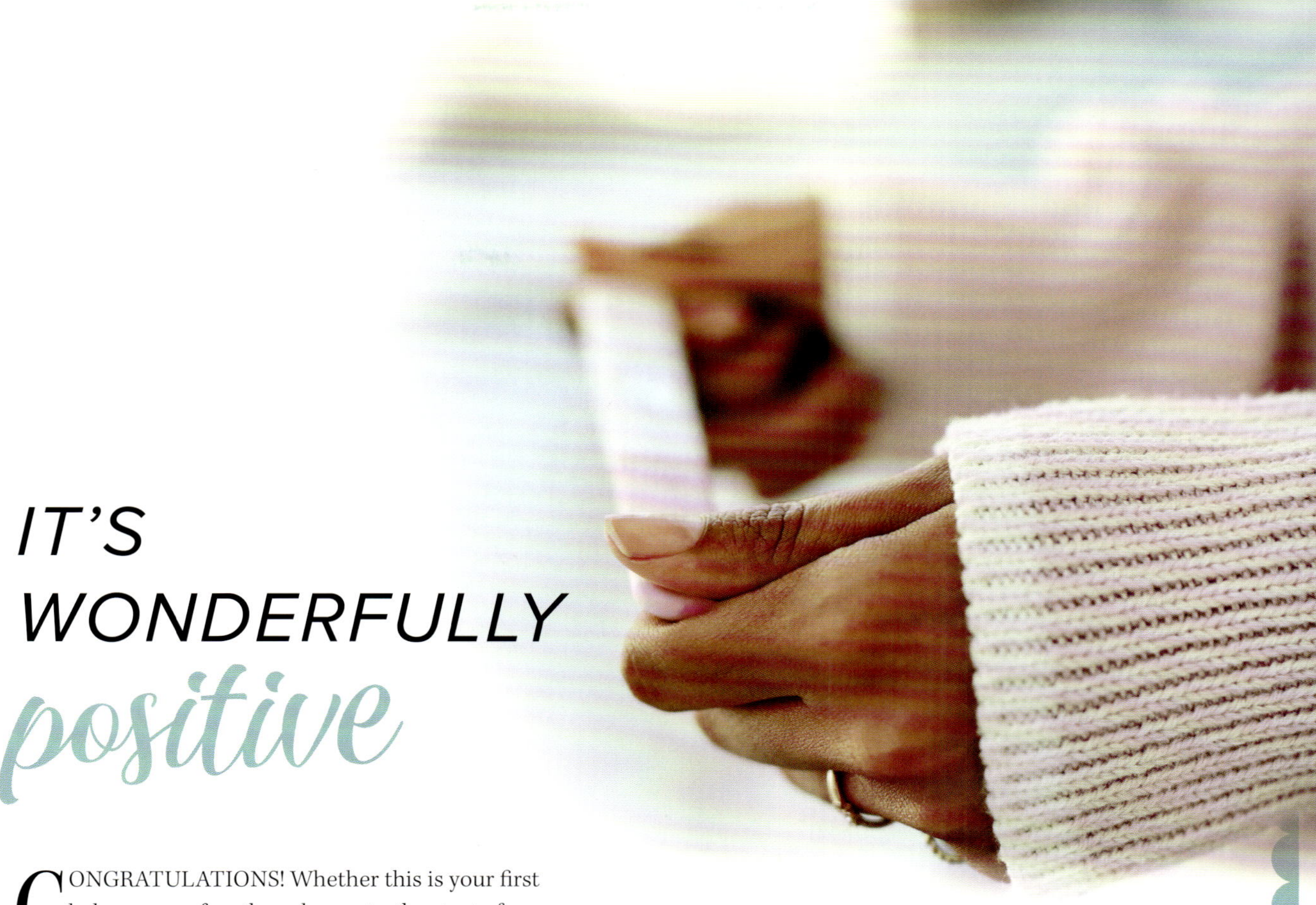

IT'S WONDERFULLY *positive*

CONGRATULATIONS! Whether this is your first baby or your fourth, welcome to the start of a new journey into motherhood!

When I told friends about my pregnancies, the first question they asked each time after congratulating me was, "How do you feel? Any nausea yet?"

Sure enough, a mere few weeks after finding out I was pregnant, I began to notice a heightening of the senses — taste and especially smell were off the charts. It's no wonder the first trimester diet often consists of strictly beige foods — crackers, toast, bagels, and pasta — limited smell and a non-offensive taste is all most newly pregnant women can handle.

It can be frustrating — you want to eat healthy meals to support your pregnancy, but you're not able to tolerate many flavours or foods. Not all women go through morning sickness, but for most women (between 50 and 80 percent) nausea and vomiting are part of the first trimester experience. Fortunately, morning sickness starts to taper off during the second trimester, with 90 percent of women reporting they are nausea-free by week 20.

The bottom line is this: when you're not feeling great, any food — whatever you crave, what you can keep down, and what makes you feel human — is the best food.

In this section, the focus is on tried-and-true tips for how and when to eat in order to set your body up for fewer days and nights of nausea. There are lots of super simple ideas and suggestions that will supercharge your bland staple food.

If you're feeling great — that's good news. There are lots of recipes that you can make depending on what looks delicious to you. However, do keep the tips about how to boost simple, comforting, and bland meals in mind — they might come in handy if you ever have an unwelcome queasy feeling.

Now let's begin!

Fighting Morning Sickness

The following tips will help you deal with nausea if and when it strikes and increase your confidence in your ability to supply your body (and your baby) with essential nutrients to support your growing needs. During this stage of pregnancy, the advice I hope you take to heart most is this: ***Be kind to yourself.*** You may not be able to incorporate any of these tips on some days, and that is okay.

- Understand the "why" behind the types of food that may make you feel better or worse with morning sickness.
- "Healthify" your go-to bland and basic staples that you can actually stomach when you're nauseous.
- Follow a "when" schedule to try to get your nausea and vomiting under control.
- Incorporate options for nutrient-dense meals that you can assemble in 10 minutes or less for times when you just can't do much in the kitchen.

Both the **timing** and **type** of meal you eat can affect how nauseous you feel (or don't feel). You will likely feel best if you do what you can to limit sugary, fried, or super-rich foods and really large meals. (This is where practising mindful eating really helps!)

We often reach for bland, carbohydrate- and sugar-rich foods (for example, crackers, bread, juice, cookies, or cereal) when we're nauseated because they feel like the only option we can stomach, and because they are what's typically recommended and immediately available in our cupboard when we have to eat — right NOW!

However, it is possible that these foods can make you feel worse because of the sharp fluctuations they cause in your blood sugar. All that energy floods into your bloodstream at once, and your body isn't equipped to deal with it. Your body activates a stress response, releasing hormones such as insulin to try to get that energy taken up into your cells right away. Then, there's nothing left, your energy wanes, your blood sugar crashes, and you feel hungry (and terrible) again quickly and rapidly.

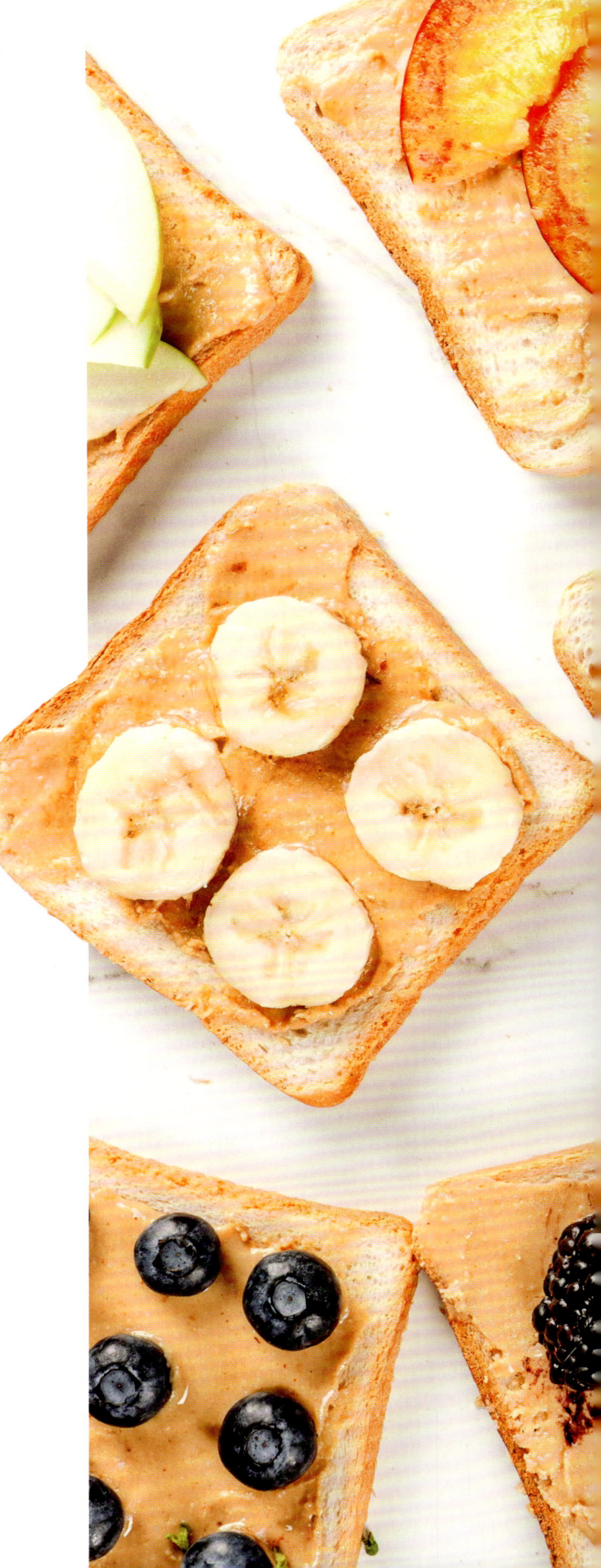

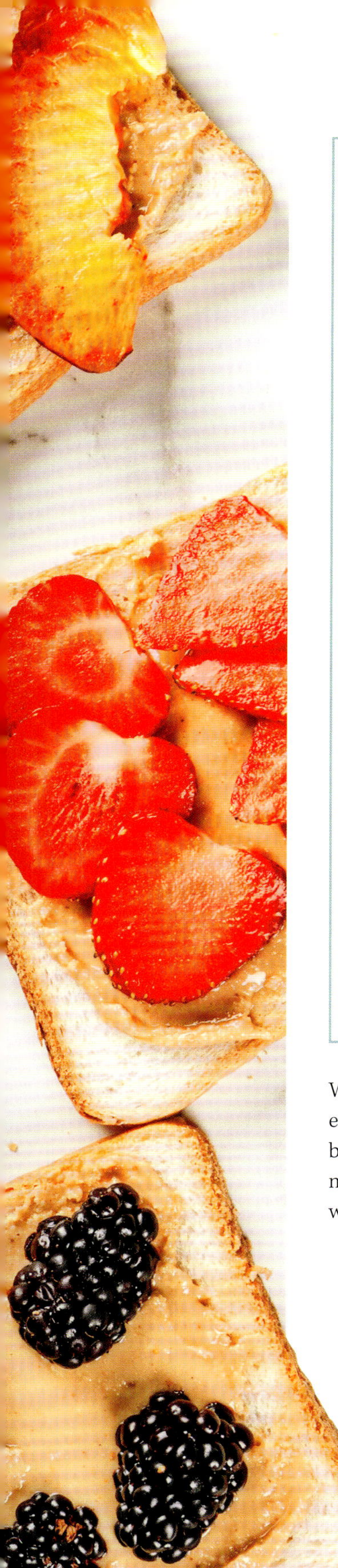

Ways to balance blood sugar to avoid nausea

Ensure all meals and snacks have a source of **fat**, **fibre**, and **protein** (for example, by adding hemp hearts to a cut-up banana or eating a piece of toast with nut butter instead of eating it plain).

Eat **regular meals** throughout the day, and have **easy-to-grab snacks** ready so that you don't get too hungry and will be less likely to reach for something sugar-packed (lots of ideas in the pages to come!).

Add **more plants** to your plate, so there will be less room for processed, refined, and sugary foods.

When you add a protein source to your meal, the energy release is slowed, leading to more stable blood sugar levels, and therefore less nausea and more steady energy. Doing this actually might be what helps you get your nausea under control.

Ways to fight morning sickness with protein

You can add protein to your go-to meal (for example, nut butter on toast, hemp hearts on fruit, or cheese on your crackers).

You can substitute your current nausea go-to food with a more nutritionally dense and protein-rich meal (for example, salted nuts instead of saltine crackers, homemade muffins instead of store-bought, or a nut-and-seed granola instead of packaged cereal).

You can follow the **No-More-Nausea Meal Schedule** (page 26) to warm yourself up to protein foods in your meals.

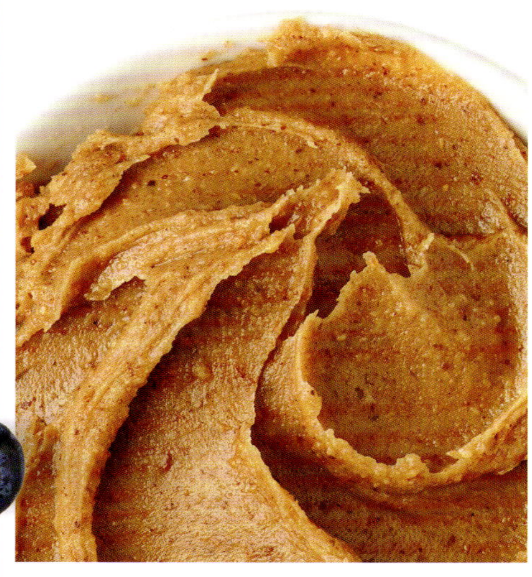

PROTEIN FOODS

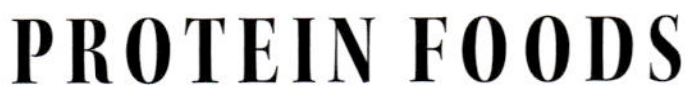

Of course, meat, fish, and eggs are all excellent sources of protein, but I know you may not feel like these often or even at all right now. (If this is not an issue, that's great — keep it up.) A tip for making meat more palatable in the first trimester is to eat it cold (for instance, shredded chicken on a salad or flatbread). Hot foods tend to taste richer and have a stronger smell, which can trigger nausea and vomiting.

Here's a quick reference chart with some wonderful protein sources. Try to add a source of protein to each of your meals and snacks to fight morning sickness.

PROTEIN SOURCE	HOW TO CHOOSE	HOW TO EAT	RECIPE INSPIRATION
Quinoa	Quinoa is one of the only vegetarian foods that has all nine essential amino acids (making it a complete protein). Buy organic quinoa, and rinse before using.	Use it on salads, as the base for Buddha bowls, in soups, or as a side with dinner.	Try the Arugula + Quinoa Steak Salad (page 149). Make a big batch, and serve yourself a scoop or two any time of day.
Seeds	Your pick: ground flaxseed, hulled hemp hearts, chia seeds, sesame seeds, pumpkin seeds, or sunflower seeds. Keep a portion in the refrigerator (especially if ground) and store leftovers in the freezer to preserve the good fats.	Sprinkle seeds on banana slices, berries, yogurt, cereal, or buttered toast. Blend into smoothies or dips, or use in a salad, pasta, or stir-fry.	Soothing Mango Green Smoothie (page 35) Amped-Up Applesauce (page 43) Bedside Granola Clusters (page 45) Apple Zucchini Oat Bowl (page 37) Strawberry Chia Jam (page 42)

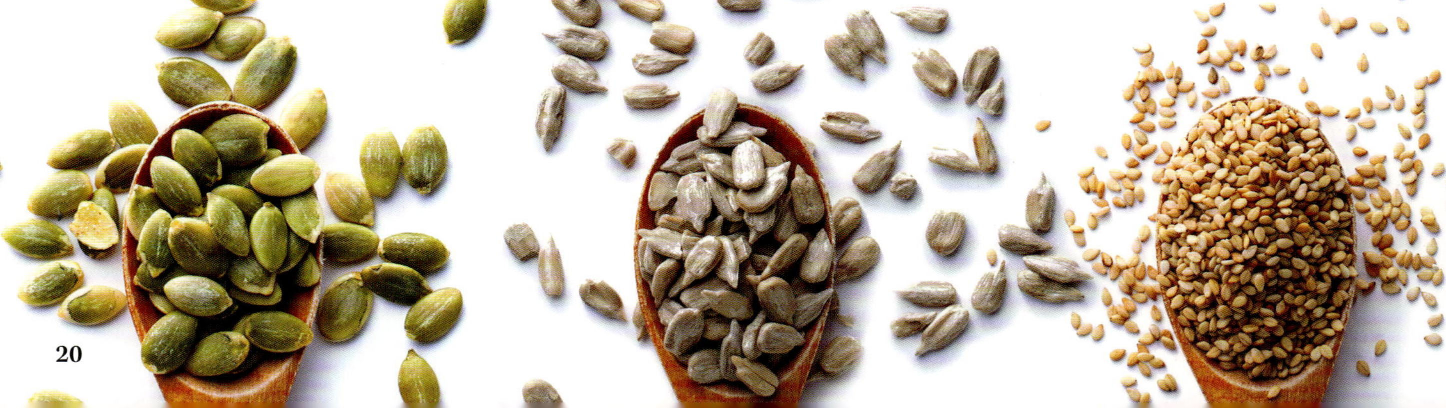

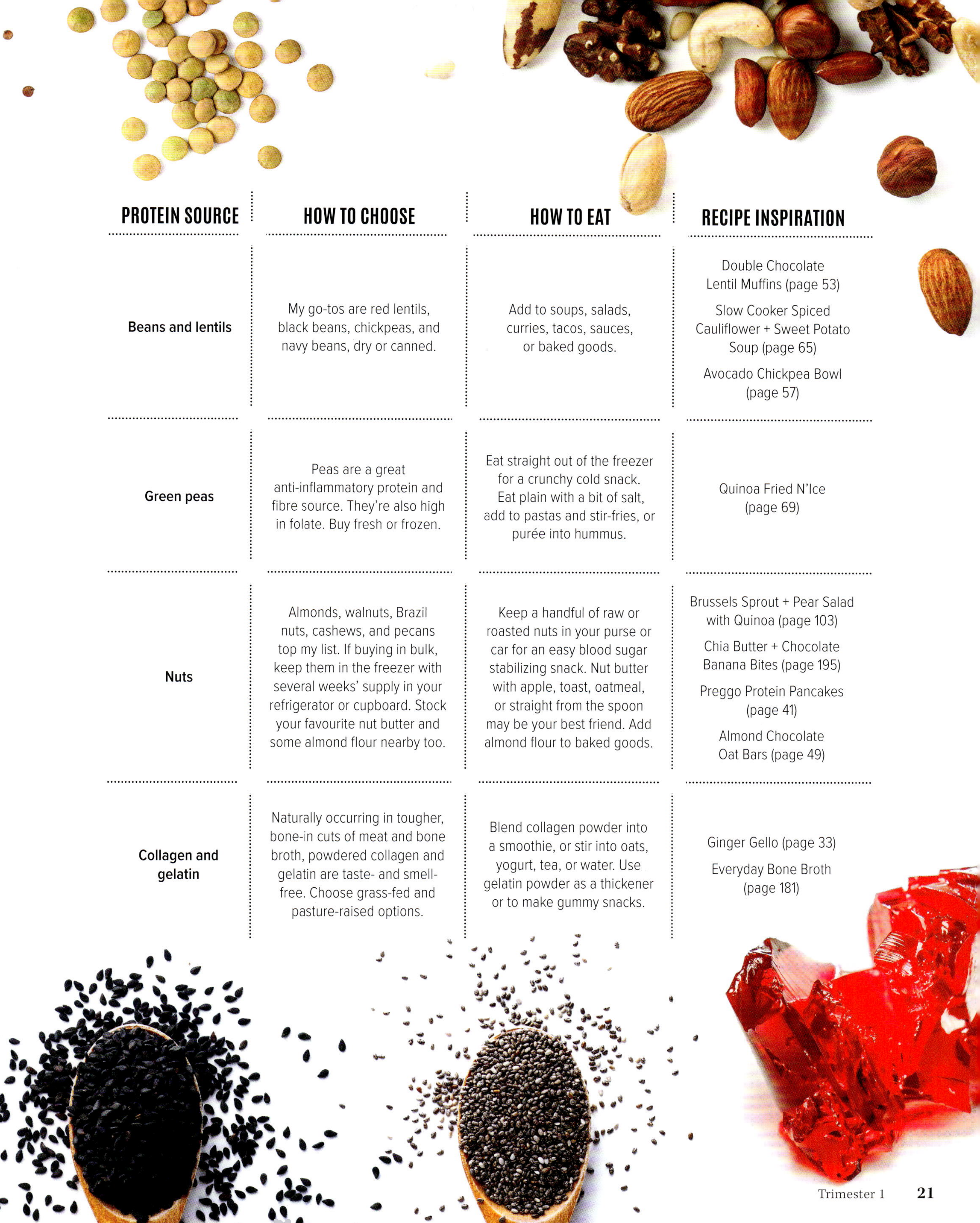

PROTEIN SOURCE	HOW TO CHOOSE	HOW TO EAT	RECIPE INSPIRATION
Beans and lentils	My go-tos are red lentils, black beans, chickpeas, and navy beans, dry or canned.	Add to soups, salads, curries, tacos, sauces, or baked goods.	Double Chocolate Lentil Muffins (page 53) Slow Cooker Spiced Cauliflower + Sweet Potato Soup (page 65) Avocado Chickpea Bowl (page 57)
Green peas	Peas are a great anti-inflammatory protein and fibre source. They're also high in folate. Buy fresh or frozen.	Eat straight out of the freezer for a crunchy cold snack. Eat plain with a bit of salt, add to pastas and stir-fries, or purée into hummus.	Quinoa Fried N'Ice (page 69)
Nuts	Almonds, walnuts, Brazil nuts, cashews, and pecans top my list. If buying in bulk, keep them in the freezer with several weeks' supply in your refrigerator or cupboard. Stock your favourite nut butter and some almond flour nearby too.	Keep a handful of raw or roasted nuts in your purse or car for an easy blood sugar stabilizing snack. Nut butter with apple, toast, oatmeal, or straight from the spoon may be your best friend. Add almond flour to baked goods.	Brussels Sprout + Pear Salad with Quinoa (page 103) Chia Butter + Chocolate Banana Bites (page 195) Preggo Protein Pancakes (page 41) Almond Chocolate Oat Bars (page 49)
Collagen and gelatin	Naturally occurring in tougher, bone-in cuts of meat and bone broth, powdered collagen and gelatin are taste- and smell-free. Choose grass-fed and pasture-raised options.	Blend collagen powder into a smoothie, or stir into oats, yogurt, tea, or water. Use gelatin powder as a thickener or to make gummy snacks.	Ginger Gello (page 33) Everyday Bone Broth (page 181)

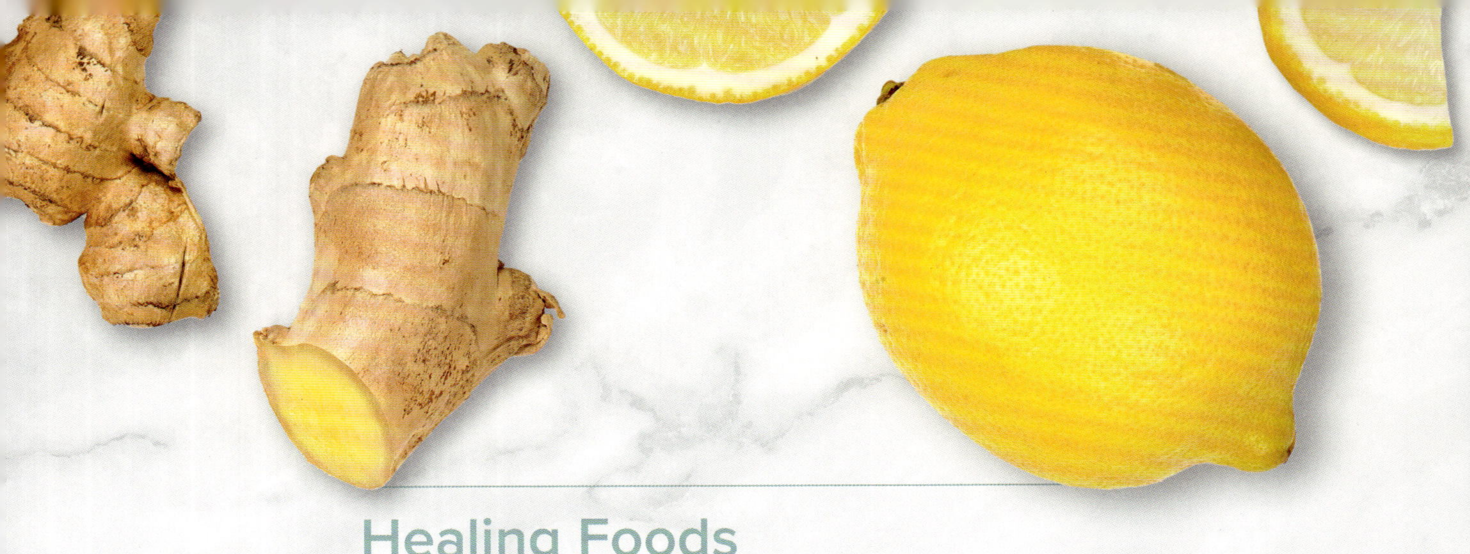

Healing Foods

In addition to getting in more protein, you can also try to incorporate into your diet the following foods, vitamins, and minerals, which act as non-pharmacological aids to reduce nausea and vomiting.

GINGER

Ginger is one of nature's most potent superfoods. It is the ingredient we look for when we are not well and want to feel better. We make ginger and lemon tea for drinking when we are sick, we eat gingery noodle soup after the flu, we use ginger chews to fight nausea, and so on. Indeed, decades of scientific research have demonstrated that ginger is effective in reducing the intensity of nausea and vomiting during pregnancy.

Don't be intimidated when prepping ginger root. Simply use a small kitchen knife to peel and slice it, or use a grater to finely shred it.

For ginger relief, try the Homemade Ginger Ale, some Ginger Tea, or the Ginger Gello (pages 32–33).

LEMON

Both ingesting lemon and being around the scent of lemon could help alleviate nausea.

Add lemon slices to your water (one big slice in the water bottle in the morning is enough for the whole day — just keep filling up with water). I like to keep a small bowl filled with lemon slices in my refrigerator at eye level — it reminds me to drink water and makes it easy for me to consume lemon all week.

Squeeze lemon over avocado toast, make lemonade ice pops, or add lemon zest into muffins or cookies. The zest of the lemon is especially good for baking. Try the Lemon + Ginger Carrot Muffins on page 51 for a delicious snack.

Harness the power of lemon in other ways too. You can use a high-quality lemon essential oil and diffuse the air around you, or add a few drops in your bath, on your pillow, or on a wool dryer ball. You could also simply slice a lemon, put it in a dish, and place it near where you work or rest.

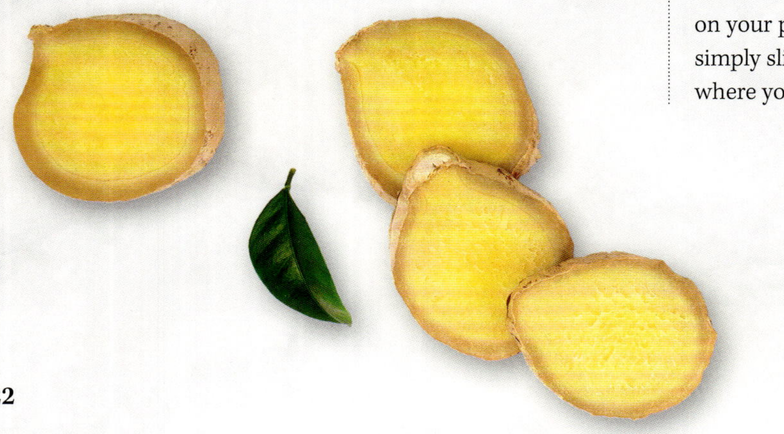

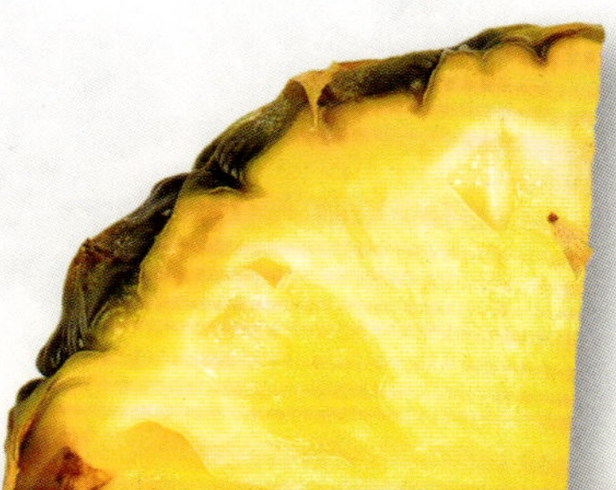

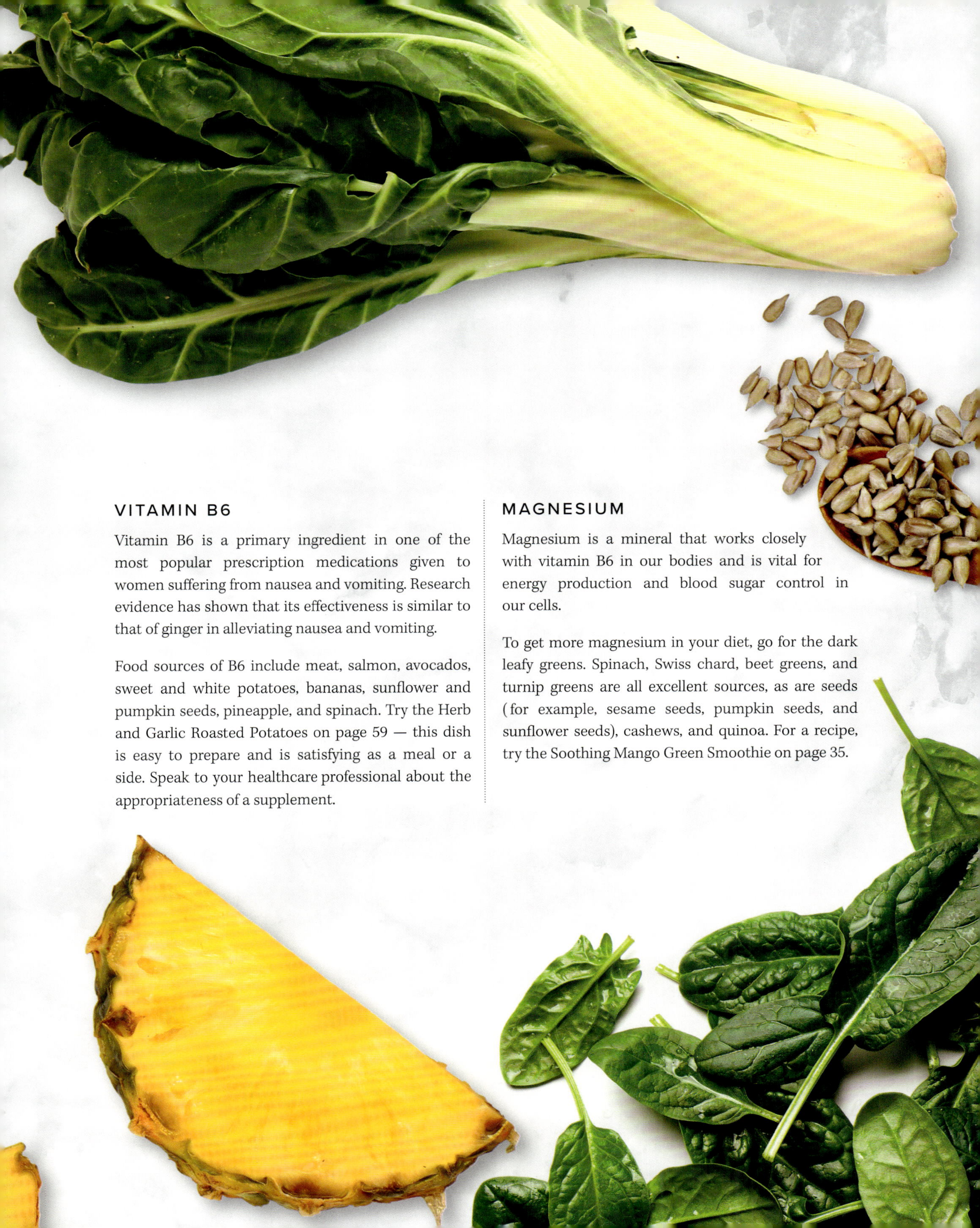

VITAMIN B6

Vitamin B6 is a primary ingredient in one of the most popular prescription medications given to women suffering from nausea and vomiting. Research evidence has shown that its effectiveness is similar to that of ginger in alleviating nausea and vomiting.

Food sources of B6 include meat, salmon, avocados, sweet and white potatoes, bananas, sunflower and pumpkin seeds, pineapple, and spinach. Try the Herb and Garlic Roasted Potatoes on page 59 — this dish is easy to prepare and is satisfying as a meal or a side. Speak to your healthcare professional about the appropriateness of a supplement.

MAGNESIUM

Magnesium is a mineral that works closely with vitamin B6 in our bodies and is vital for energy production and blood sugar control in our cells.

To get more magnesium in your diet, go for the dark leafy greens. Spinach, Swiss chard, beet greens, and turnip greens are all excellent sources, as are seeds (for example, sesame seeds, pumpkin seeds, and sunflower seeds), cashews, and quinoa. For a recipe, try the Soothing Mango Green Smoothie on page 35.

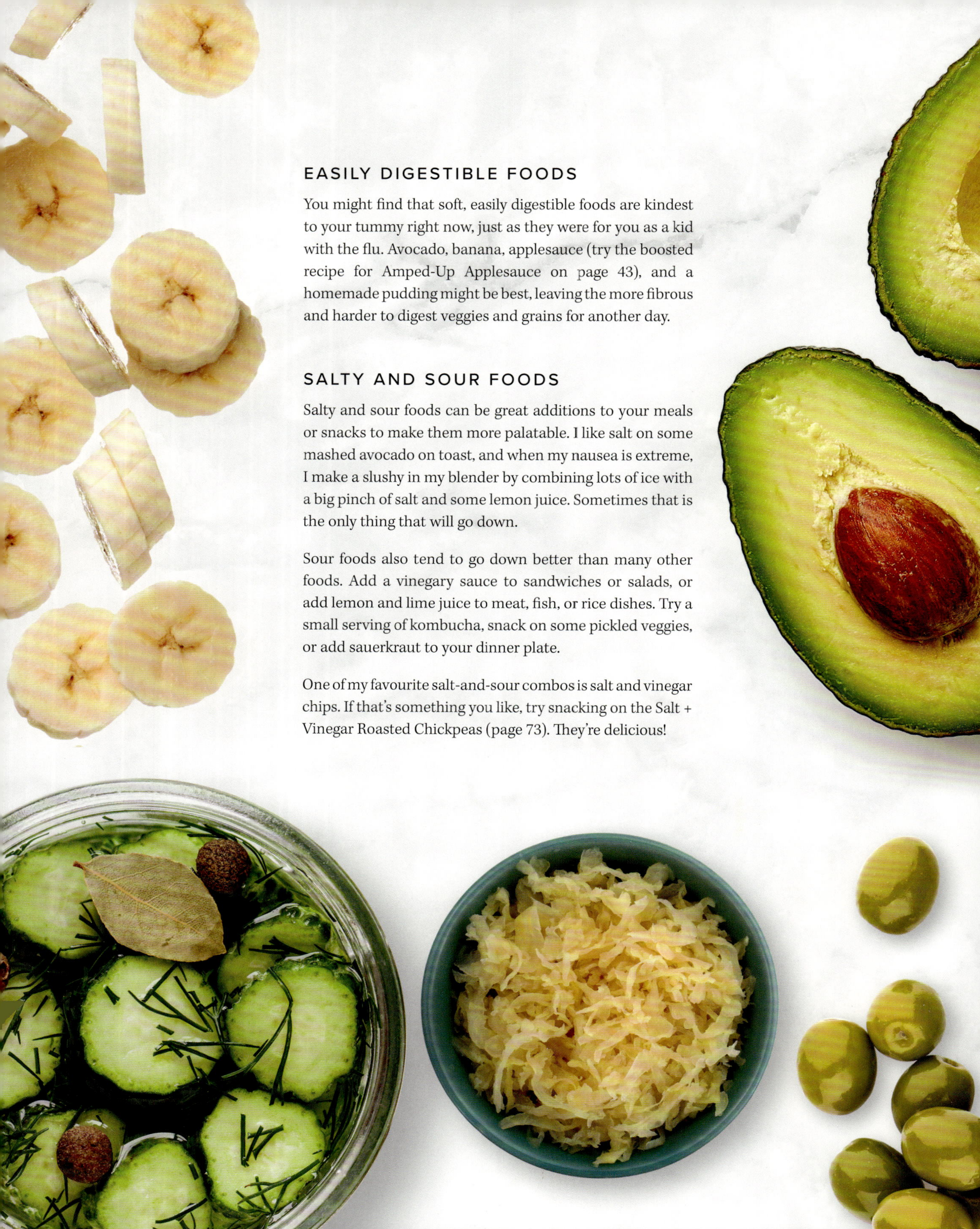

EASILY DIGESTIBLE FOODS

You might find that soft, easily digestible foods are kindest to your tummy right now, just as they were for you as a kid with the flu. Avocado, banana, applesauce (try the boosted recipe for Amped-Up Applesauce on page 43), and a homemade pudding might be best, leaving the more fibrous and harder to digest veggies and grains for another day.

SALTY AND SOUR FOODS

Salty and sour foods can be great additions to your meals or snacks to make them more palatable. I like salt on some mashed avocado on toast, and when my nausea is extreme, I make a slushy in my blender by combining lots of ice with a big pinch of salt and some lemon juice. Sometimes that is the only thing that will go down.

Sour foods also tend to go down better than many other foods. Add a vinegary sauce to sandwiches or salads, or add lemon and lime juice to meat, fish, or rice dishes. Try a small serving of kombucha, snack on some pickled veggies, or add sauerkraut to your dinner plate.

One of my favourite salt-and-sour combos is salt and vinegar chips. If that's something you like, try snacking on the Salt + Vinegar Roasted Chickpeas (page 73). They're delicious!

Deciding When to Eat

I would usually suggest listening to your body for cues on when to eat, but when you're experiencing nausea and vomiting, you might find that waiting until you're hungry to eat gives you the jitters, makes you nauseous, and triggers vomiting. I suggest eating before you get to that point, every two to three hours. Experiment and see what works best for you.

BEING READY FOR HUNGER

After I gave birth for the first time, my midwife advised me to "stay ahead of the pain" by taking pain relievers before I really started to feel pain again. This made a difference — I was definitely pain-free more often when I took my meds by the clock instead of waiting for the pain to get bad enough that I really needed them. The same practice applies to eating when you're trying to control nausea.

Planning for and eating smaller, regular meals throughout the day can help keep your body feeling balanced and less nauseous. I recommend the No-More-Nausea Meal Schedule on page 26 if you feel nauseous often and regularly find that you can't eat many of the healthy foods you wish you could.

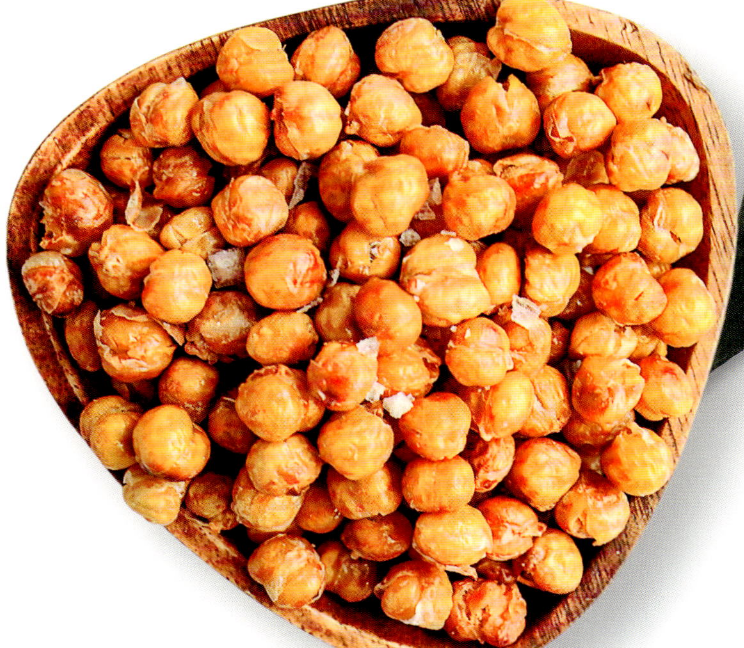

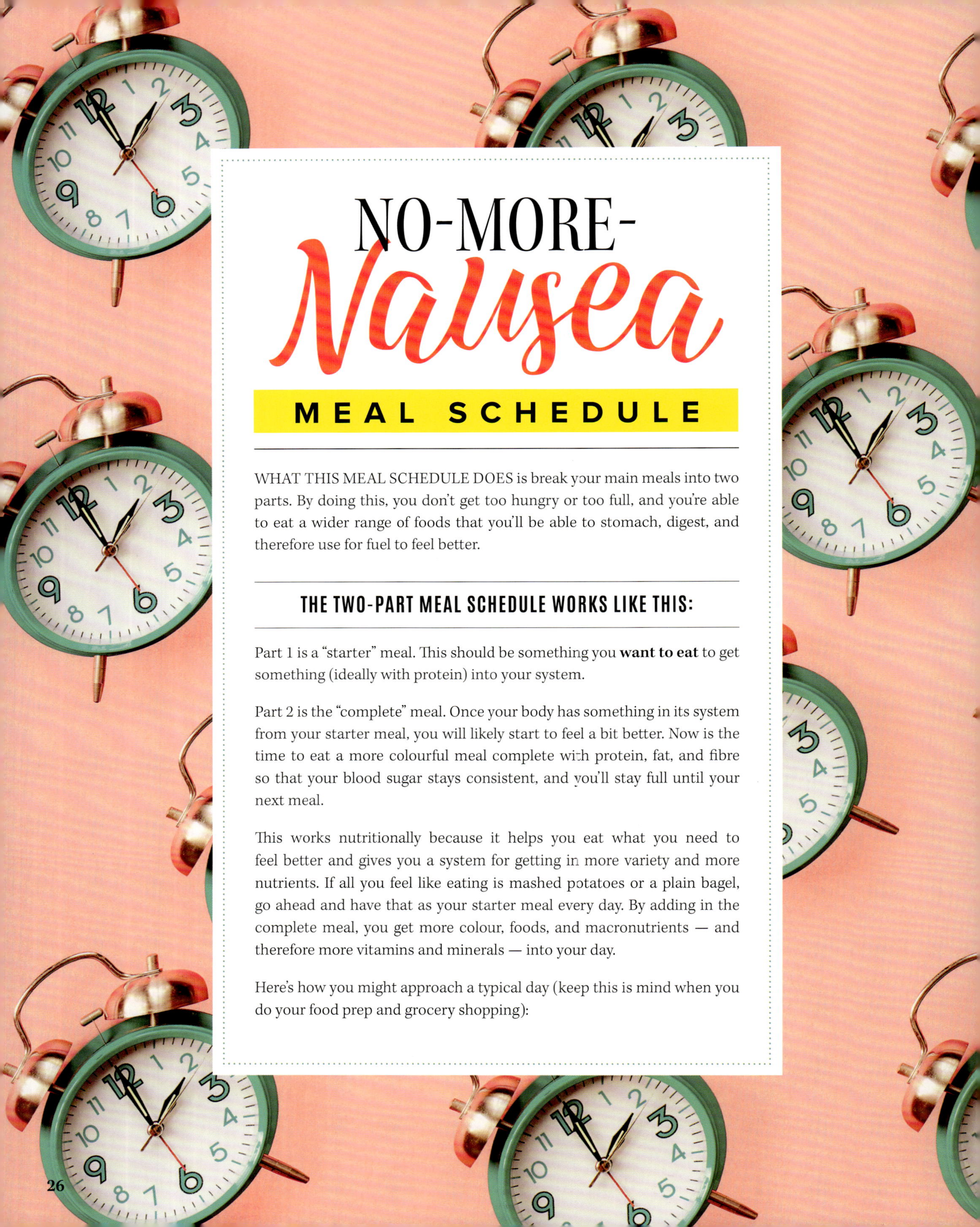

NO-MORE-*Nausea*

MEAL SCHEDULE

WHAT THIS MEAL SCHEDULE DOES is break your main meals into two parts. By doing this, you don't get too hungry or too full, and you're able to eat a wider range of foods that you'll be able to stomach, digest, and therefore use for fuel to feel better.

THE TWO-PART MEAL SCHEDULE WORKS LIKE THIS:

Part 1 is a "starter" meal. This should be something you **want to eat** to get something (ideally with protein) into your system.

Part 2 is the "complete" meal. Once your body has something in its system from your starter meal, you will likely start to feel a bit better. Now is the time to eat a more colourful meal complete with protein, fat, and fibre so that your blood sugar stays consistent, and you'll stay full until your next meal.

This works nutritionally because it helps you eat what you need to feel better and gives you a system for getting in more variety and more nutrients. If all you feel like eating is mashed potatoes or a plain bagel, go ahead and have that as your starter meal every day. By adding in the complete meal, you get more colour, foods, and macronutrients — and therefore more vitamins and minerals — into your day.

Here's how you might approach a typical day (keep this is mind when you do your food prep and grocery shopping):

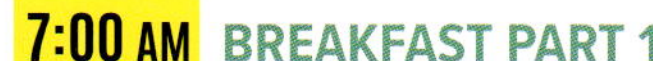

7:00 AM BREAKFAST PART 1

Upon waking (in bed)

Wake up at least 15 minutes before you need to get out of bed to give your body some time to stabilize. Your blood sugar is going to be at its lowest when you wake up because you have gone without food overnight, so plan to eat Part 1 of your breakfast before you get out of bed.

Keep something on your nightstand that doesn't need to be refrigerated: salted nuts, a homemade muffin, or my favourite, the Bedside Granola Clusters (page 45). Alternatively, ask your partner to grab something from the refrigerator or freezer and bring it to you, for example, an apple with almond butter, a Chia Yogurt Bite (page 47), or a cold pancake or waffle.

7:45 AM BREAKFAST PART 2

Within an hour of getting out of bed

Who doesn't love a second breakfast? Hopefully your snack in bed has made you feel better and ready to eat a more fulsome breakfast.

In Part 2, go for some oats with seeds and berries, toast with almond butter, eggs the way you like them, or a smoothie. Try the Apple Zucchini Oat Bowl (page 37), the Cravings Breakfast Sandwich (page 87), or the Soothing Mango Green Smoothie (page 35).

10:00 AM LUNCH PART 1

Mid-to-late morning

Go for some fruit and mixed nuts, a chia pudding (page 135), or an Almond Chocolate Oat Bar (page 49). A little sweet homemade baked snack might be just what you need if you're starting to feel woozy again.

12:30 PM LUNCH PART 2

Early afternoon

For many pregnant women, this is the time of day they feel at their best. For that reason, plan to have a veggie-loaded meal here: perhaps a big green salad with wild salmon or chopped chicken and quinoa topped with your favourite veggies and dressing — something like the Mango Chopped Chicken Salad (page 55).

3:00 PM DINNER PART 1

Late afternoon

I like to snack on Salt + Vinegar Roasted Chickpeas (page 73) at my desk — the combination of salty and crunchy works for me. Alternatively, pair some chopped veggies with a couple of Seed Strong Chocolate Energy Balls (page 159). This may be your last snack before you wrap up work and commute home, so the bonus of a snack high in healthy fats is that it will keep you full until you can eat dinner.

6:00 PM DINNER PART 2

Early evening

If you're still feeling pretty good around now, go for a home-run dinner such as wild salmon and zucchini noodles, a lentil-based pasta and meatballs in the Goodness Me Tomato Sauce (page 61), or some roasted chicken on top of a roasted veggie salad.

If you tend to feel nauseated again around dinnertime, don't feel that you need to have a big dinner. Eat your veggie-loaded meal with a good protein at lunch if that's a better time for you, and eat something easy and simple for dinner.

9:00 PM DINNER PART 3*

Before bed

*Recommended if you wake up feeling nauseous

A before-bed snack can be helpful for waking up in the morning feeling less nauseous. The night is the longest time your body goes without food, which means you're waking up with low blood sugar. This could lead many women to feel pretty awful in the morning.

Having a high-protein bedtime snack can reduce your morning discomfort. The protein will help slow down the release of energy throughout the night, keeping your blood sugar levels balanced. Have a homemade granola bar dipped in almond butter (try the Apple Pie Oat Bars, page 196) with a smoothie, or make yourself several Late-Night Protein Packs (page 72), store them in the refrigerator, and grab one before bed or in the middle of the night if you need to.

MEAL IDEAS FOR WHEN YOU JUST CAN'T COOK

There are days when cooking is not in the cards or when all you can manage is a one-step, one-pot, zero-effort meal. Here are some suggestions for meals that should take no longer than 10 minutes to prepare. Each includes options for bump boosters that can upgrade a simple bland meal into one with way more nutritional power.

IDEAS	WHAT YOU NEED	BUMP BOOSTERS
Granola with milk and berries	**Prep for it:** Keep a big glass jar with ready-to-go granola in your cupboard, with extra in the freezer (try the Bedside Granola Clusters on page 45), and berries on hand in the refrigerator. No granola prepped? Make a two-minute raw-nola by throwing a handful of two or three of these bump boosters into a bowl, topped with milk or your choice of yogurt.	Oats Seeds (pumpkin, sunflower, hemp, flax, chia) Chopped nuts (walnuts, almonds, pecans) Berries Cinnamon and/or nutmeg
Oatmeal	**Prep for it:** As soon as you get home from the grocery store, use your cheese grater, and pick one of the veggie boosters listed to grate and keep in a small container in your refrigerator. Oatmeal makes a great meal any time of day. Just remember to add your protein and fat source (nut butter, nuts, seeds, or melted coconut oil).	Grated zucchini, carrot, squash, or apple Nuts and seeds (sliced almonds or Brazil nuts, pumpkin seeds, flax seeds, chia seeds, and sunflower seeds are all great choices) Berries or Strawberry Chia Jam (page 42) Melted coconut oil
Loaded sweet potato	**Prep for it:** On the day that works best for you to do some food prep for the week, throw some sweet potatoes (pricked all over with a fork) in the oven at 425°F (220°C) for 45 to 60 minutes while you're doing something else.	Top with beans, herbs, and veggies Eat it with some coconut oil or ghee, and cinnamon Chop and add to quesadillas, bowls, or soups
Eggs and toast	**Shop for it:** Read the ingredient list on your loaf of bread. Prioritize those breads made with sprouted whole grains, and ignore those packed with additives and preservatives.	Add veggies to your eggs. If you don't get around to chopping and cooking them in the pan before you add your eggs, just cut up a few veggies (cherry tomatoes, herbs, onion, spinach) while the eggs are cooking, and throw them on top of the cooked eggs in a bowl. A few slices of avocado Butter or ghee Kimchee or sauerkraut

IDEAS	WHAT YOU NEED	BUMP BOOSTERS
Buddha bowl	**Prep for it:** When you do feel up to cooking (or when you have a partner or a friend cooking for you), always make extras: extra protein, extra veggies, and extra beans, lentils, and grains. Give yourself at least one night in the week where you have a B.O.W.L. (bunch of whole-food leftovers). Just grab those miscellaneous leftovers, and put them in a bowl. Top with a dip or salad dressing from your refrigerator (hummus, green goddess dip, hot sauce, tzatziki), and sprinkle on some seeds, chopped nuts, or fresh herbs.	If you have no protein sources on hand, open and rinse a can of beans, and add a ¼ cup serving to your bowl; or defrost some frozen edamame or peas. Prepare in advance for leftovers by making up a pot of quinoa for the week on days you feel up to cooking. Add kimchee or sauerkraut. Drizzle olive oil, avocado oil, or coconut oil on top.
Boxed pasta with sauce	**Shop for it:** Buy a variety of pastas made of lentils, peas, quinoa, and beans. You're getting in way more protein with this simple and comforting dish. **Prep for it:** Make large batches of your favourite sauce, and keep several individual servings in freezer-safe jars or containers in your freezer. Try the Goodness Me Tomato Sauce on page 61.	Add some spiralized zucchini, sweet potato, or squash. Stir in some hemp hearts. Purée your jar of tomato sauce with a handful of leftover roasted veggies or lentils. Wilt a handful of spinach in the sauce for the last few minutes to heat it up.
Picnic plate	**Shop for it:** Easy-to-assemble foods you enjoy, for example, fruit, cheese, nuts and seeds, pretzels and dips, and a few different veggies (cucumbers, peppers, snap peas, or carrots).	Dress up your cheese — roll it up in big pieces of lettuce for extra crunch and a serving of greens, or make mini cucumber sandwiches with it by slicing a cucumber horizontally. Top your hummus with a sprinkling of sesame and chia seeds. Add any veggies you like to the plate!
Freezer pancakes or waffles	**Prep for it:** Whip up a double or triple batch on a day you're feeling good, or ask your partner or support person to do it for you. Keep the pancakes or waffles in the freezer, separating them with squares of parchment or waxed paper. These make an easy meal or snack — simply defrost and pop in your toaster. If you have kids at home, this also makes an easy grab-and-go staple for lunch boxes. Try the Preggo Protein Pancakes recipe (page 41).	Almond butter Ghee, butter, or coconut oil Berries, apples and cinnamon, clementines, pomegranates, or chia jam Flax or hemp hearts

Maximizing Nutrition Through Aversions

Food aversions got you down? Here's how you can cope *and* maximize your nutrition.

Aversion to Meat: This is among the most common food-related complaints of early pregnancy. A food aversion to meat can result in a lower than normal level of heme iron (the super-absorbable iron we get from animal products).

Iron deficiency and anemia are common in pregnancy (up to 20 percent of women will experience it by the third trimester). Anemia can make you feel unwell — weak, exhausted, dizzy — and may increase the risk of preterm birth. However, if meat is off the table for you — no fear! Non-heme iron, or iron from plant sources, is much less absorbable than heme iron, but the amount absorbed by your body can be increased significantly by cleverly combining different foods. Here's the secret: *Pair top plant sources of iron with foods high in vitamin C.*

PLANT SOURCE OF IRON		VITAMIN C FOOD		PERFECT PAIRING
Seeds (hemp hearts or pumpkin seeds)	+	Orange	→	Combine in a smoothie, salad, or sprinkle seeds on orange slices
Lentils	+	Broccoli	→	Combine in a warming soup, or roast together in the oven
Oats	+	Strawberries	→	Combine in oatmeal, pancakes, or a smoothie
Spinach	+	Red Bell Peppers	→	Combine in a salad, omelette, or stir-fry

Aversion to Eggs: We can get around that too. Some people can handle eggs hidden in a recipe — for example, in a pancake or crepe. Try the Preggo Protein Pancakes on page 41 for the nutrition without the taste of eggs.

Although it's hard to replace the valuable DHA, choline, and vitamin B12 in eggs when you can't eat them, try adding more beans, lentils, nuts, and seeds to your diet. Nuts, seeds (and lentils!) can be added to a smoothie, or sprinkled on toast, fruit, salad, or roasted veggies.

If you're strongly averse to eggs, you can replace them in baking recipes with a flax egg. Simply mix 1 tbsp of ground flaxseed with 2.5 tbsp of warm water. Then let it sit for 5 to 10 minutes before adding it to your recipe.

You may have other aversions — to green vegetables, garlic, or anything with a strong smell. It's not easy! *Just remember — these aversions are likely short-lived, so be kind to yourself at this stage.*

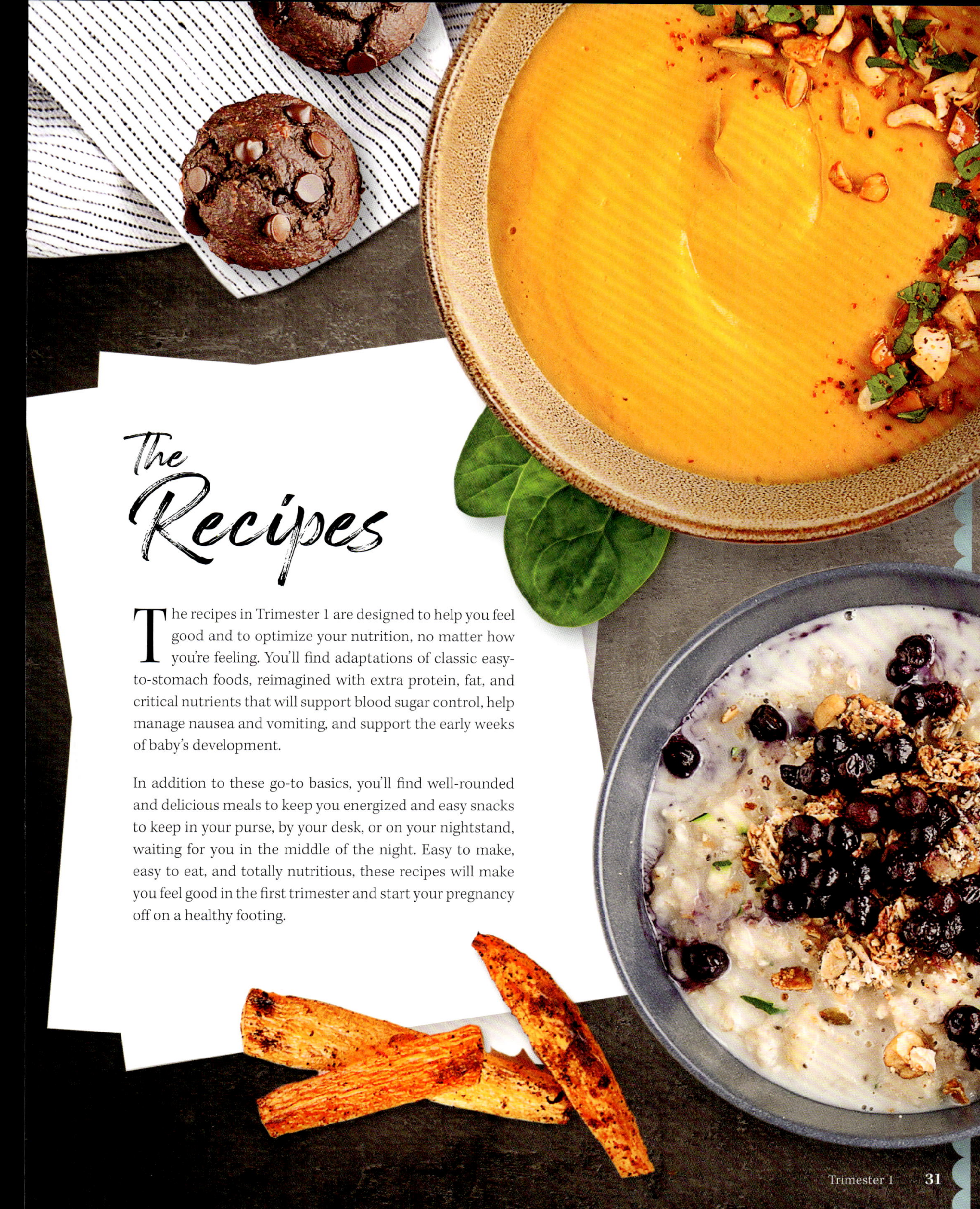

The Recipes

The recipes in Trimester 1 are designed to help you feel good and to optimize your nutrition, no matter how you're feeling. You'll find adaptations of classic easy-to-stomach foods, reimagined with extra protein, fat, and critical nutrients that will support blood sugar control, help manage nausea and vomiting, and support the early weeks of baby's development.

In addition to these go-to basics, you'll find well-rounded and delicious meals to keep you energized and easy snacks to keep in your purse, by your desk, or on your nightstand, waiting for you in the middle of the night. Easy to make, easy to eat, and totally nutritious, these recipes will make you feel good in the first trimester and start your pregnancy off on a healthy footing.

Dairy-Free • Gluten-Free • Grain-Free • Nut-Free

Ginger Tonic 3 Ways

HOMEMADE GINGER ALE OR GINGER TEA

Without the high-fructose corn syrup and preservatives found in the store-bought variety, homemade ginger ale is a bubbly, soothing tonic that harnesses the power of ginger to alleviate nausea during morning sickness. If you'd rather make tea, simply eliminate the sparkling water, and enjoy the drink hot after stirring in the lemon juice and honey.

5 MINUTES PREPPING • 20 MINUTES COOKING • MAKES 3 SERVINGS

WHAT YOU NEED:

- 2 to 4 tbsp (30 to 60 mL) peeled and sliced ginger
- 4 cups (1 L) water
- 2 tbsp (30 mL) lemon juice
- 2 to 3 tbsp (30 to 45 mL) honey
- Sparkling water, to taste

HOW TO MAKE IT:

1. Place ginger in a medium pot with the water, and heat to a boil.
2. Reduce heat to low, and simmer for 20 minutes, covered.
3. Remove from heat, strain out ginger pieces, and stir in lemon juice and honey. Let cool. Transfer to a storage container, and chill in the refrigerator (or drink as is if you're in the mood for tea).
4. Once cold, add to a glass, and top with sparkling water.

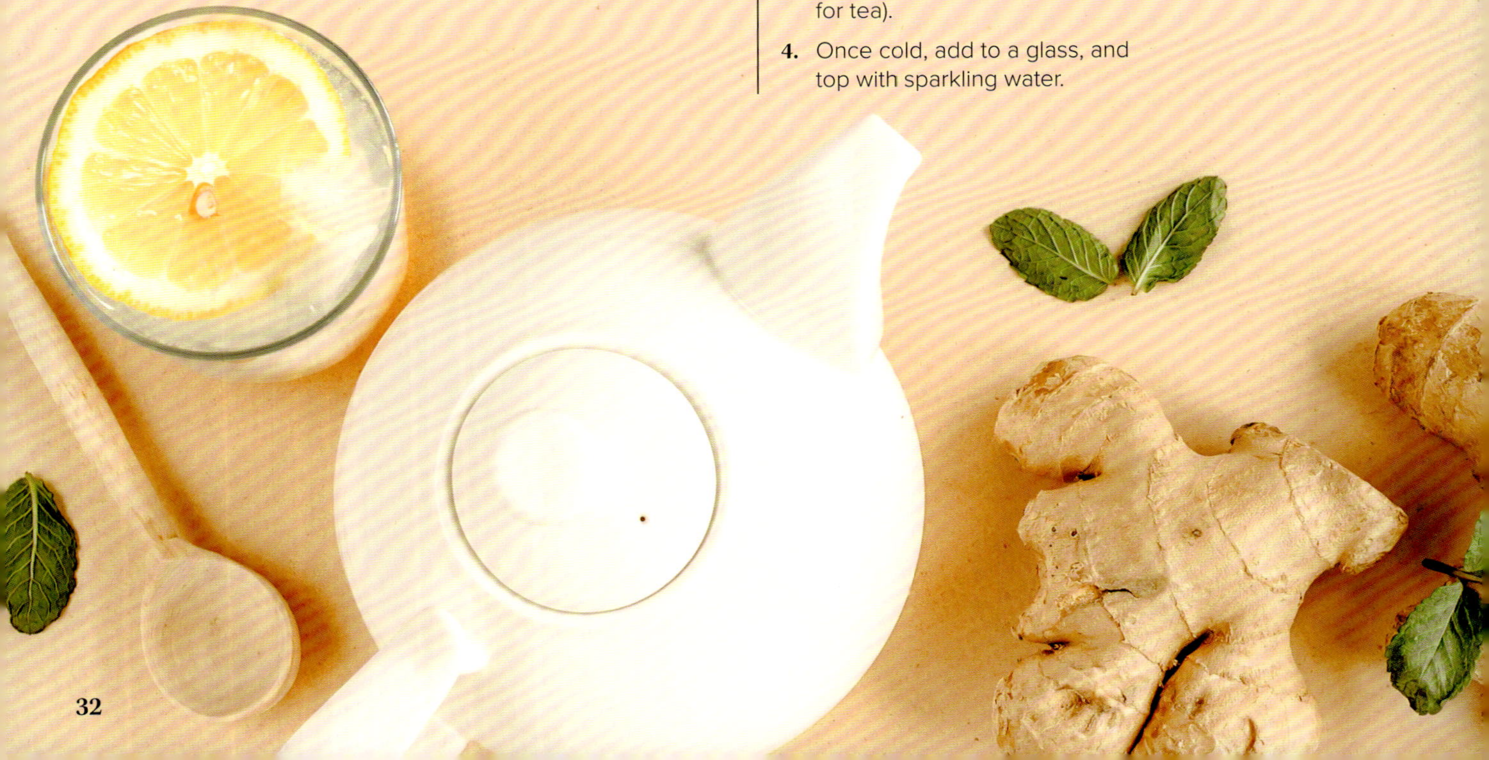

GINGER GELLO

Here is a soothing and mild honey and ginger snack to try on those days you don't feel like much else. Gelatin is more than just the thing that makes your bowl jiggle. It is full of essential amino acids, making it a rich protein source (gelatin is one of the reasons bone broth is so nutritious). Gelatin may also aid in digestion, help with skin elasticity, ease joint pain, and promote restful sleep (win, win, win, win).

I like to keep some brewed tea or juice in the refrigerator most of the time. This easy snack can come together in just a couple of minutes. Make sure to warm up your base liquid before whisking in the gelatin for a nice smooth consistency as the gelatin can set too quickly if it is immersed in cold liquid.

Looking to change up the flavour? Use this simple formula: 2 cups of your favourite juice or tea (warm) + 2 tbsp gelatin.

5 MINUTES PREPPING • 3 HOURS COOLING • MAKES 1 PAN

WHAT YOU NEED:	HOW TO MAKE IT:
2 cups (500 mL) prepared ginger tea (use homemade or store-bought) 1 tbsp (15 mL) honey (if using store-bought tea) 2 tbsp (30 mL) grass-fed gelatin powder	1. Pour warm ginger tea into an 8 × 8-inch (2L) pan, and whisk in the honey (if using). 2. Slowly sprinkle in the gelatin powder, whisking to incorporate constantly as you pour. 3. Cover and let cool in the refrigerator, about 3 hours, or until set (and jiggly).

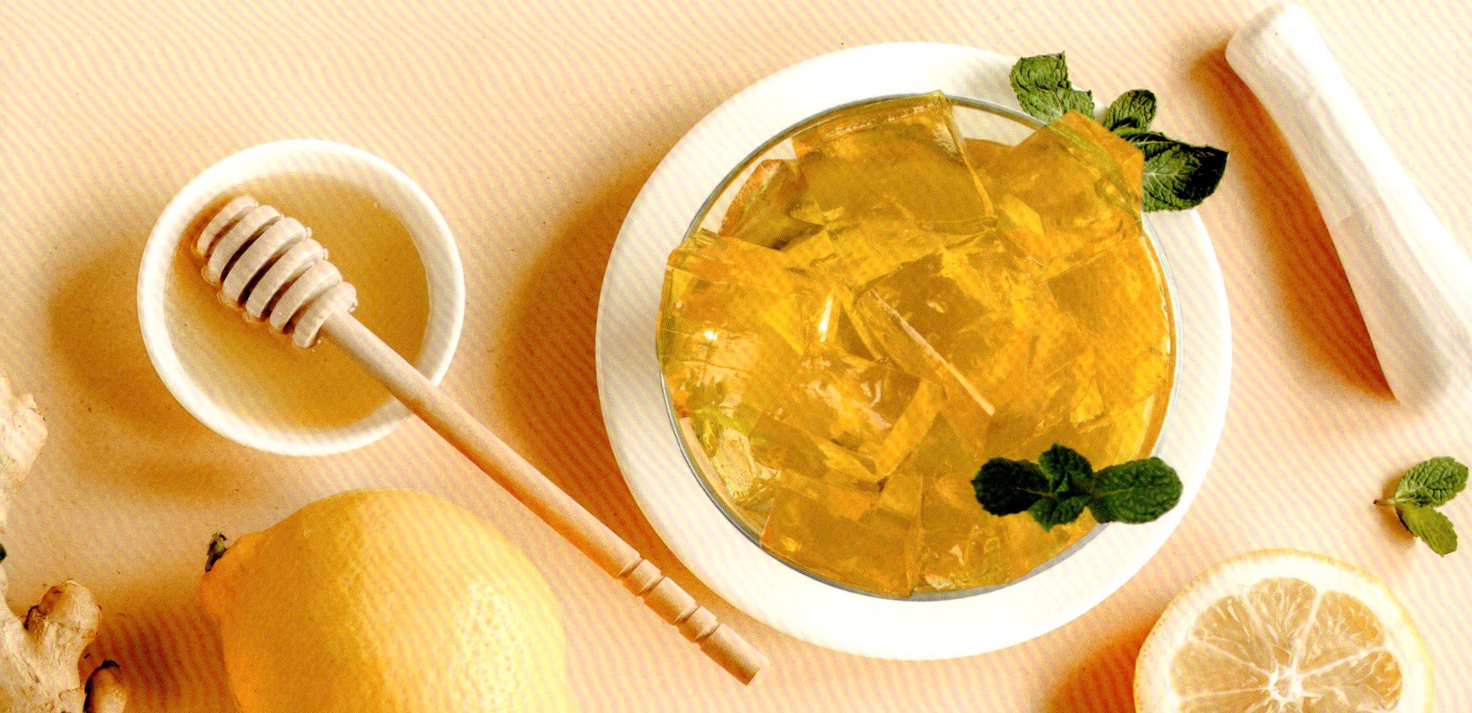

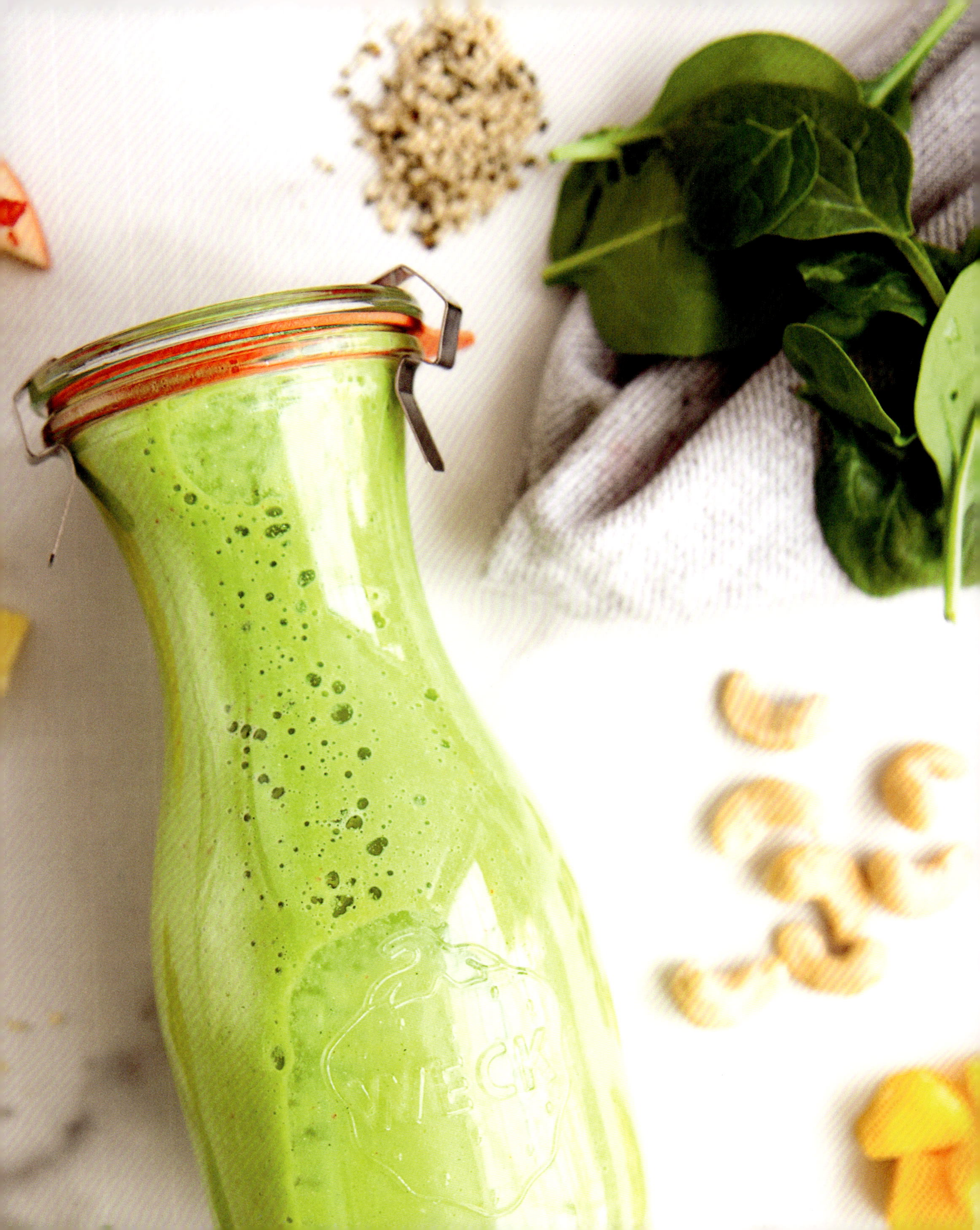
WECK

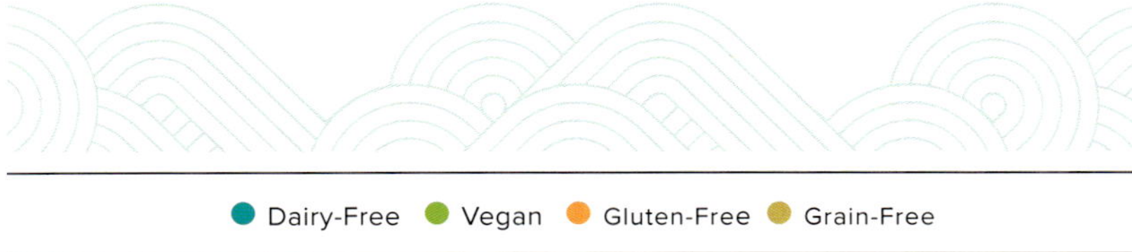

Dairy-Free · Vegan · Gluten-Free · Grain-Free

Soothing Mango Green Smoothie

This mango-sweetened green smoothie is an easy light breakfast or morning snack that packs in lots of nutrients and, thanks to the hemp hearts and cashews, has the protein you need to keep your blood sugar stable. If you don't have a high-powered blender, soak cashews in a dish of water in the refrigerator to soften them and help them blend easily.

10 MINUTES PREPPING • MAKES 1 LARGE OR 2 SMALL SMOOTHIES

WHAT YOU NEED:	HOW TO MAKE IT:
1 ½ cups (375 mL) water 1 cup (250 mL) spinach, lightly packed 1 tbsp (15 mL) hemp hearts 1 apple, cored and roughly chopped 1 small piece of fresh ginger, peeled and sliced (approx. 1 tsp/5 mL) ½ tsp (2 mL) fresh lemon juice 8 raw cashews 1 cup (250 mL) frozen mango	**1.** Add all ingredients to a high-powered blender, and blend on high until smooth, about 30 seconds. **2.** Taste and adjust ingredients as needed, adding water to thin, ice to cool, more cashews to thicken, or more mango to sweeten.

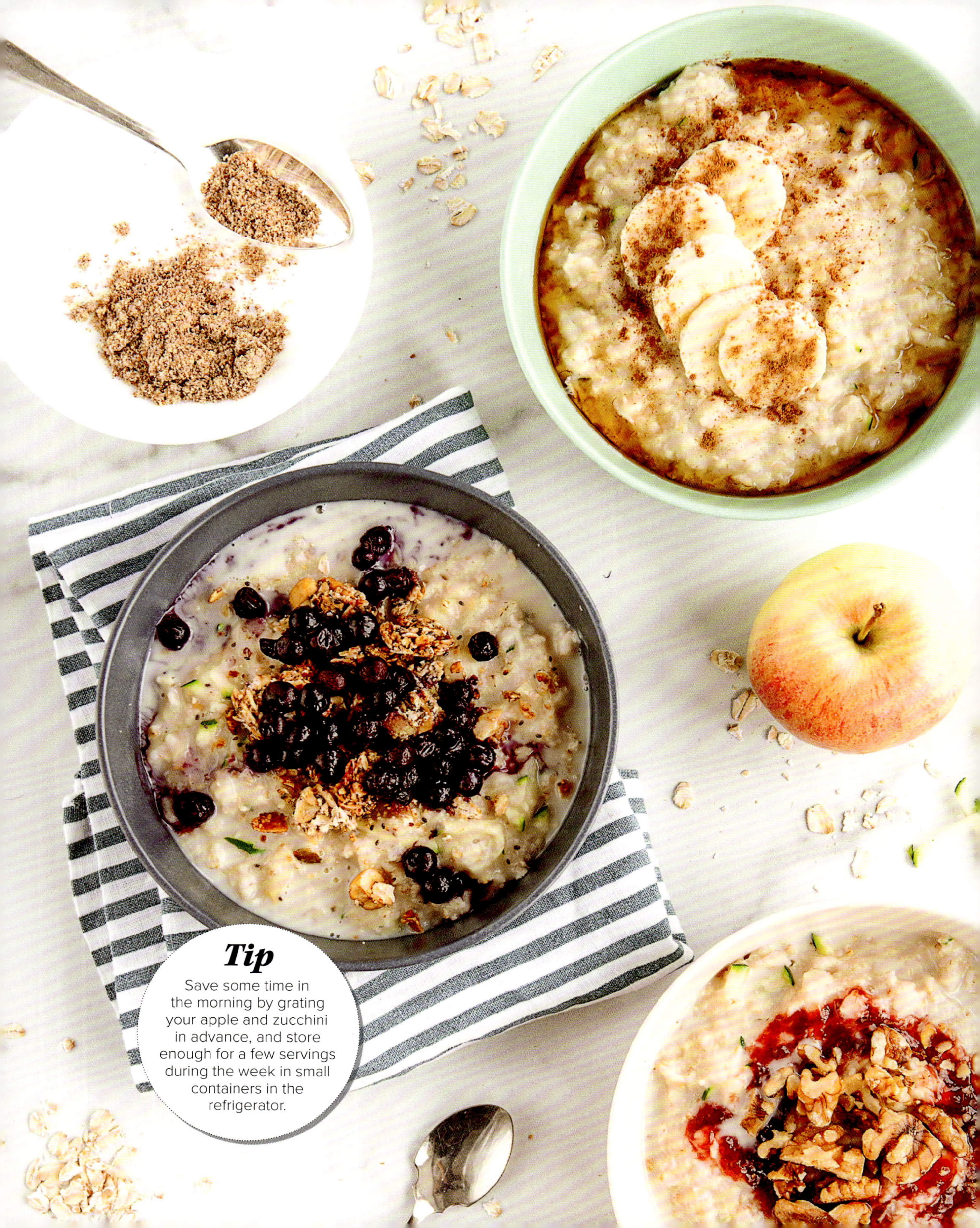

Tip

Save some time in the morning by grating your apple and zucchini in advance, and store enough for a few servings during the week in small containers in the refrigerator.

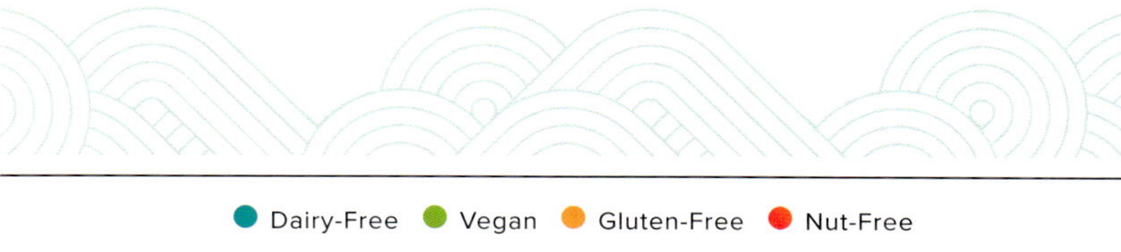

Dairy-Free • Vegan • Gluten-Free • Nut-Free

Apple Zucchini Oat Bowl

Comforting and warming cinnamon-packed oats hide a serving of vegetables and fruit that you won't even notice. No zucchini on hand? Use carrots, squash, or sweet potato instead. No ground flaxseed? Use hemp hearts or chia seeds instead.

5 MINUTES PREPPING • 10 MINUTES COOKING • MAKES 2 SERVINGS

WHAT YOU NEED:

- 1 cup (250 mL) rolled oats
- ½ cup (125 mL) non-dairy milk of choice
- 1 ½ cups (375 mL) water
- ½ large apple, grated
- ¼ cup (60 mL) zucchini, grated
- 1 tsp (5 mL) cinnamon
- 2 tbsp (30 mL) ground flaxseed
- Maple syrup and melted coconut oil, for serving

HOW TO MAKE IT:

1. Add oats, milk, and water to a medium pan, and bring to a boil.
2. Lower heat to a simmer, and stir in the grated apple and zucchini.
3. Let oats cook about 7 minutes, or until they reach your desired consistency.
4. Turn off the heat, and stir in the cinnamon, ground flaxseed, maple syrup, and coconut oil (if using).

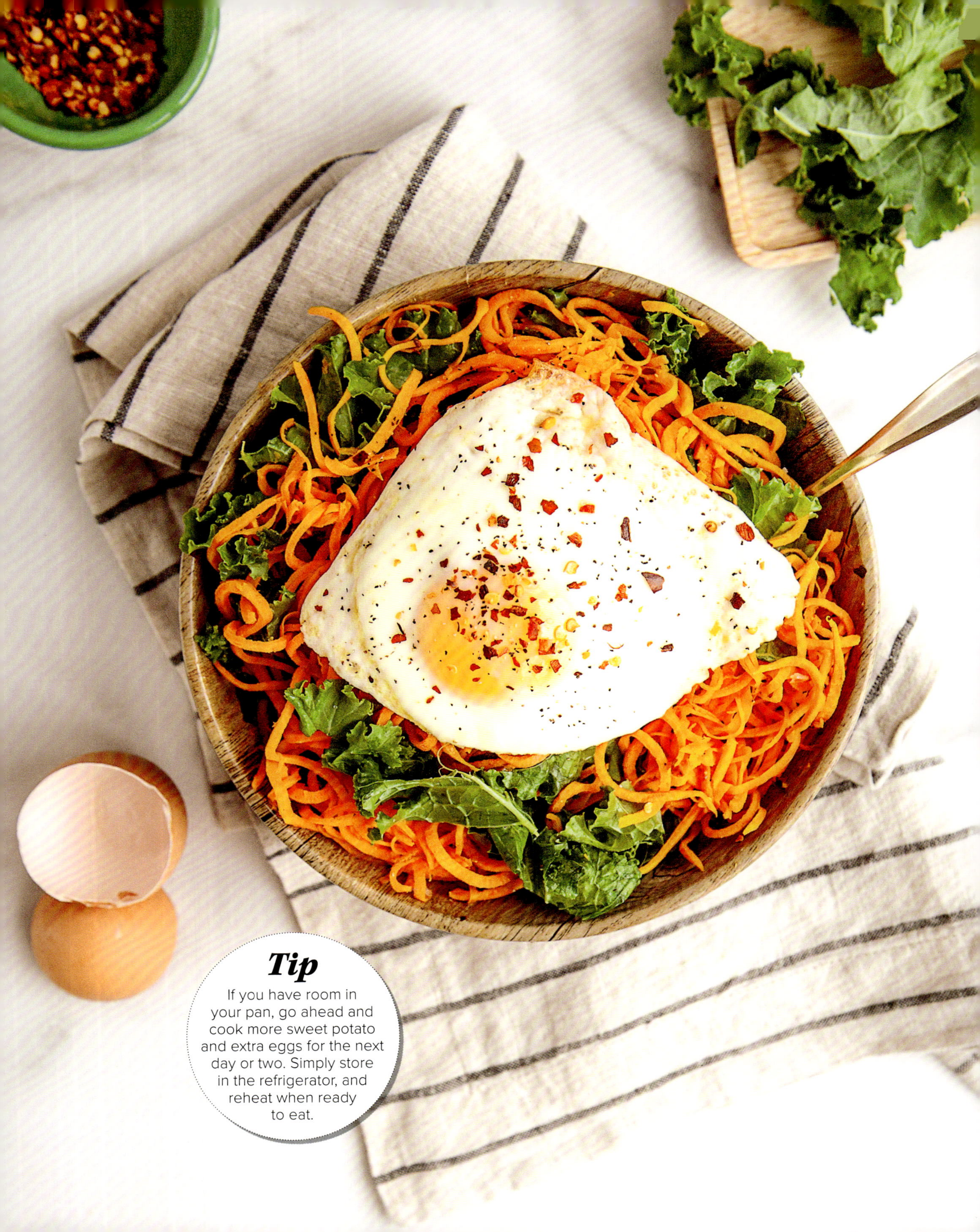

Tip

If you have room in your pan, go ahead and cook more sweet potato and extra eggs for the next day or two. Simply store in the refrigerator, and reheat when ready to eat.

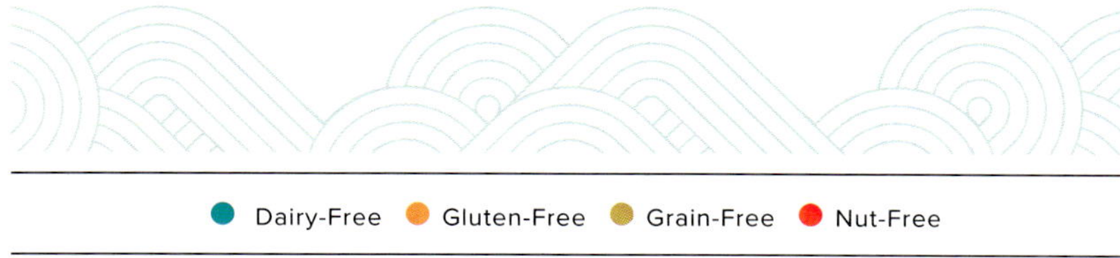

Dairy-Free • Gluten-Free • Grain-Free • Nut-Free

7-Minute Ultimate Breakfast Bowl

The ultimate morning fuel, this is like a prenatal vitamin in a bowl. This breakfast won't make your blood sugar soar, but it will give you balanced, steady energy all morning long. Feel free to change up the greens too. Spinach, bok choy, Swiss chard, or other greens are just as tasty and are good substitutes.

5 MINUTES PREPPING • 7 MINUTES COOKING • MAKES 1 SERVING

WHAT YOU NEED:

½ sweet potato, peeled and spiralized (or large handful if buying already spiralized)

2 large kale leaves, stemmed and roughly chopped or ripped

1 egg

1 tbsp (15 mL) olive oil

Sea salt, pepper, and chili flakes to taste

HOW TO MAKE IT:

1. Heat a large pan over low-medium heat, and add olive oil to lightly coat bottom of pan.
2. Add sweet potato, stirring to coat in olive oil, and cook for 3 minutes.
3. Move sweet potato to one side of the pan, crack egg onto half of the remaining part of the pan, and then add kale in the empty spot, quickly tossing the leaves to coat in remaining oil.
4. Cover the pan, and let cook for 4 minutes, or until egg yolk is fully cooked.
5. Transfer to a plate, and sprinkle with sea salt, pepper, and chili flakes to taste.

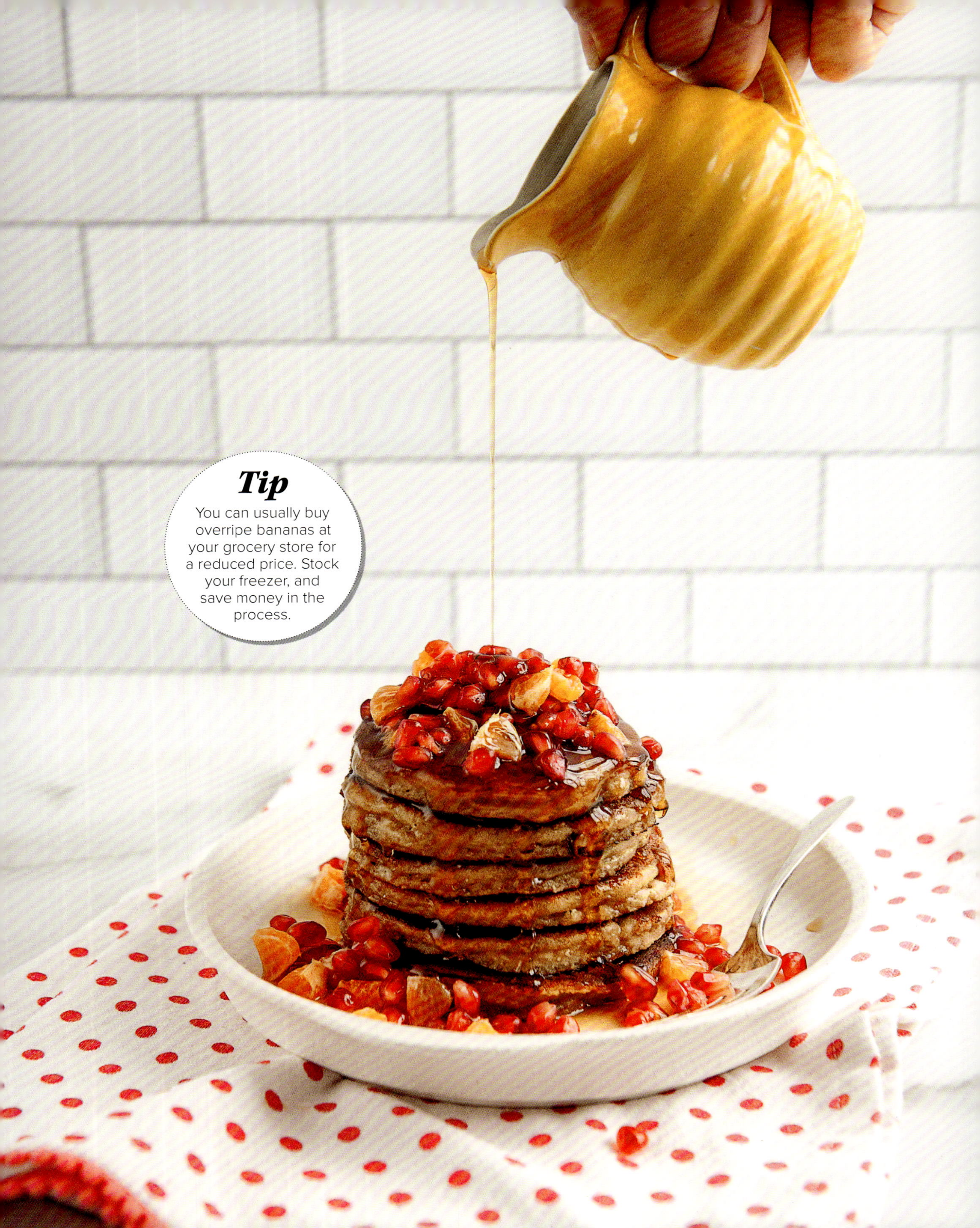

Tip

You can usually buy overripe bananas at your grocery store for a reduced price. Stock your freezer, and save money in the process.

Dairy-Free · Gluten-Free · Grain-Free · Freezer-Friendly

Preggo Protein Pancakes

Naturally sweetened, high-protein, grain-free pancakes are the perfect protein-powered breakfast (or dinner). I always make extras to freeze — simply defrost and eat them cold (especially good for those days you don't feel very well), or pop them into the toaster, and top with some almond butter and hemp hearts. Almond flour is essential for this recipe. If it isn't readily available at your local store, you can make your own by processing raw almonds in your food processor.

10 MINUTES PREPPING • 20 MINUTES COOKING • MAKES 12 PANCAKES

WHAT YOU NEED:

2 ½ cups (625 mL) almond flour

½ tsp (2 mL) baking soda

½ tsp (2 mL) sea salt

3 eggs

⅔ cup (150 mL) coconut milk (full fat, from a can)

1 ripe banana, puréed or mashed

2 tsp (10 mL) vanilla

1 tbsp (15 mL) coconut oil for the pan

Toppings (optional):

Pomegranate arils (the ruby red seeds), sliced clementines, and poppy seeds

Fresh or frozen berries

Maple syrup

Melted coconut oil

Chopped nuts or seeds

HOW TO MAKE IT:

1. Combine dry ingredients in a large bowl. In a medium-sized bowl, whisk eggs, then stir in coconut milk, banana, and vanilla, and mix until smooth.
2. Pour wet ingredients over dry, and mix to combine.
3. Coat a large skillet with coconut oil, and turn to medium-low heat.
4. Add batter to pan in small scoops, pressing lightly to thin slightly. Cook until bubbles start to form and the underside is golden brown, then flip. Repeat with remaining batter.

NOTE

When you open your can of coconut milk, you will likely find that the cream and water have separated. Give it a quick stir before you measure out the ⅔ cup for the batter. Use the rest in a smoothie or as a yogurt substitute in the **Chia Yogurt Bites** (page 47).

For a shortcut, place all of the wet ingredients (eggs through to vanilla) in a blender, and blend until smooth.

Dairy-Free · Gluten-Free · Grain-Free · Nut-Free · Freezer-Friendly

Strawberry Chia Jam

This refined sugar-free, gut-loving jam packs in the fibre and protein, helping you say goodbye to stomach complaints and nausea. We love this on toast, stirred into oats, as the fruity middle of the Chia Yogurt Bites (page 47) — or on top of some ice cream. For the most delicious and flavourful strawberries, buy in season, and freeze on a parchment-lined baking tray overnight, transferring to a freezer bag or container to enjoy in the off-season.

5 MINUTES PREPPING • 10 MINUTES COOKING • MAKES 2 CUPS (500 ML)

WHAT YOU NEED:

- 2 cups (500 mL) strawberries (frozen or fresh)
- 2 tbsp (30 mL) chia seeds
- 1 tbsp (15 mL) lemon juice
- 1 tbsp (15 mL) honey

HOW TO MAKE IT:

1. Add berries to a small saucepan, and cook over medium heat for 5 to 10 minutes, until berries have softened and have begun to release their juices.
2. Mash berries with a potato masher or wooden spoon in the pot until they reach your preferred jam texture.
3. Remove pot from heat, and stir in lemon juice, chia seeds, and honey. Let sit until thickened, stirring occasionally, about 10 minutes. Transfer to a glass jar, and keep in the refrigerator for 2 weeks or the freezer for 3 months.

Tip

If berries aren't in season, opt for frozen berries. They'll be cheaper, fresher, and more flavourful since they were likely frozen right after picking.

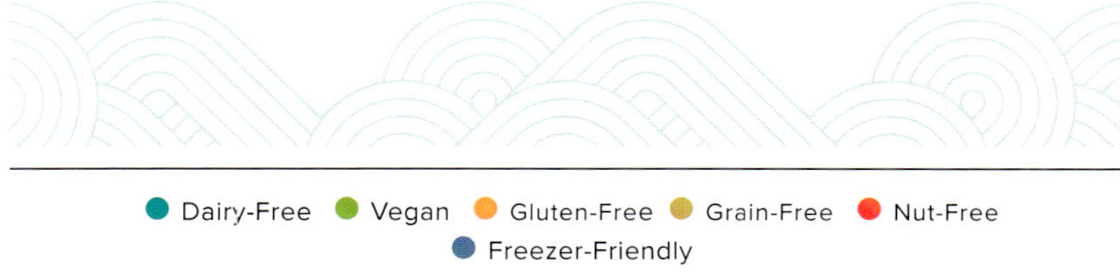

Dairy-Free · Vegan · Gluten-Free · Grain-Free · Nut-Free · Freezer-Friendly

Amped-Up Applesauce

Applesauce has always been a go-to food for sick days since it ticks all the boxes: soft, sweet, and easy to digest. The addition of hemp hearts and coconut oil brings protein and fat to this sweet treat, making it a balanced snack at any time of day.

5 MINUTES PREPPING • 25 MINUTES COOKING • MAKES 2 CUPS (500 ML)

WHAT YOU NEED:

- 5 apples, cored and chopped
- ⅔ cup (150 mL) of water
- Juice of ½ a lemon
- 1 to 2 tbsp (15 to 30 mL) hemp hearts
- ½ tsp (2 mL) cinnamon
- ¼ tsp (1 mL) fresh nutmeg
- 1 tbsp (15 mL) coconut oil, melted (for serving) (optional)

HOW TO MAKE IT:

1. Set a medium-sized pot to medium-high heat, and add the apples, water, lemon juice, and spices.
2. Simmer apples until they are soft and getting mushy, about 20 minutes.
3. Pour apple mixture into the blender, add the hemp hearts, and then purée until smooth.
4. Stir in melted coconut oil (if using), and enjoy.

Tip

McIntosh is the go-to apple for applesauce, but for pretty pink sauce, add some sweet red apples such as Cortland or Empire.

Link-up

Double up on your applesauce and use it to make the **Lemon + Ginger Carrot Muffins** (page 51).

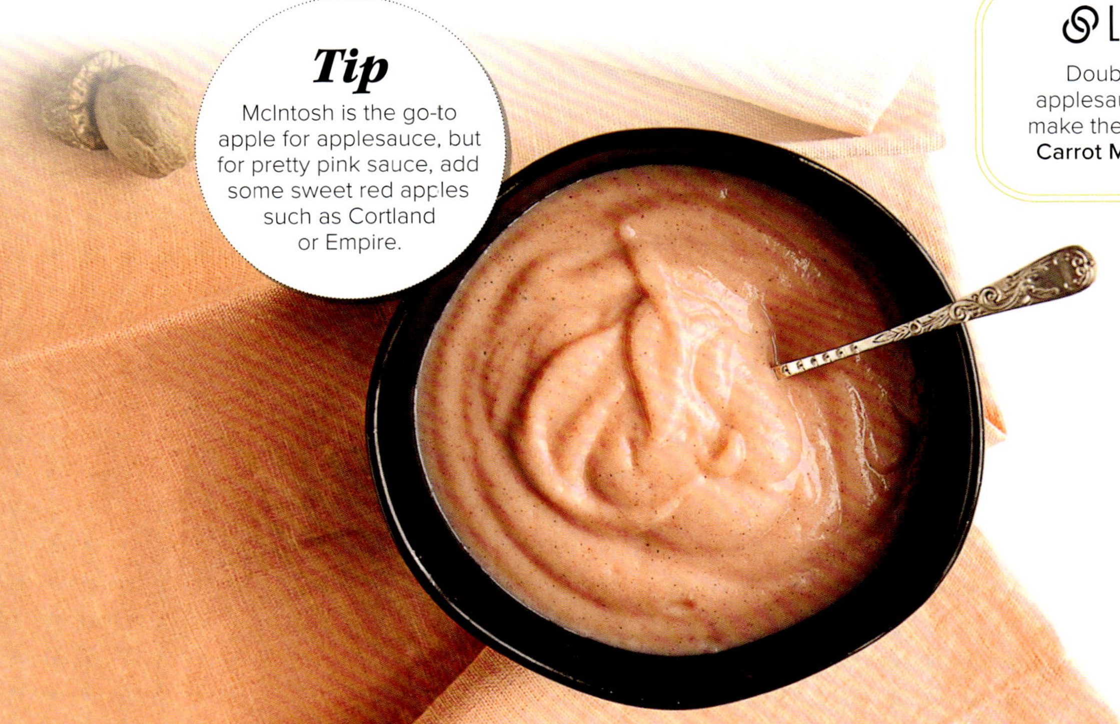

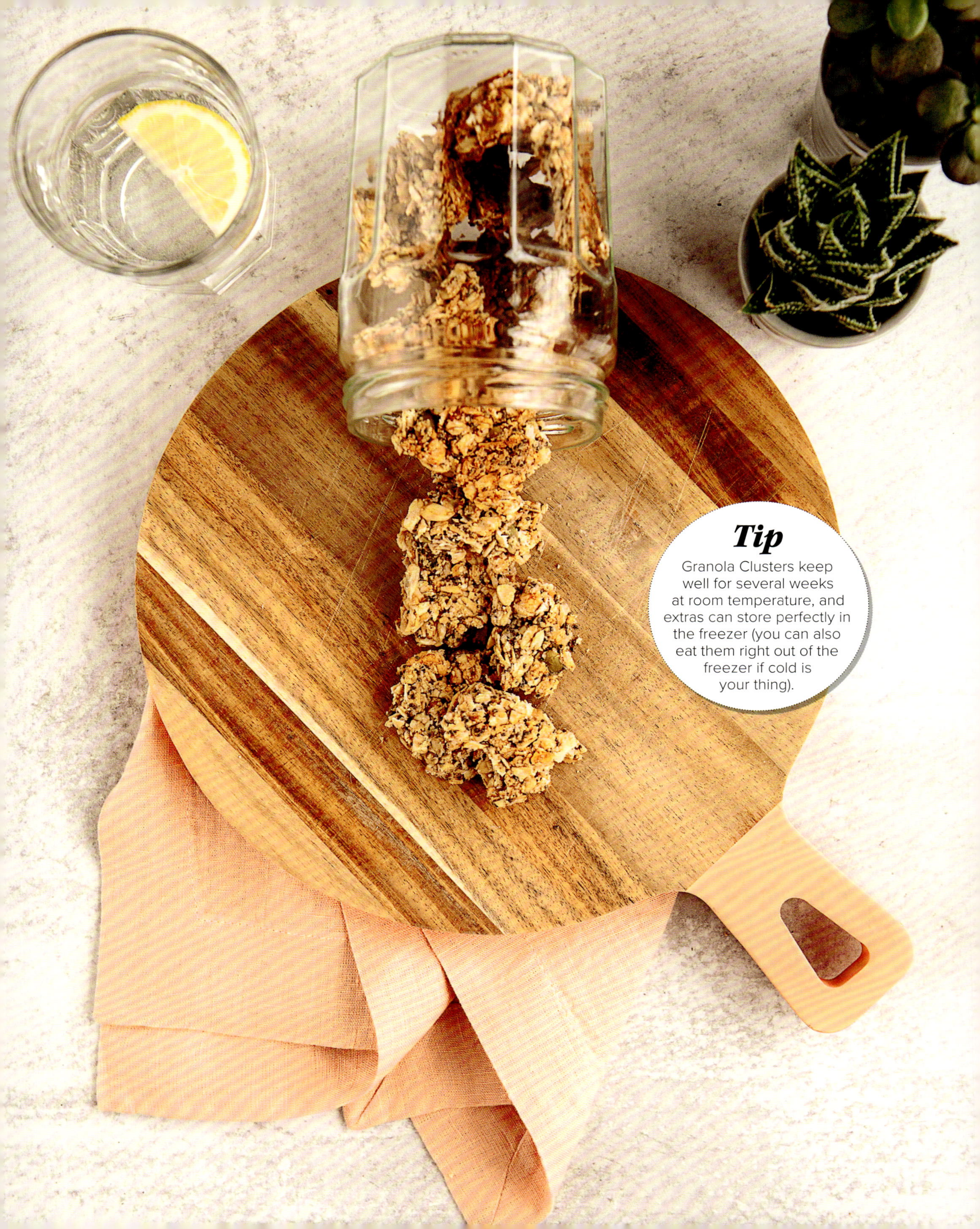

Tip

Granola Clusters keep well for several weeks at room temperature, and extras can store perfectly in the freezer (you can also eat them right out of the freezer if cold is your thing).

Dairy-Free • Gluten-Free • Freezer-Friendly

Bedside Granola Clusters

The perfect crunchy, satisfying, and stomach-settling snack to keep in your nightstand to eat in the middle of the night or early morning. Swap out the nuts and seeds depending on what you have, and add an extra pinch of salt if salt helps you feel good right now.

10 MINUTES PREPPING • 10 MINUTES COOKING • MAKES 1 TRAY FULL

WHAT YOU NEED:

For the flax eggs

⅓ cup (75 mL) warm water

2 tbsp (30 mL) ground flaxseed

Dry ingredients

2 cups (500 mL) oat flour

3 cups (750 mL) rolled oats

1 cup (250 mL) salted cashews, chopped

1 cup (250 mL) almonds, chopped

1 cup (250 mL) seeds of choice (pumpkin, sunflower, chia)

1 tsp (5 mL) cinnamon

½ tsp (2 mL) sea salt

Wet ingredients

½ cup (125 mL) coconut oil, melted

½ cup (125 mL) honey

1 tsp (5 mL) vanilla

HOW TO MAKE IT:

1. Preheat oven to 375°F (190°C), and line a baking tray with parchment paper.
2. Combine the water and ground flaxseed in a small bowl, and let sit (this makes flax eggs, an alternative to eggs).
3. In a medium bowl, combine wet ingredients.
4. In a large bowl, combine dry ingredients.
5. Pour wet mixture over dry mixture, and stir to combine. Add your flax eggs, and stir to thoroughly combine.
6. Transfer mixture to prepared baking tray, and pack firmly together with spatula by pressing down across pan.
7. Bake for 10 minutes, then turn off oven, and let the granola sit overnight, or for 4 to 8 hours.
8. Remove from oven, and break into pieces, transferring to a sealed storage container.

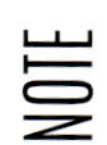

The key to keeping the clusters formed like mini granola bars is leaving the sheet of granola packed together and untouched overnight.

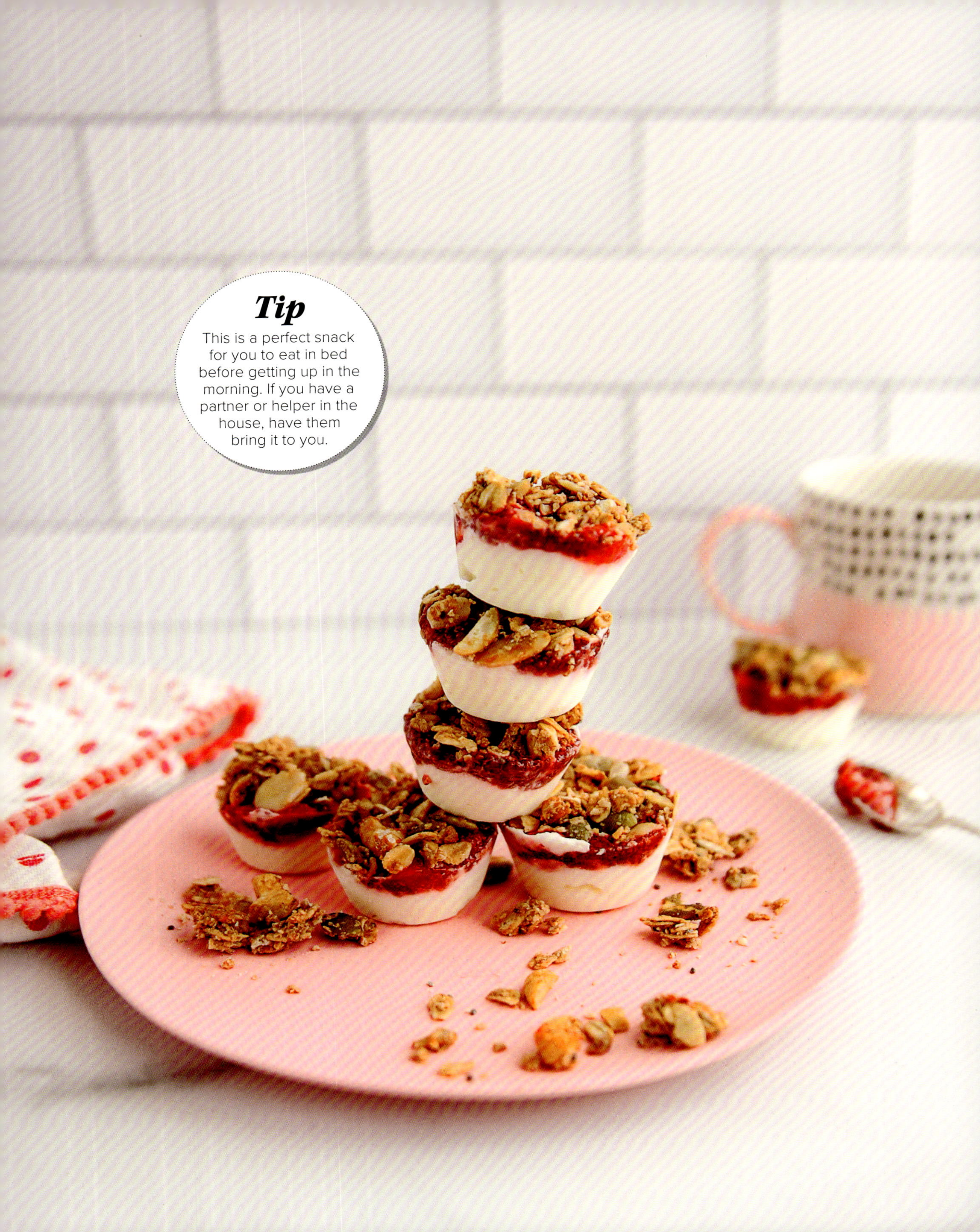
Tip
This is a perfect snack for you to eat in bed before getting up in the morning. If you have a partner or helper in the house, have them bring it to you.

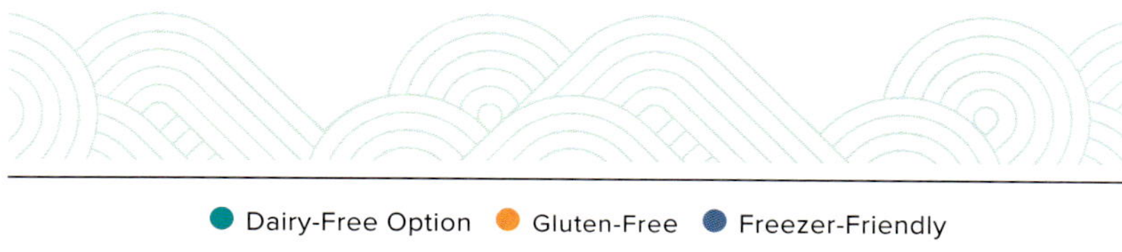

● Dairy-Free Option ● Gluten-Free ● Freezer-Friendly

Chia Yogurt Bites

Relieve any early-morning nausea with these nutritious freezer bites. This cold treat is likely to help soothe your stomach and has a balanced ratio of fat, fibre, and protein to help stabilize your blood sugar.

If you don't have a mini muffin pan, you can make frozen chia yogurt bark by adding the ingredients in the order listed to a parchment-lined tray before transferring to the freezer. Simply break the mixture up into pieces once frozen, and transfer the pieces to a freezer bag so that you can grab a piece each time you need a pick-me-up.

5 MINUTES PREPPING • 2 HOURS FREEZING • MAKES 12 BITES

WHAT YOU NEED:	HOW TO MAKE IT:
¾ cup (175 mL) yogurt of choice 1 tbsp (15 mL) coconut oil or ghee (optional) 1 tbsp (15 mL) collagen powder (optional) ¼ cup (60 mL) prepared Strawberry Chia Jam (page 42) or store-bought jam ¼ cup (60 mL) prepared Bedside Granola Clusters (page 45) or store-bought granola	**1.** Mix your coconut oil/ghee and collagen powder into the yogurt, if using them. **2.** Into each space in a silicone mini muffin pan, scoop 2 heaping tsp (12 mL) of yogurt, followed by 1 tsp (5 mL) chia jam and about 1 tsp (5 mL) crumbly granola; then place in the freezer for about 2 hours.

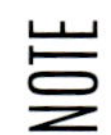

If using non-dairy yogurt (e.g., coconut milk yogurt) or low-fat yogurt, you will need to stir approximately 1 tbsp coconut oil or ghee into the yogurt before adding it to the muffin tray to ensure the bites are creamy and don't turn hard like ice.

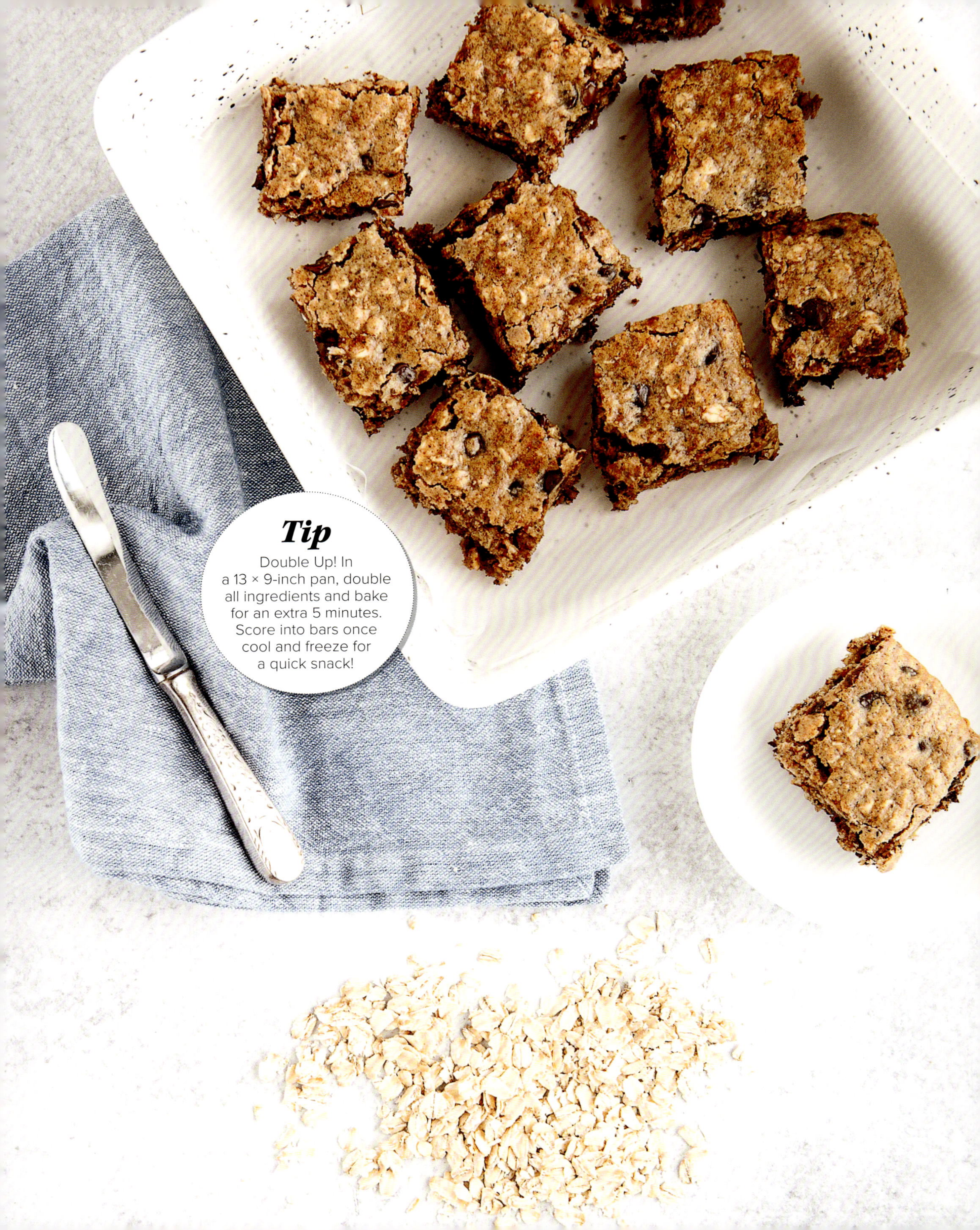
Tip
Double Up! In
a 13 × 9-inch pan, double
all ingredients and bake
for an extra 5 minutes.
Score into bars once
cool and freeze for
a quick snack!

● Dairy-Free Option ● Gluten-Free ● Freezer-Friendly

Almond Chocolate Oat Bars

These soft, chocolate-filled oat bars are free of all of the additives and refined sugar found in store-bought versions. These slightly sweet bars are full of protein and are perfect for a bite at your desk or as a late-night snack.

10 MINUTES PREPPING • 25 TO 30 MINUTES COOKING • MAKES ONE 8 × 8-INCH PAN

WHAT YOU NEED:

Dry ingredients

1 cup (250 mL) rolled oats

½ cup (125 mL) almond flour

2 tbsp (30 mL) ground flaxseed

½ tsp (2 mL) cinnamon

½ tsp (2 mL) sea salt

¼ tsp (1 mL) baking soda

Wet ingredients

2 eggs

½ cup (125 mL) almond butter

¼ cup (60 mL) maple syrup

3 tbsp (45 mL) coconut oil, melted

½ tsp (2 mL) vanilla

Mix-in

⅓ cup (75 mL) chocolate chips (dairy-free or regular)

HOW TO MAKE IT:

1. Preheat oven to 350°F (180°C), and line an 8 × 8-inch pan with parchment paper.
2. Mix dry ingredients together in a large bowl.
3. Whisk eggs in a medium bowl, and stir in the almond butter, maple syrup, coconut oil, and vanilla.
4. Pour the wet mixture over dry ingredients, and mix until the oats are covered and look wet. Fold in chocolate chips.
5. Pour mixture into parchment-lined pan. Use spatula or another piece of parchment paper to press down and smooth out mixture so that it fills pan evenly.
6. Bake for 25 to 30 minutes, or until the centre springs back up after a light touch. Allow to cool in the pan, then cut into bars, and store in an airtight container.

Link-up

Put your bag of almond flour to use by making the **Grain-Free Chicken Fingers** (page 106), **Preggo Protein Pancakes** (page 41), or **Blueberry Zucchini Muffins** (page 92).

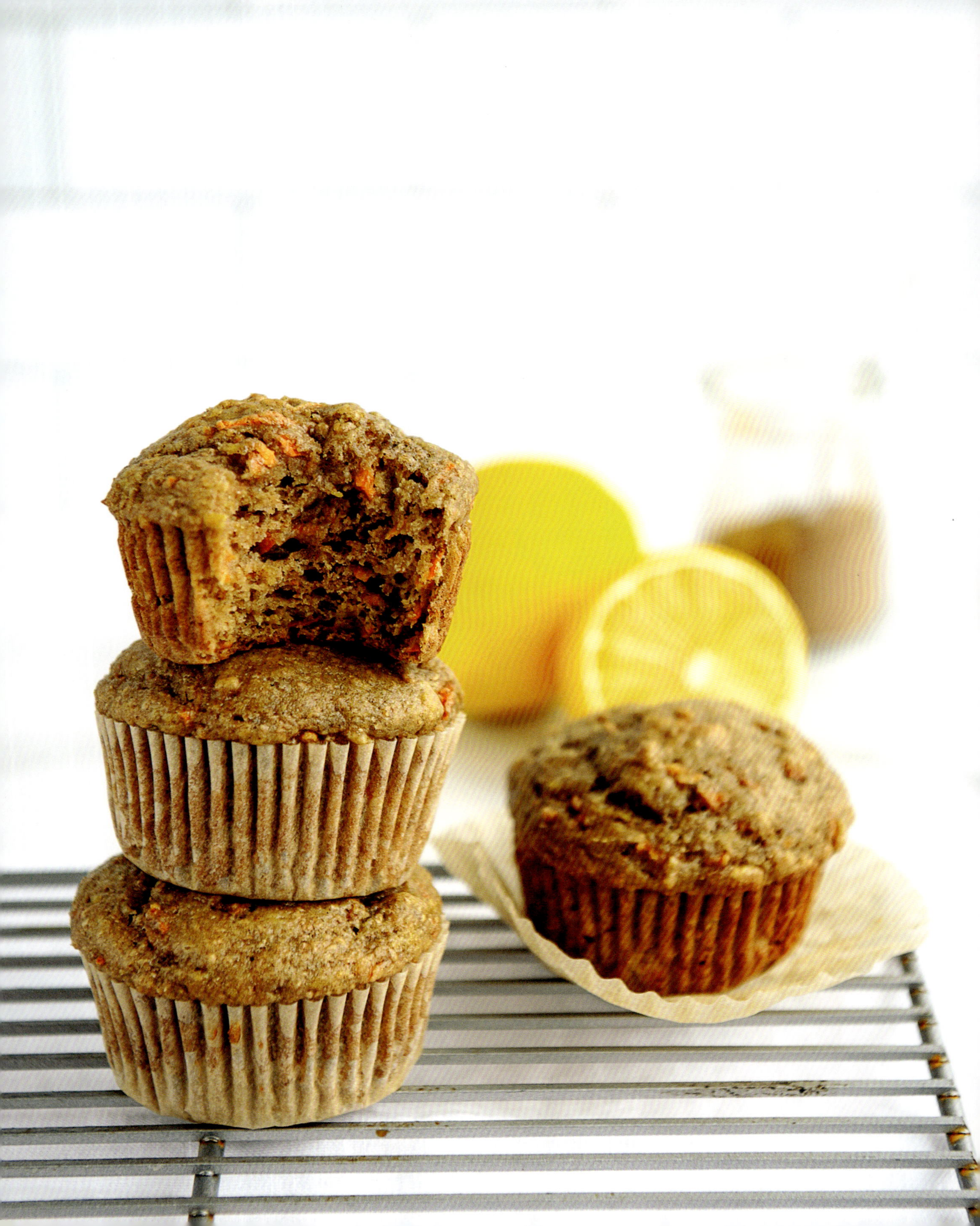

● Dairy-Free Option ● Vegan Option ● Gluten-Free Option ● Nut-Free ● Freezer-Friendly

Lemon + Ginger Carrot Muffins

The best carrot muffins you've ever had, made even better with two of the most potent natural anti-nausea foods — lemon and ginger! You're going to want to make a double batch — enjoy some for the week and keep the rest in the freezer for next time. These can stay on the counter for a couple of days, in the refrigerator for about a week, or in the freezer for several months.

15 MINUTES PREPPING • 20 MINUTES COOKING • MAKES 10 MUFFINS

WHAT YOU NEED:

Dry ingredients

1 ½ cups (375 mL) oat flour (or substitute whole wheat for non-GF)

1 tsp (5 mL) baking soda

1 tsp (5 mL) cinnamon

1 tsp (5 mL) ground ginger

¼ tsp (1 mL) sea salt

Mix-in

1 cup (250 mL) grated carrot

1 heaping tbsp (20 mL) lemon zest

Wet ingredients

2 tbsp (30 mL) ghee or butter, melted

1 egg, beaten

1 cup (250 mL) applesauce

½ cup (125 mL) maple syrup or honey

1 tsp (5 mL) vanilla extract

HOW TO MAKE IT:

1. Preheat oven to 350°F (180°C), and grease muffin pan with avocado oil or butter.
2. Sift dry ingredients together in a large mixing bowl.
3. Combine wet ingredients in a medium bowl, then pour over the dry ingredients, stirring to combine.
4. Fold in carrots and lemon zest.
5. Scoop into prepared muffin pans using an ice cream scoop, and bake for 16 to 20 minutes, or until the tops of the muffins spring back up when pressed with your finger.

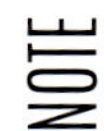

For a dairy-free and vegan option, use coconut oil in place of the butter, a flax egg (1 tbsp ground flaxseed mixed with 2 ½ tbsp warm water) in place of the egg, and maple syrup instead of honey.

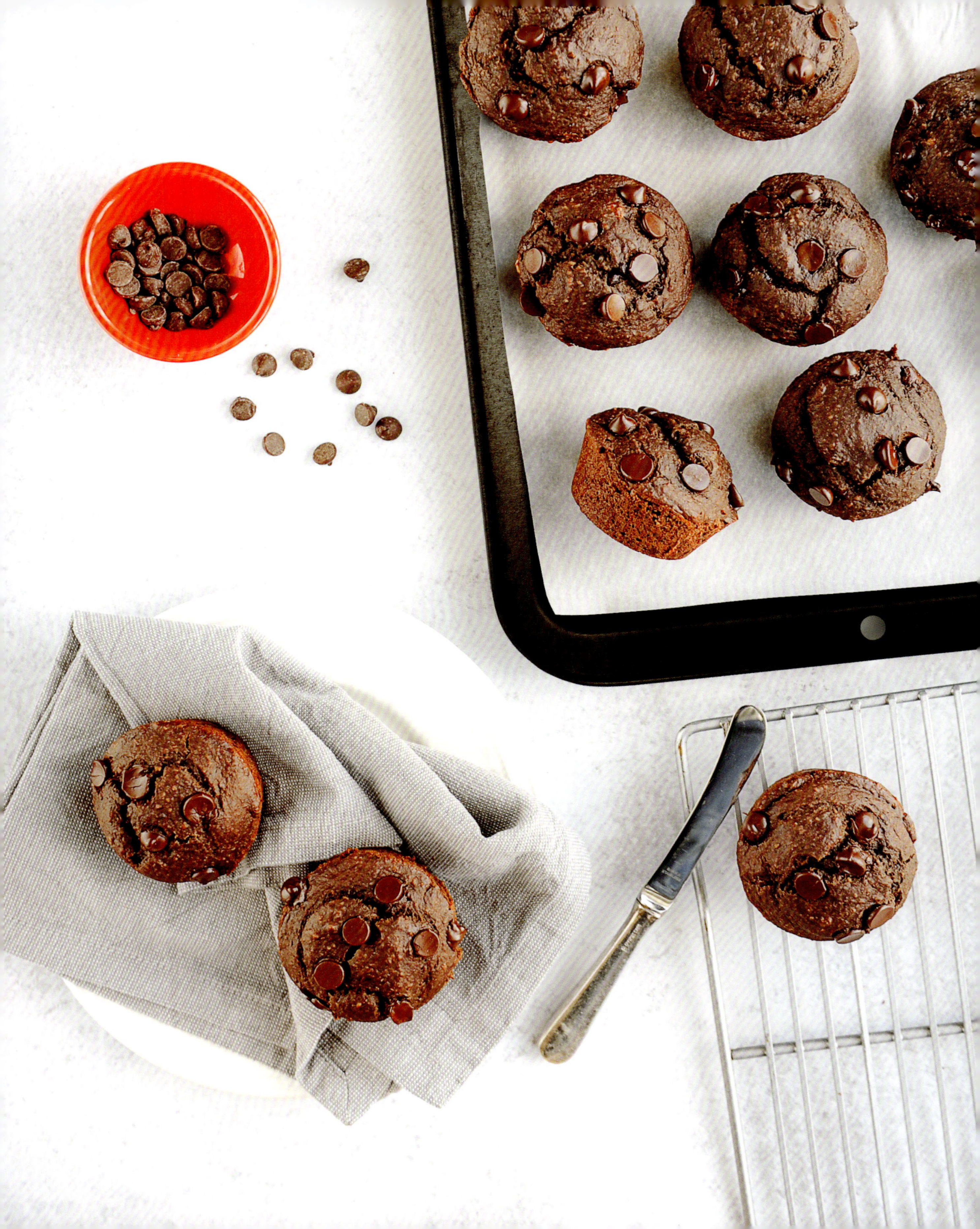

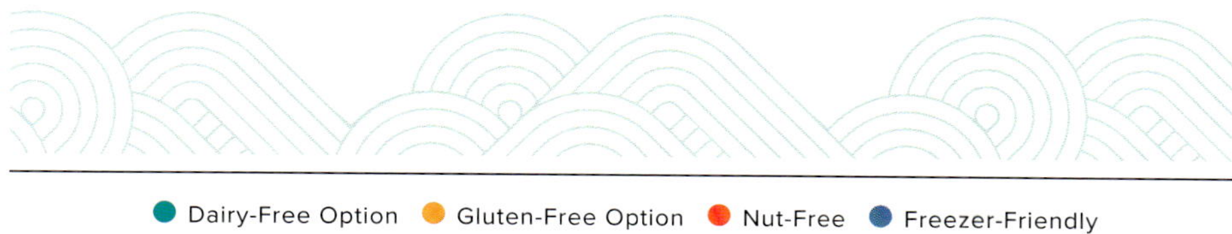

Dairy-Free Option · Gluten-Free Option · Nut-Free · Freezer-Friendly

Double Chocolate Lentil Muffins

Go with me on this one. Lentils are one of the best food sources of folate, an essential nutrient for early pregnancy. These are the perfect chocolate muffins that happen to have a hefty serving of lentils baked right in — and they taste nothing like lentils. Get ready for a surprise!

10 MINUTES PREPPING • 15 TO 17 MINUTES COOKING • MAKES 12 MUFFINS

WHAT YOU NEED:

Dry ingredients

1 ½ cups (375 mL) oat flour (or substitute whole wheat flour for non-GF)

⅓ cup (75 mL) cacao powder

⅓ cup (75 mL) coconut sugar

1 tsp (5 mL) baking powder

1 tsp (5 mL) baking soda

½ tsp (2 mL) salt

Mix-in

½ to ⅔ cup (125 to 150 mL) chocolate chips (dairy-free or regular)

Wet ingredients

1 cup (250 mL) cooked red lentils (this can be made several days in advance)

1 cup (250 mL) ripe banana, mashed

1 egg

¼ cup (60 mL) coconut oil, melted

3 tbsp (45 mL) maple syrup

1 tsp (5 mL) vanilla extract

HOW TO MAKE IT:

1. Preheat oven to 350°F (180°C) and grease a muffin tin with coconut oil or avocado oil.
2. In a food processor or blender, process the wet ingredients until smooth.
3. In a large bowl, sift together the dry ingredients.
4. Combine the wet and dry ingredients by pouring the wet mix into the dry bowl and stirring to combine.
5. Fold in the chocolate chips with a spatula, and using an ice cream scoop, portion muffin mix into prepared muffin tin. Top each muffin with a few extra chocolate chips if desired.
6. Bake muffins for 15 to 17 minutes, or until the middle springs back when pressed with a finger.

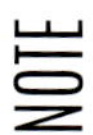

How to cook dried red lentils: Combine ½ cup lentils and 1 cup of water in a small saucepan. Bring to a boil, reduce heat to low, cover, and cook, about 20 minutes, or until lentils are very soft and water is absorbed. Remove from heat and cool. Consider making double and freezing half for use next time.

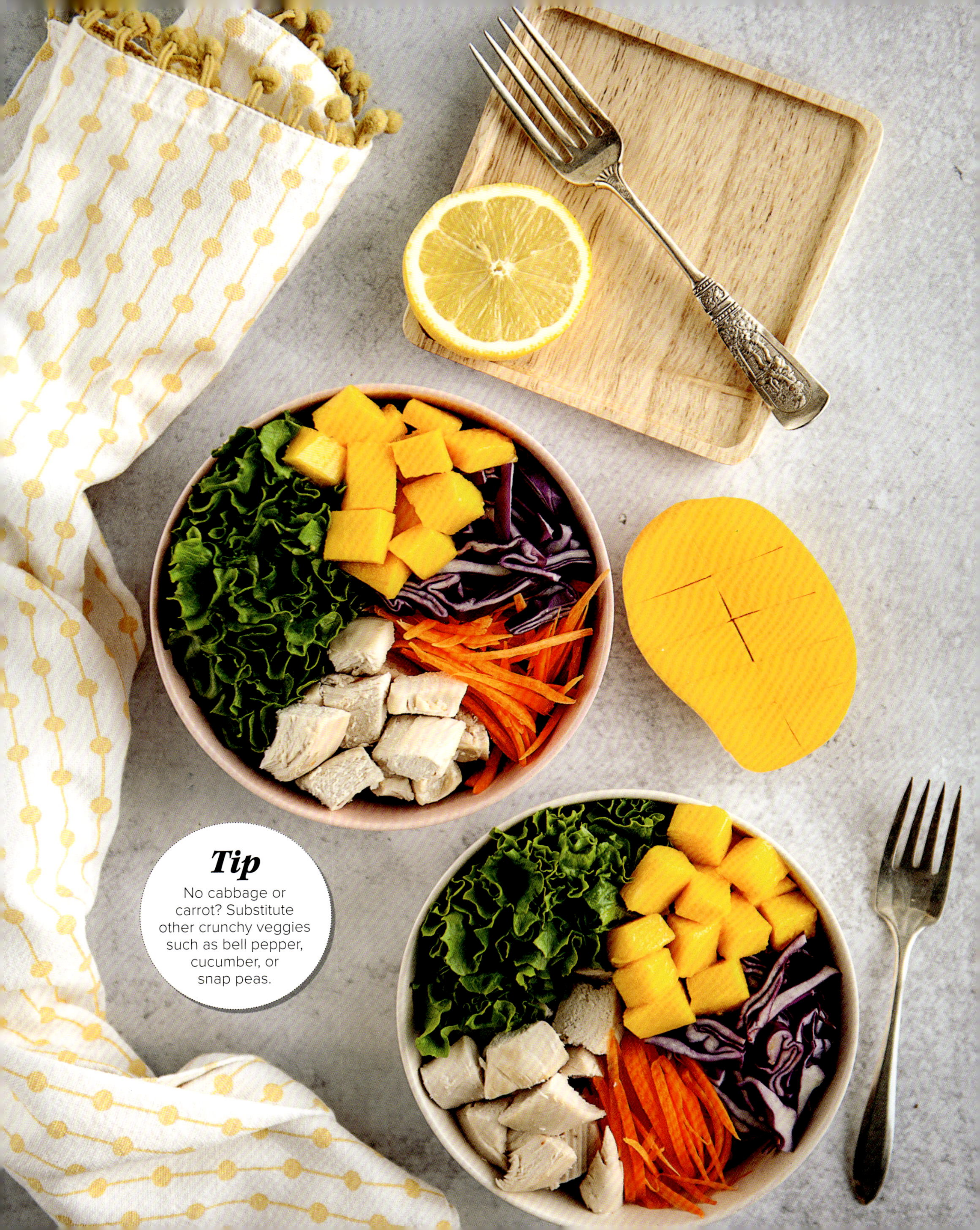
Tip
No cabbage or carrot? Substitute other crunchy veggies such as bell pepper, cucumber, or snap peas.

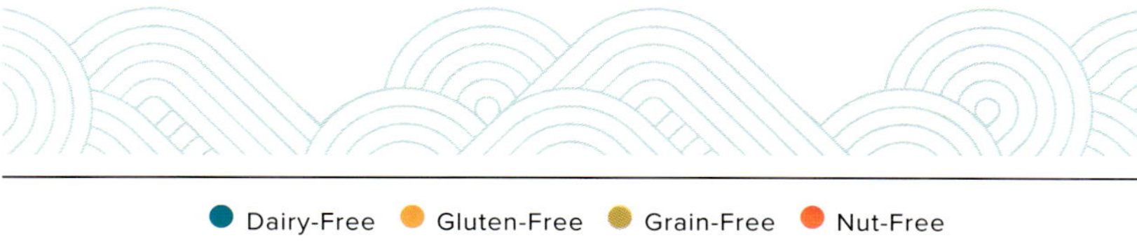

● Dairy-Free ● Gluten-Free ● Grain-Free ● Nut-Free

Mango Chopped Chicken Salad with Lemon Vinaigrette

This cold and sweet salad explodes with colour and gives a satisfying crunch for those days when you're not in the salad mood. Not in the mood for chicken? Substitute it with salted cashews, chickpeas, or cooked quinoa.

20 MINUTES PREPPING • MAKES 2 SERVINGS

WHAT YOU NEED:

For the salad

4 cups (1 L) lettuce of choice, roughly chopped

1 cup (250 mL) carrots, julienned

1 cup (250 mL) red cabbage, thinly sliced

1 cup (250 mL) cooked chicken, chopped

1 mango, cubed

For the lemon vinaigrette

¼ cup (60 mL) extra virgin olive oil

2 tbsp (30 mL) apple cider vinegar

2 tbsp (30 mL) lemon juice

½ tbsp (7 mL) honey

¼ tsp (1 mL) sea salt

Pinch of pepper

HOW TO MAKE IT:

1. Add all vinaigrette ingredients to a small glass jar, and shake to combine.
2. To a large bowl, add the lettuce, carrots, cabbage, chicken, and mango. Pour on dressing until the salad is coated to your liking, and toss to combine. If you're making this for a packed lunch, hold off adding the dressing until it's time to eat.

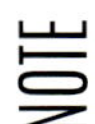

For the salad, in place of the cooked chicken, I like using **Greek Chicken Skewers** leftovers (page 150).

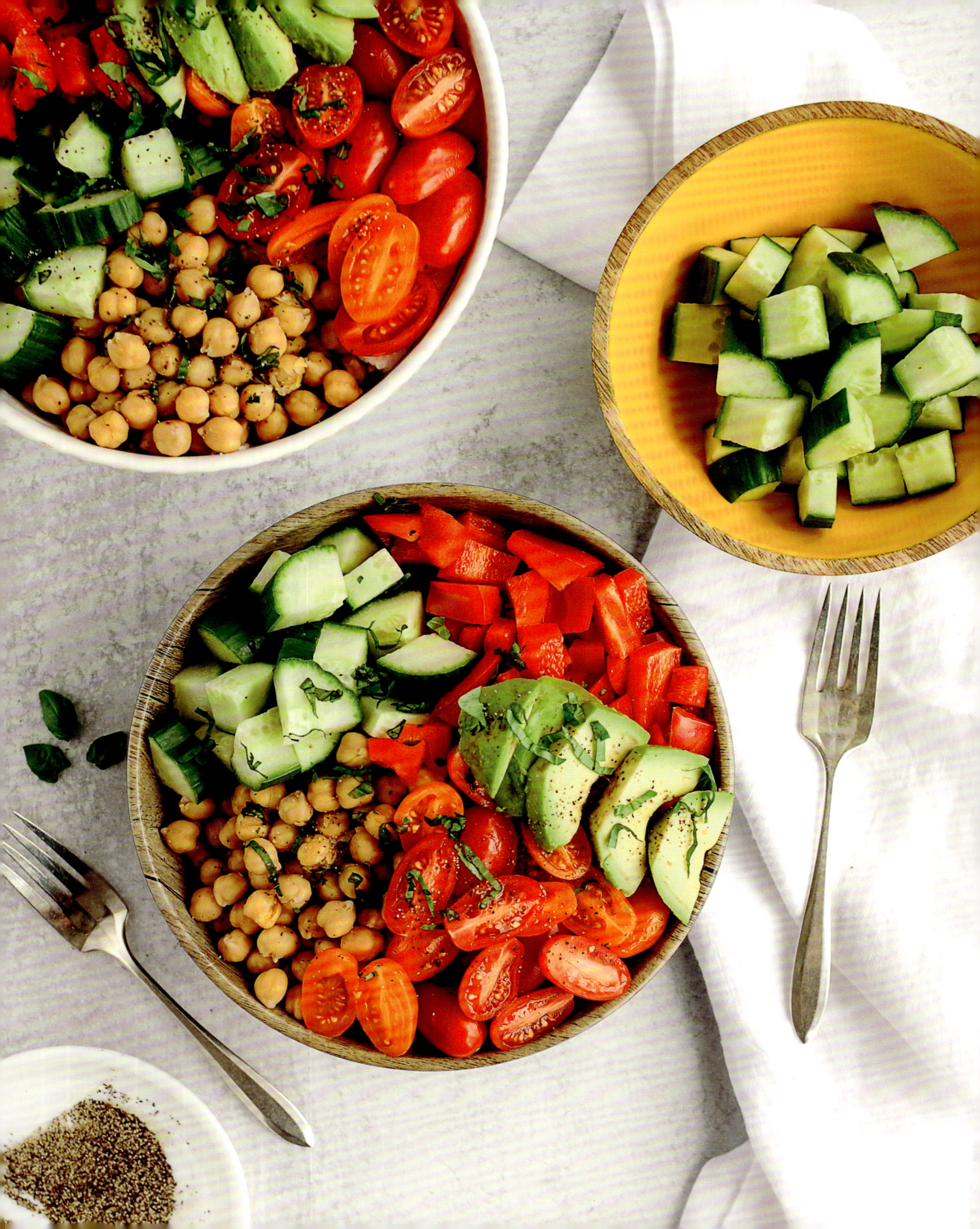

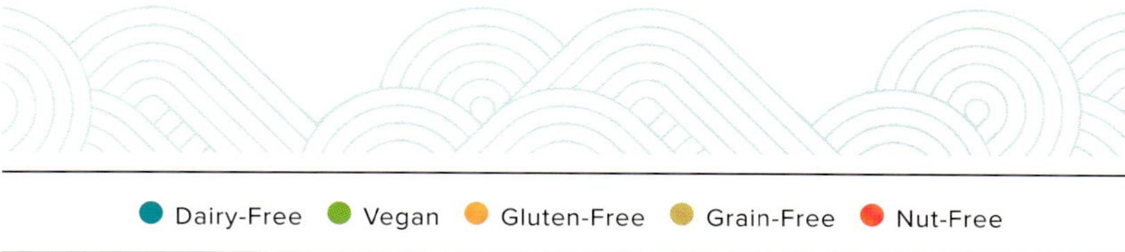

Dairy-Free • Vegan • Gluten-Free • Grain-Free • Nut-Free

Avocado Chickpea Bowl

Bowls such as this are a meal-prep staple for me. They're easy to make and keep well in the refrigerator for a couple of days, making them the perfect nutritious lunch. Customize this recipe from week to week by replacing the chickpeas with lentils or chopped chicken, or adding quinoa, millet, kale, or rice.

15 MINUTES PREPPING • MAKES 2 TO 3 SERVINGS

WHAT YOU NEED:

For the bowl

2 cups (500 mL) cherry tomatoes, halved

1 cup (250 mL) chickpeas

1 avocado, sliced

1 large cucumber, quartered and sliced

1 red pepper, chopped

1 green onion, chopped

1 tbsp (15 mL) fresh basil, chopped

For the vinaigrette

⅓ cup (75 mL) extra virgin olive oil

3 tbsp (45 mL) apple cider vinegar

1 clove garlic, minced

¼ tsp (1 mL) sea salt

Pinch of pepper

HOW TO MAKE IT:

1. In a large bowl, combine all the bowl ingredients.
2. In a medium bowl or small glass jar, combine the vinaigrette ingredients, and whisk or shake to combine.
3. Pour vinaigrette over bowl ingredients until the ingredients are coated to your liking. Enjoy immediately.
4. Transfer extras to glass storage jars for ready-made lunches (keeps well for 2 days).

Link-up

Leftover chickpeas? Try roasting them! Check out the **Salt + Vinegar Roasted Chickpeas**, page 73.

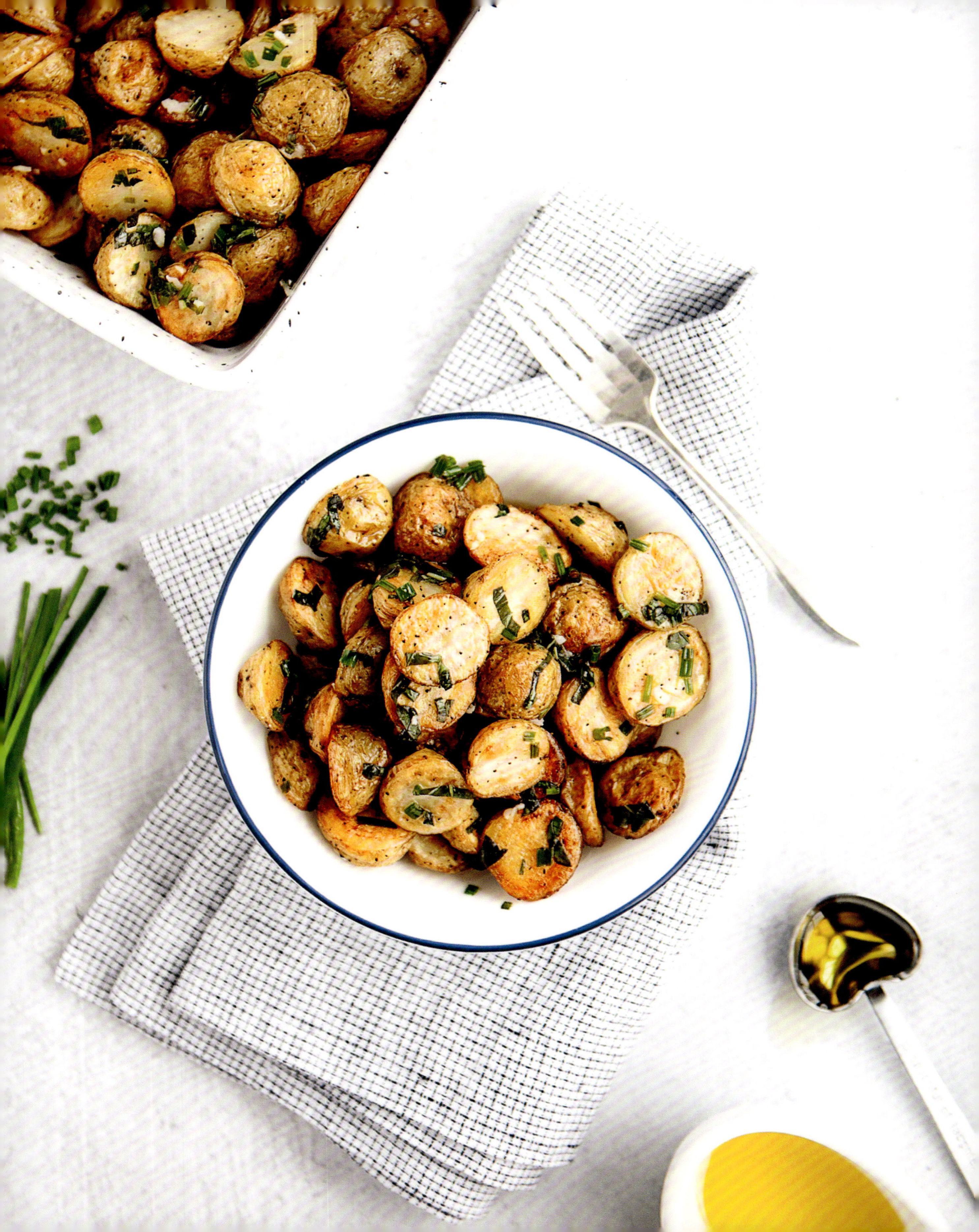

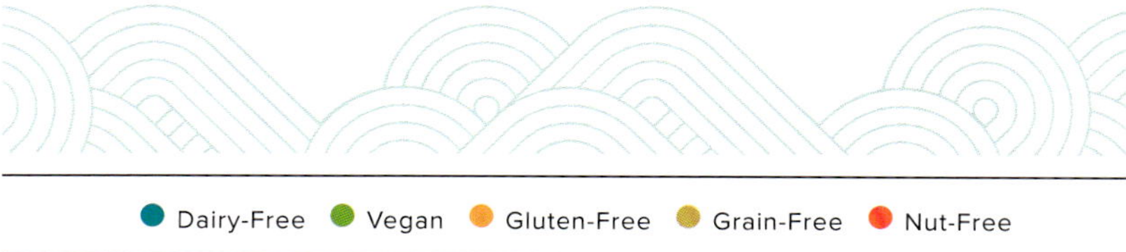

Dairy-Free · Vegan · Gluten-Free · Grain-Free · Nut-Free

Herb + Garlic Roasted Potatoes

This counts as salad in your first trimester — even if you just eat the potatoes and hold the herbs. This is a satisfyingly delicious side to any meal, and I have been known to eat a heaping bowl as a meal here and there. The herb and garlic drizzle is a fan favourite, and I often double the recipe to use on top of bowls, as a salad dressing, or on salmon.

10 MINUTES PREPPING • 25 MINUTES COOKING • MAKES 2 TO 3 SERVINGS

WHAT YOU NEED:

For the potatoes

1 ½ lb (680 g) baby potatoes, halved or quartered if large

1 ½ tbsp (22 mL) avocado oil

Pinch of salt and pepper

For the herb and garlic drizzle

¼ cup (60 mL) extra virgin olive oil

1 tbsp (15 mL) white wine vinegar

1 clove garlic, minced

1 tbsp (15 mL) fresh basil, finely chopped

1 tbsp (15 mL) chives, finely chopped

¼ tsp (1 mL) sea salt

Pinch of pepper

HOW TO MAKE IT:

1. Heat oven to 450°F (230°C), and line a baking tray with parchment paper.
2. Add chopped potatoes to baking tray, and coat with avocado oil, salt, and pepper. Mix together, and arrange potatoes cut side down. Move tray to oven.
3. While potatoes roast, prepare the herb and garlic drizzle. Add the drizzle ingredients to a medium bowl or small mason jar, and whisk or shake to combine.
4. Potatoes are done after about 22 to 25 minutes, or when the potato bottoms look golden brown and the inside is creamy.
5. Pour herb and garlic drizzle over potatoes until coated to your liking, and enjoy!

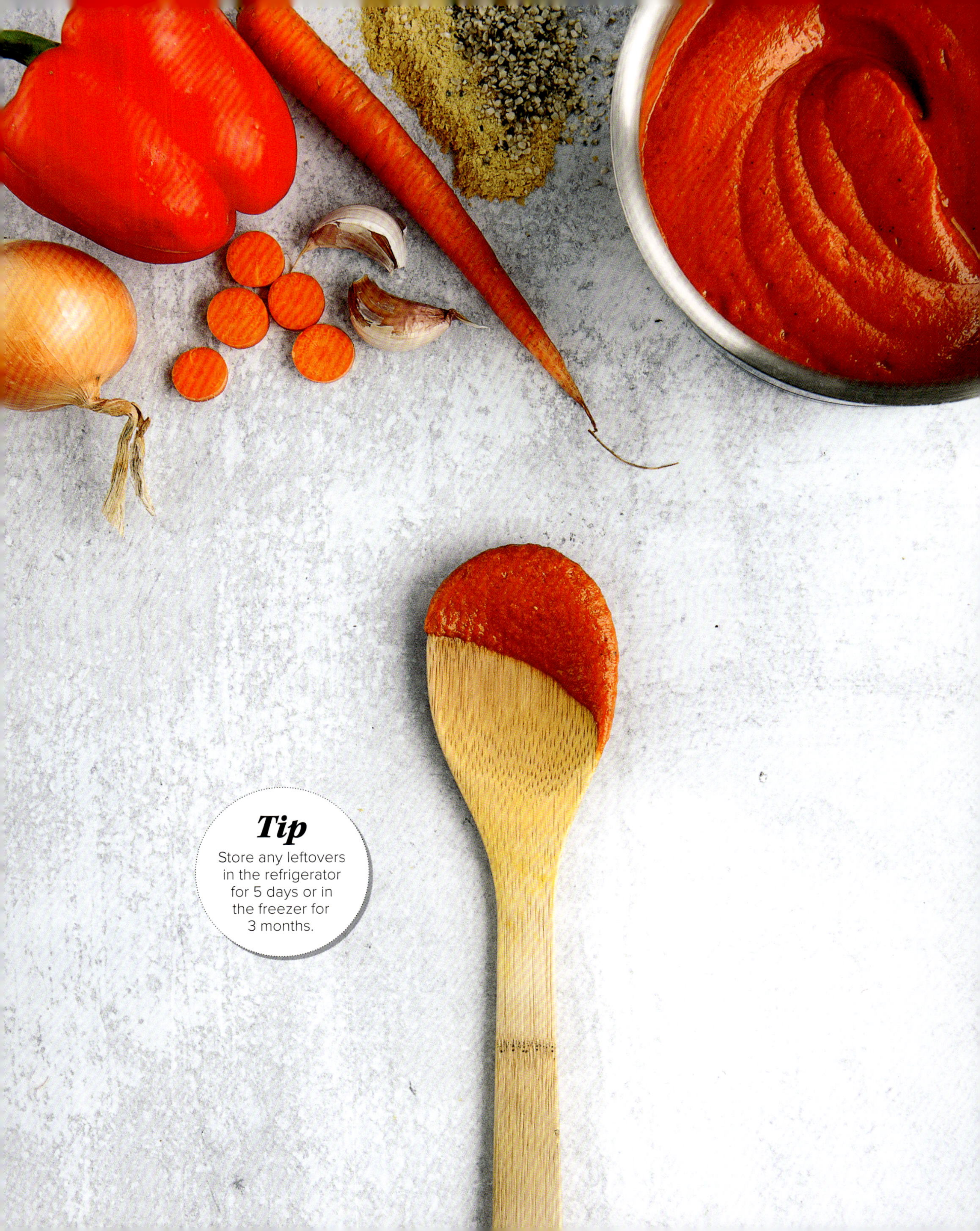

Tip

Store any leftovers in the refrigerator for 5 days or in the freezer for 3 months.

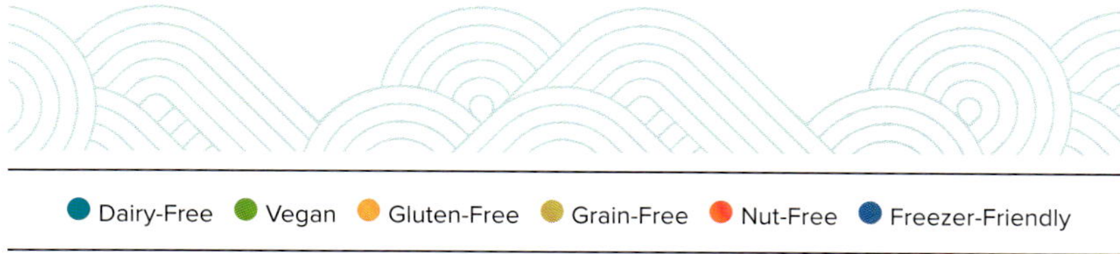

● Dairy-Free ● Vegan ● Gluten-Free ● Grain-Free ● Nut-Free ● Freezer-Friendly

Goodness Me Tomato Sauce

A flavourful and caramelized veggie-packed tomato sauce that easily turns a basic staple into a meal packed with veggie goodness. Pair it with a lentil- or quinoa-based pasta and meatballs, or use it to make a delicious shakshuka (page 91).

SUMMER VERSION:

Roast a tray full of halved plum tomatoes with 6 garlic cloves, a drizzle of olive oil, and a handful of chopped onions at 400°F (205°C) for 30 minutes. When cooled, purée the tomatoes in batches with a handful of fresh basil. Summer sauce awaits!

5 MINUTES PREPPING • 50 MINUTES COOKING • MAKES 4 CUPS

WHAT YOU NEED:	HOW TO MAKE IT:
1 small onion, cut into big pieces 2 cloves garlic, peeled 1 red pepper, cut into 4 pieces 2 carrots, roughly chopped 1 tbsp (15 mL) avocado oil 1 (24 fl oz/680 mL) jar of passata (strained tomatoes) ½ tsp (2 mL) dried oregano ¼ tsp (1 mL) sea salt ½ cup (125 mL) water 1 heaping tbsp (20 mL) hemp hearts (optional) 1 heaping tbsp (20 mL) nutritional yeast (optional)	1. Preheat oven to 400°F (205°C), and line a baking pan with parchment paper. 2. Roughly chop the onion, red pepper, and carrots, peel the garlic, and toss with the avocado oil on the parchment-lined pan. 3. Roast veggies for about 20 minutes, or until they are caramelized. 4. Transfer veggies to a medium pot set to medium heat, and add the passata, sea salt, and oregano. Fill the empty passata bottle with about a ½ cup (125 mL) water, give it a shake to get the last of the tomato, and add to the pot. 5. Simmer for 25 minutes, then turn off the heat. Add the hemp hearts and nutritional yeast (if using), and then purée the sauce to the desired consistency.

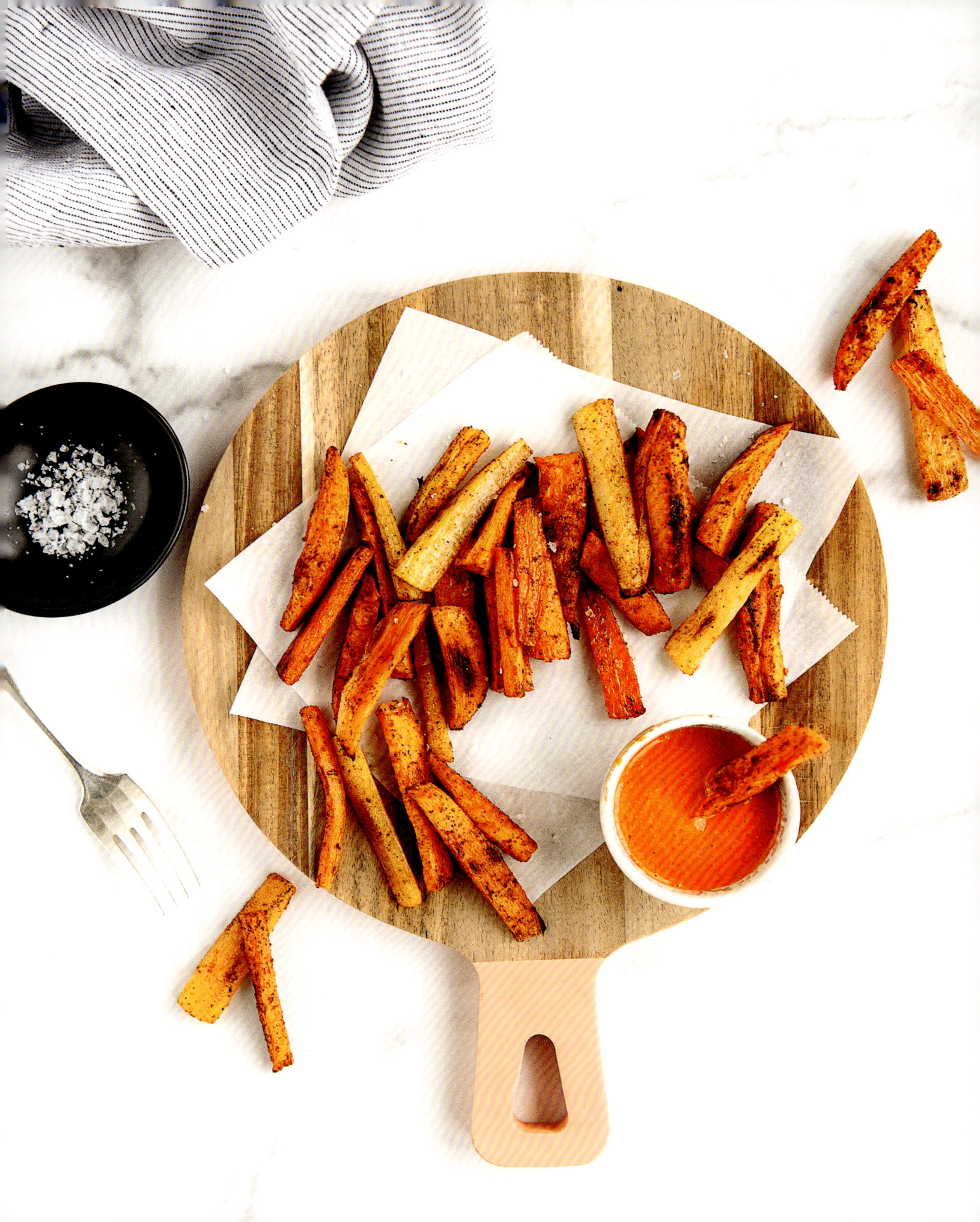

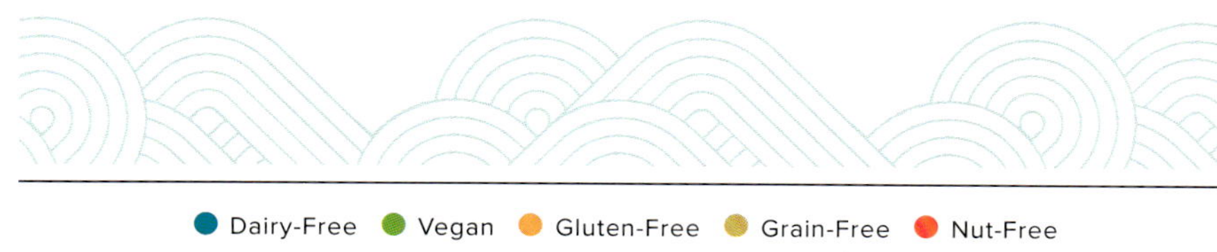

● Dairy-Free ● Vegan ● Gluten-Free ● Grain-Free ● Nut-Free

Smoky Sweet Potato + Carrot Fries with Roasted Red Pepper Dipping Sauce

Orange vegetables, including sweet potatoes and carrots, are excellent sources of beta carotene, which the body uses to make vitamin A. Vitamin A is crucial for the functional development of baby's organs and immune system. Pairing beta-carotene-rich vegetables with a high-quality fat, such as avocado oil, helps the body take in as much of this important micronutrient as possible. And also ... fries are delicious. ***Orange you glad fries are part of a healthy pregnancy diet?***

15 MINUTES PREPPING • 25 MINUTES COOKING • MAKES 1 TRAY

WHAT YOU NEED:

For the fries

1 ½ tbsp (22 mL) avocado oil

2 small sweet potatoes

4 medium carrots

1 ½ tsp (7.5 mL) smoked paprika

½ tsp (2 mL) sea salt

½ tsp (2 mL) cumin

For the dipping sauce

¼ cup (60 mL) extra virgin olive oil

2 or 3 roasted red peppers (from a jar)

2 tbsp (30 mL) tahini

Juice from 1 lemon

1 tbsp (15 mL) minced garlic

¼ tsp (1 mL) sea salt

HOW TO MAKE IT:

1. Preheat oven to 450°F (230°C), and line a baking tray with parchment paper.
2. Peel and chop carrots and sweet potatoes into finger-sized pieces. For carrots: cut into 2 or 3 pieces, then halve each lengthwise. For sweet potatoes: cut into quarters, halve each piece, then make half-inch slices lengthwise, slicing in half again to desired size.
3. Add carrots and sweet potatoes to prepared baking tray, and coat with avocado oil and spices. Mix and evenly coat each piece, doing your best to give each piece its own space on the tray before putting the fries in the oven.
4. While carrots and sweet potatoes are in the oven, add all dipping sauce ingredients to food processor or blender, and pulse until smooth.
5. Bake for 25 minutes, until fries begin to get crisp but stay soft on the inside. Sprinkle with another pinch of sea salt, and enjoy.

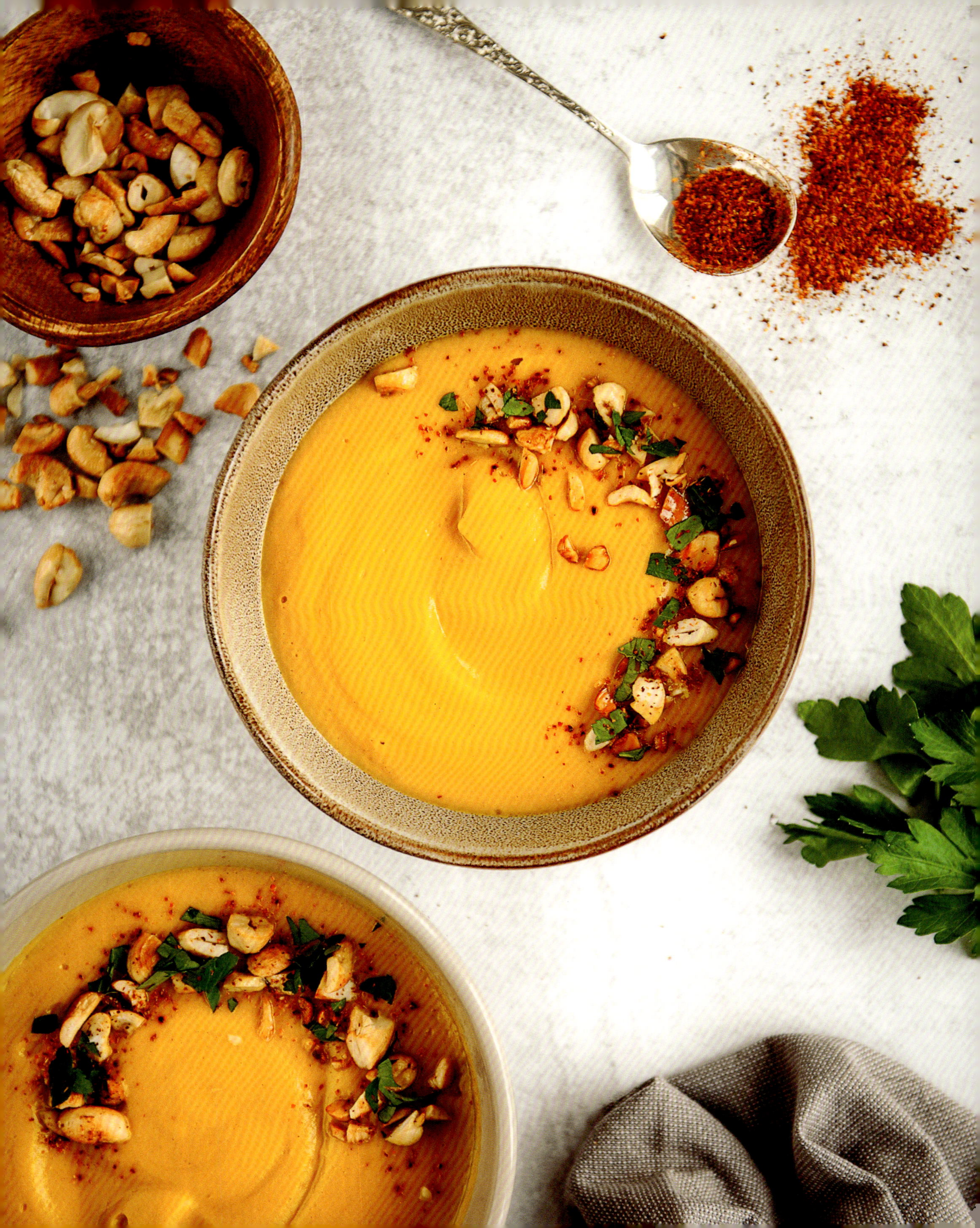

Dairy-Free · Gluten-Free · Grain-Free · Freezer-Friendly

Slow Cooker Spiced Cauliflower + Sweet Potato Soup

One of my all-time go-tos, this soup takes only 10 minutes of hands-on time. The fantastic thing about this recipe (besides the taste!) is that the cooking time doesn't matter very much. Since you'll be puréeing all of the veggies, it doesn't matter if they get too soft. Just set the slow cooker to low, go about your day, then purée the soup when it's time to eat. The addition of red lentils and cashews to this soup makes it silky and more substantial, adding to the nutrients provided by the veggies with lots of protein, folate, and fabulous fats.

10 MINUTES PREPPING • 3 TO 8 HOURS COOKING • MAKES 5 TO 6 SERVINGS

WHAT YOU NEED:

½ medium cauliflower, roughly chopped into florets

2 medium sweet potatoes, peeled and roughly chopped

1 red onion, roughly chopped

2 cloves garlic, peeled

6 to 7 cups (1.5 to 1.75 L) chicken broth

½ cup (125 mL) raw cashews

½ cup (125 mL) uncooked red lentils, rinsed

1 tsp (5 mL) paprika

½ tsp (2 mL) turmeric

½ tsp (2 mL) cinnamon

¼ tsp (1 mL) salt

¼ tsp (1 mL) pepper

HOW TO MAKE IT:

1. Add all ingredients to a slow cooker or a multicooker set to low/slow cook mode for 6 to 8 hours or high for 3 hours, and leave it to cook.
2. Once the veggies appear nice and soft (or when you get around to it), purée the soup with an immersion blender, or transfer the soup in batches to a blender and blend until smooth.

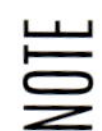

This recipe halves well, if you prefer to make a smaller batch of soup. If you do make the full batch, note that this soup freezes perfectly in glass jars (ensure you leave an inch (2.5 cm) of space at the top).

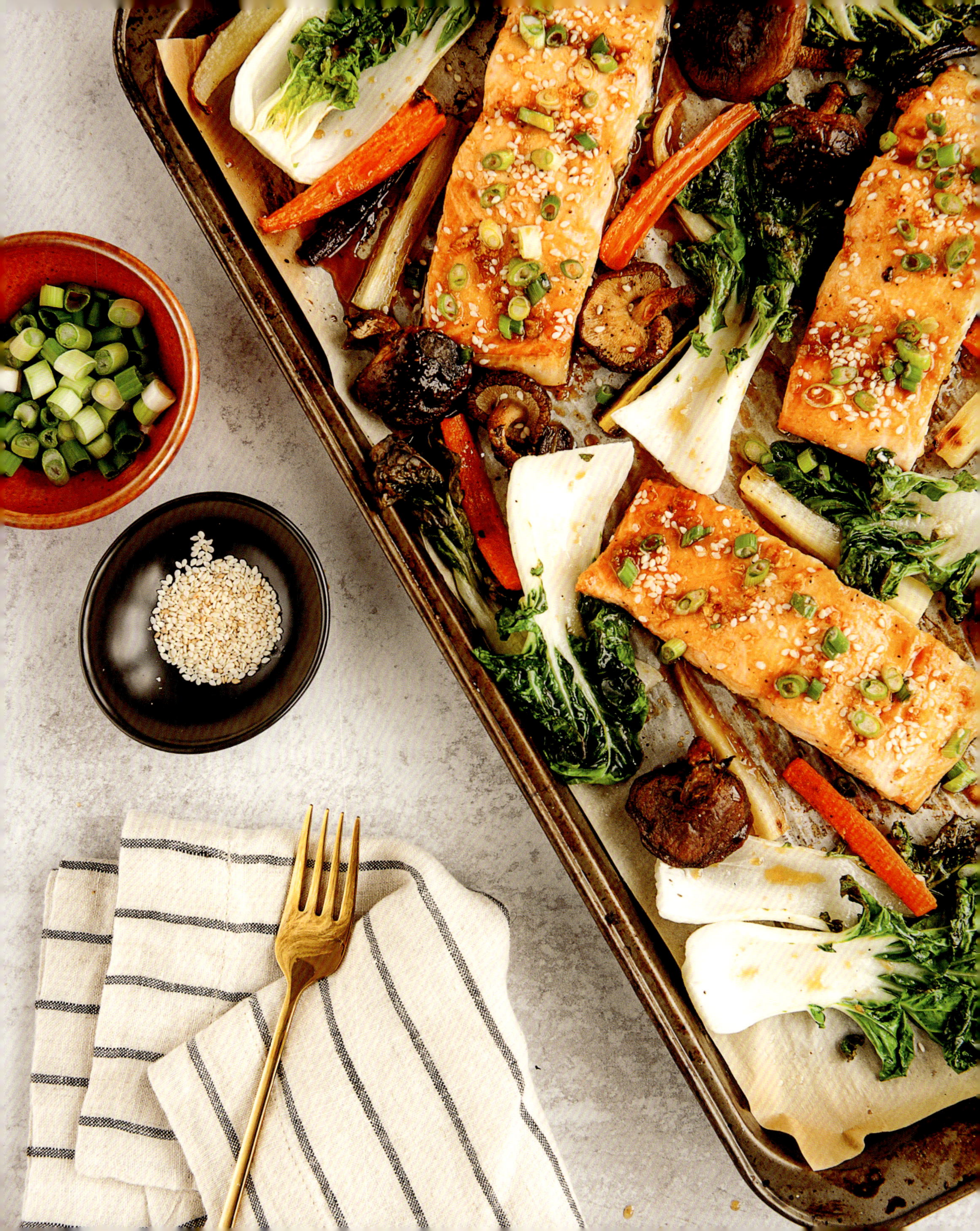

Dairy-Free · Gluten-Free · Grain-Free · Nut-Free

Sheet Pan Maple Sesame + Shiitake Salmon

DHA (a type of omega-3 fatty acid) is an especially important building block in supporting baby's brain development. DHA helps ensure a baby's brain, eyes, and nervous system develop optimally. It's not just about baby, either. Getting in enough omega-3 fatty acids, including DHA, may lower the risk of postpartum depression. Fish and seafood are major real-food sources of DHA, and salmon is a perfect choice. Serve on top of quinoa or rice, and enjoy the baby brain boost!

20 MINUTES PREPPING • 20 MINUTES COOKING • MAKES 3 TO 4 SERVINGS

WHAT YOU NEED:

3 to 4 salmon fillets

15 shiitake mushrooms (or mushrooms of choice), cleaned and dried with a paper towel

3 carrots, sliced into thin strips

5 baby bok choy, washed and sliced in half

2 tbsp (30 mL) avocado oil, divided

A pinch of salt and pepper

2 green onions, chopped

1 tbsp (15 mL) sesame seeds

Marinade

¼ cup (60 mL) maple syrup

2 tbsp (30 mL) tamari (or soy sauce for non-GF)

1 tbsp (15 mL) sesame oil

2 cloves garlic, minced

½ tsp (2 mL) ground ginger

Pinch of pepper

HOW TO MAKE IT:

1. Combine marinade ingredients in a bowl, and heat oven to 450°F (230°C).
2. Place salmon in a shallow dish, and cover with about ¼ cup (60 mL) of the marinade (reserving the rest). Cover, and let marinate in the refrigerator.
3. Transfer carrots and mushrooms to a 18 × 13-inch sheet pan lined with parchment paper. Pour 1 tbsp (15 mL) of the avocado oil on top, add the salt and pepper, and mix to coat veggies. Bake for about 10 minutes. Remove tray from oven, add salmon and bok choy, and brush with the remaining 1 tbsp (15 mL) of avocado oil. Bake another 10 minutes, or until salmon flakes when pressed with a fork. Drizzle reserved marinade on top of dish, garnishing with green onions and sesame seeds.

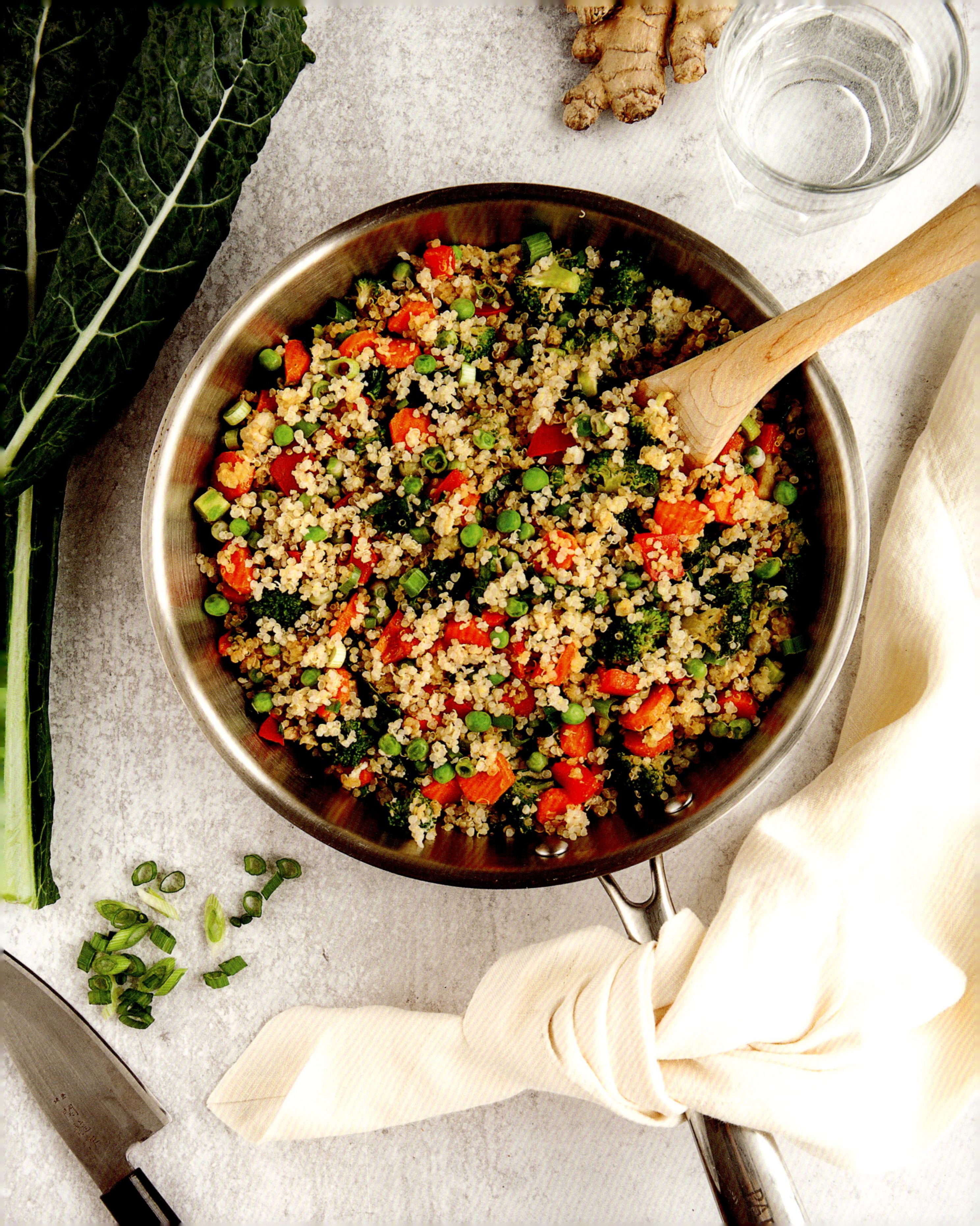

Dairy-Free · Gluten-Free · Grain-Free · Nut-Free

Quinoa Fried Nice

Chances are, you've got a crisper full of half-used-up veggies. Am I right? Put them to good use in this reimagined version of the classic fried rice that uses protein-rich quinoa instead of rice, includes eggs (outside of breakfast) for a dose of the essential mineral choline, and incorporates some dark leafy greens for extra prenatal folate, vitamin C, potassium, and magnesium. All the flavour of take-out with veggie-packed nutrition!

15 MINUTES PREPPING • 10 MINUTES COOKING • MAKES 3 MEAL-SIZED SERVINGS

WHAT YOU NEED:

1 tbsp (15 mL) extra virgin olive oil

1 tbsp (15 mL) minced fresh ginger

2 cloves garlic, minced

5 to 6 cups (1.25 to 1.5 L) veggies of choice, chopped small (you can use what I list below or make this your own)

- 2 medium carrots, chopped
- ½ crown of broccoli, chopped into bite-sized florets
- ½ red pepper, chopped
- 1 cup (250 mL) frozen peas
- 3 to 4 kale leaves, stemmed and chopped small
- 2 green onions, sliced

3 eggs

2 cups (500 mL) cooked quinoa

2 tbsp (30 mL) tamari (or soy sauce for non-GF)

2 tbsp (30 mL) sesame oil

HOW TO MAKE IT:

1. Add olive oil to a large pan over medium heat. Add garlic, ginger, and veggies (reserving the kale and green onions if using), and cook 5 minutes.
2. Move veggies over to one half of the pan, and add eggs. Scramble for 2 to 3 minutes until eggs are cooked.
3. Add kale and green onion and mix to combine, follow with the cooked quinoa, and then the tamari and sesame oil. Cook 2 to 3 minutes more until everything is warm and kale has softened and turned bright green.
4. Taste and add more sesame oil or tamari to taste, and enjoy!

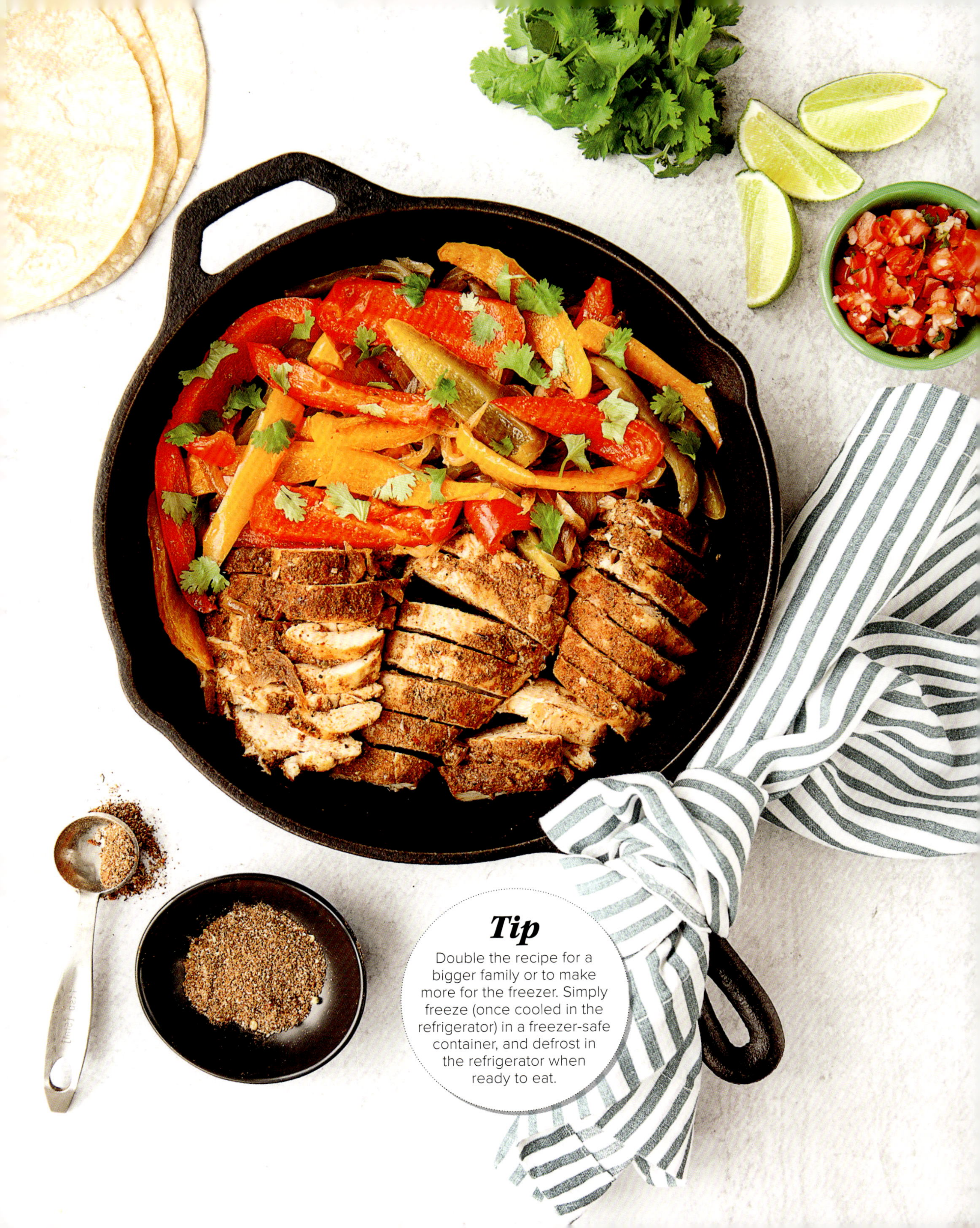

Tip

Double the recipe for a bigger family or to make more for the freezer. Simply freeze (once cooled in the refrigerator) in a freezer-safe container, and defrost in the refrigerator when ready to eat.

Dairy-Free Option · Gluten-Free · Grain-Free Option · Nut-Free · Freezer-Friendly

Slow Cooker Chicken Fajitas

One of my all-time favourite weeknight meals, this recipe takes only a few minutes of hands-on time, and the slow cooker does the rest. If you're making this for a work-night dinner, consider throwing everything into the slow cooker the evening before. It can cook for two hours while you go about your evening, and then dinner for the next night is good to go! To make the recipe even more hands-off, you can add the peppers to the slow cooker at the same time you add everything else, if you don't mind your peppers a little softer.

Why not make your own fajita spice mix? You will avoid food preservatives, plus you can customize it to your taste, adding extra garlic, extra spice, or more herbs — it's your choice.

10 MINUTES PREPPING • 2 HOURS COOKING • MAKES 2 TO 3 SERVINGS

WHAT YOU NEED:

Fajitas

3 tbsp (45 mL) butter or ghee (or substitute avocado oil for dairy-free)

2 chicken breasts or 1 ½ lb (680 g) chicken thighs

1 large onion, sliced

3 bell peppers, sliced

1 ½ tbsp (22 mL) fajita spice mix

6 small corn tortillas (or substitute a large package of mixed greens for grain-free)

Optional fajita toppings: avocado, pico de gallo, cilantro, hot sauce, or whatever your heart desires!

Fajita spice mix

1 tbsp (15 mL) chili powder

½ tbsp (7 mL) smoked paprika

½ tbsp (7 mL) cumin

1 tsp (5 mL) garlic powder

1 tsp (5 mL) onion powder

1 tsp (5 mL) red pepper flakes

1 tsp (5 mL) oregano

½ tsp (2 mL) sea salt

½ tsp (2 mL) pepper

Mix in a small bowl, and store in an empty spice jar or small storage container. Double the recipe if this is one you use often.

HOW TO MAKE IT:

1. Add butter or ghee, chicken, onion, and fajita spice mix to the slow cooker (reserving the peppers).
2. Turn the slow cooker to high, and cook for 1 hour. Add peppers to the slow cooker, then cover and cook another hour, or until chicken is cooked through.
3. Using tongs or a fork, remove chicken from the slow cooker, and slice or shred it, returning to the slow cooker once done.
4. Using a slotted spoon or tongs, scoop out the fajita mixture, and place in a serving bowl, discarding the remaining liquid.
5. Enjoy on corn tortillas with avocado, pico de gallo, and cilantro, or serve on a bed of greens for a fajita salad.

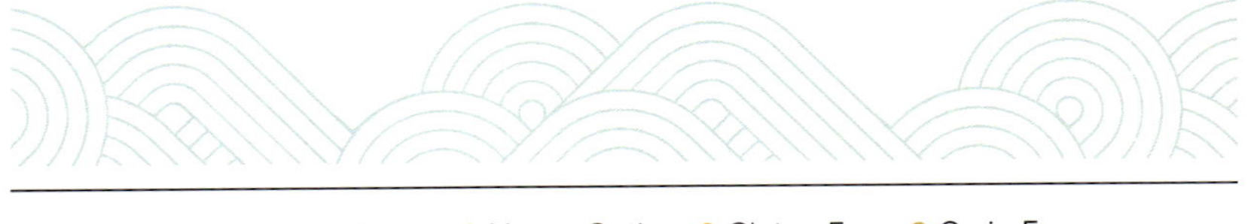

● Dairy-Free Option ● Vegan Option ● Gluten-Free ● Grain-Free

Late-Night Protein Packs

If you are waking up feeling nauseous, a protein-packed late-night snack is a good idea as it will help your body release energy slowly throughout the night, leading to more balanced blood sugar levels. I recommend making up several protein packs and storing them in the refrigerator for when hunger strikes. Then grab one, enjoy, and feel good taking in healthy fat from the almond butter, fibre from the cucumber, apple, and chickpeas, and protein from the chickpeas and almond butter.

10 MINUTES PREPPING • MAKES 3 PROTEIN PACKS

WHAT YOU NEED:	HOW TO MAKE IT:
3 apples, cored and sliced (or substitute another dippable fruit such as banana or pear) ¾ cup (175 mL) Salt + Vinegar Roasted Chickpeas (page 73) or store bought (or substitute with another high-protein snack such as organic cheddar, trail mix, slices of meat, or edamame) 3 tbsp (45 mL) almond butter (or substitute with another dip, e.g., hummus, roasted red pepper, or baba ghanouj) 2 mini cucumbers, sliced (or substitute with your favourite snacking veggie, e.g., sliced bell peppers, snap peas, carrots, or radishes)	1. Divide the apples, roasted chickpeas, almond butter, and cucumbers equally into 3 snack containers. 2. Store in the refrigerator for 2 to 3 days.

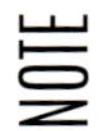

NOTE

If using perishable foods, such as meat, cheese, or hummus, do not leave Protein Packs out of the refrigerator for more than 2 hours.

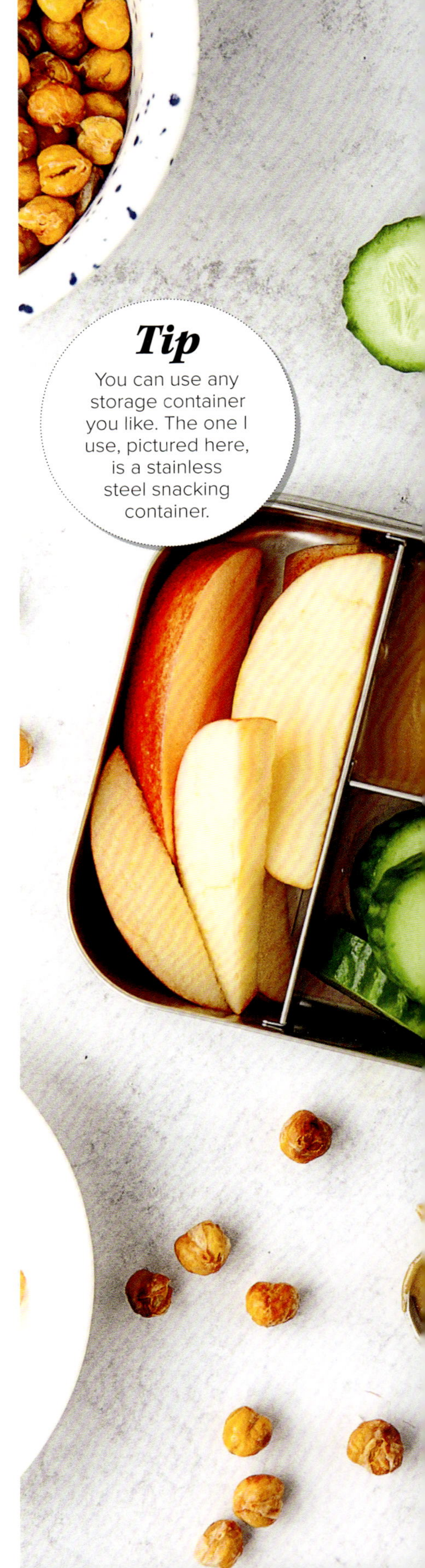

Tip

You can use any storage container you like. The one I use, pictured here, is a stainless steel snacking container.

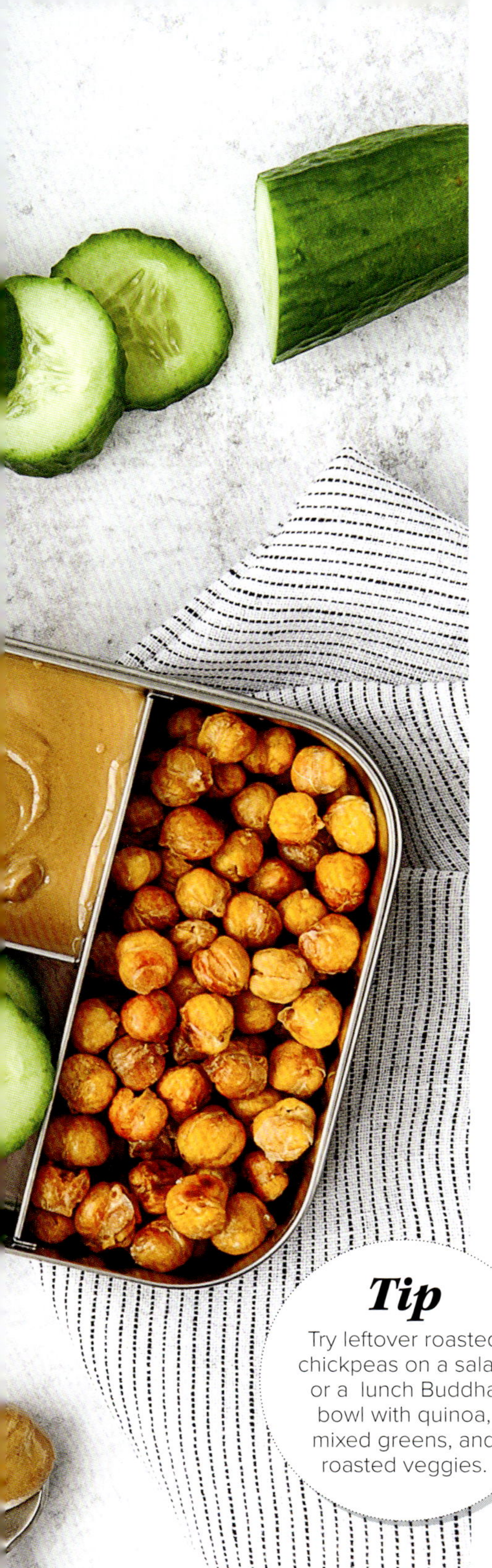

Tip

Try leftover roasted chickpeas on a salad or a lunch Buddha bowl with quinoa, mixed greens, and roasted veggies.

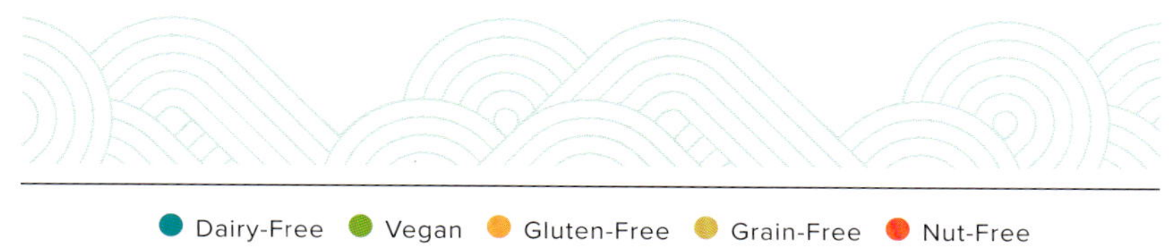

Dairy-Free • Vegan • Gluten-Free • Grain-Free • Nut-Free

Salt + Vinegar Roasted Chickpeas

Try this upgrade to classic salt and vinegar chips that gives you protein, fibre, folate, and iron all wrapped up as a perfect TV snack. It's got taste. It's got crunch. You'll want to have it all in one sitting.

5 MINUTES PREPPING • 2 HOURS SOAKING + 40 MINUTES COOKING • MAKES 2 CUPS (500 ML)

WHAT YOU NEED:

- 1 (19 oz/540 mL) can chickpeas, rinsed
- 4 cups (1 L) white vinegar
- 1 ¼ tsp (6 mL) sea salt
- 1 ½ tbsp (22 mL) olive oil

HOW TO MAKE IT:

1. Soak rinsed chickpeas in a covered bowl with the vinegar for 2 to 3 hours in the refrigerator.
2. Line a baking sheet with parchment paper. Heat oven to 350°F (180°C).
3. Drain chickpeas, and transfer to the parchment-lined baking sheet. Top chickpeas with olive oil and sea salt, and mix well using a spoon.
4. Roast for 40 to 50 minutes, shaking and turning pan halfway through and checking often after the 40-minute mark to prevent chickpeas from burning. Chickpeas are done when they are golden and crispy to the touch.
5. Let chickpeas cool on pan, then transfer to a storage container with the lid resting on top but not snapped closed (this will help them stay crispy). Store on counter for 2 to 3 days.

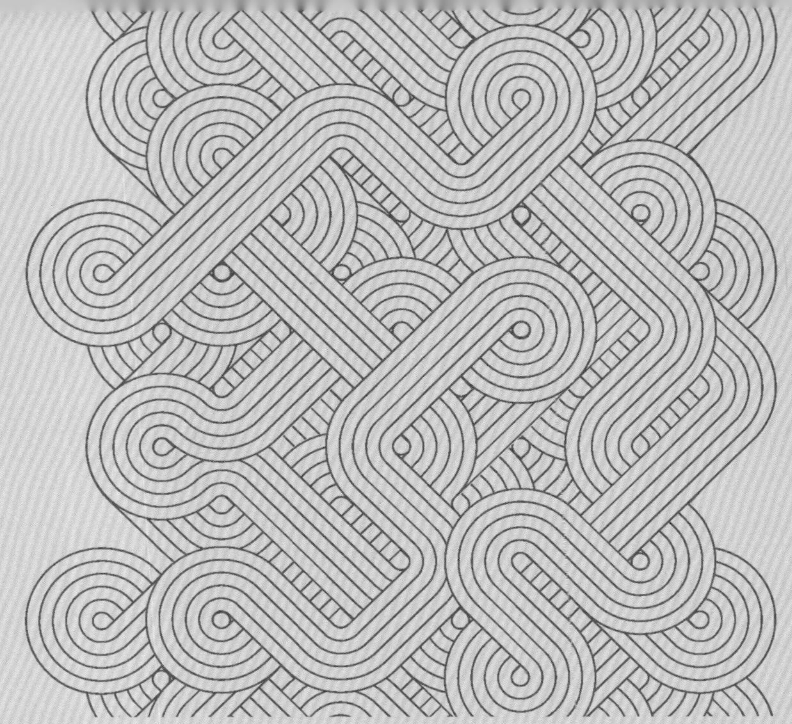

TRIMESTER 2

(WEEKS 13–28)

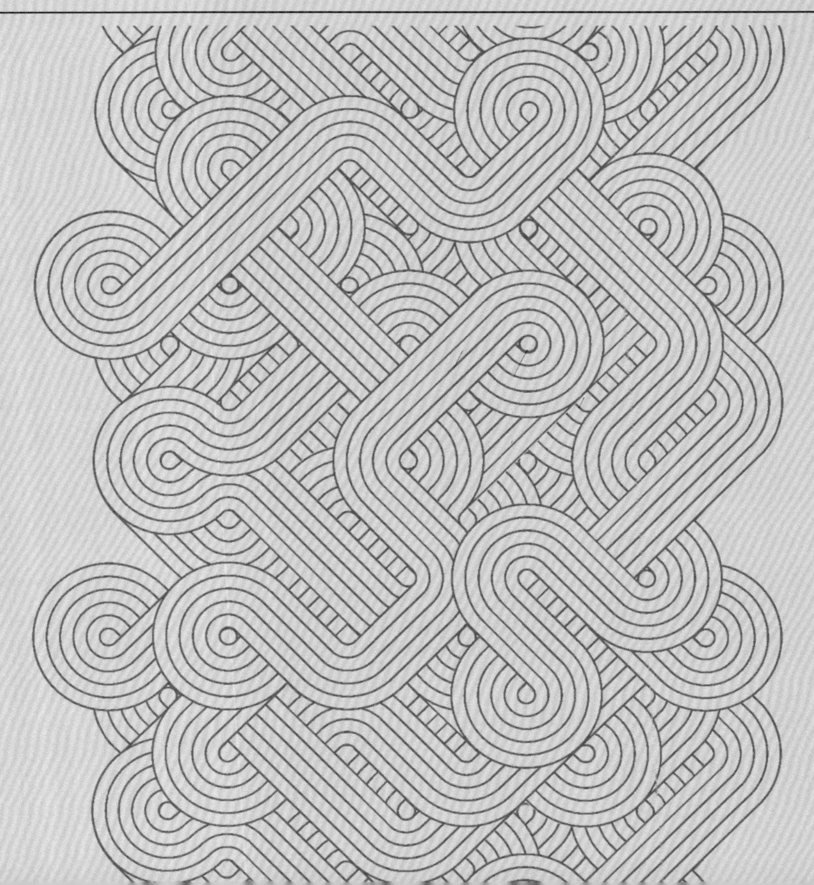

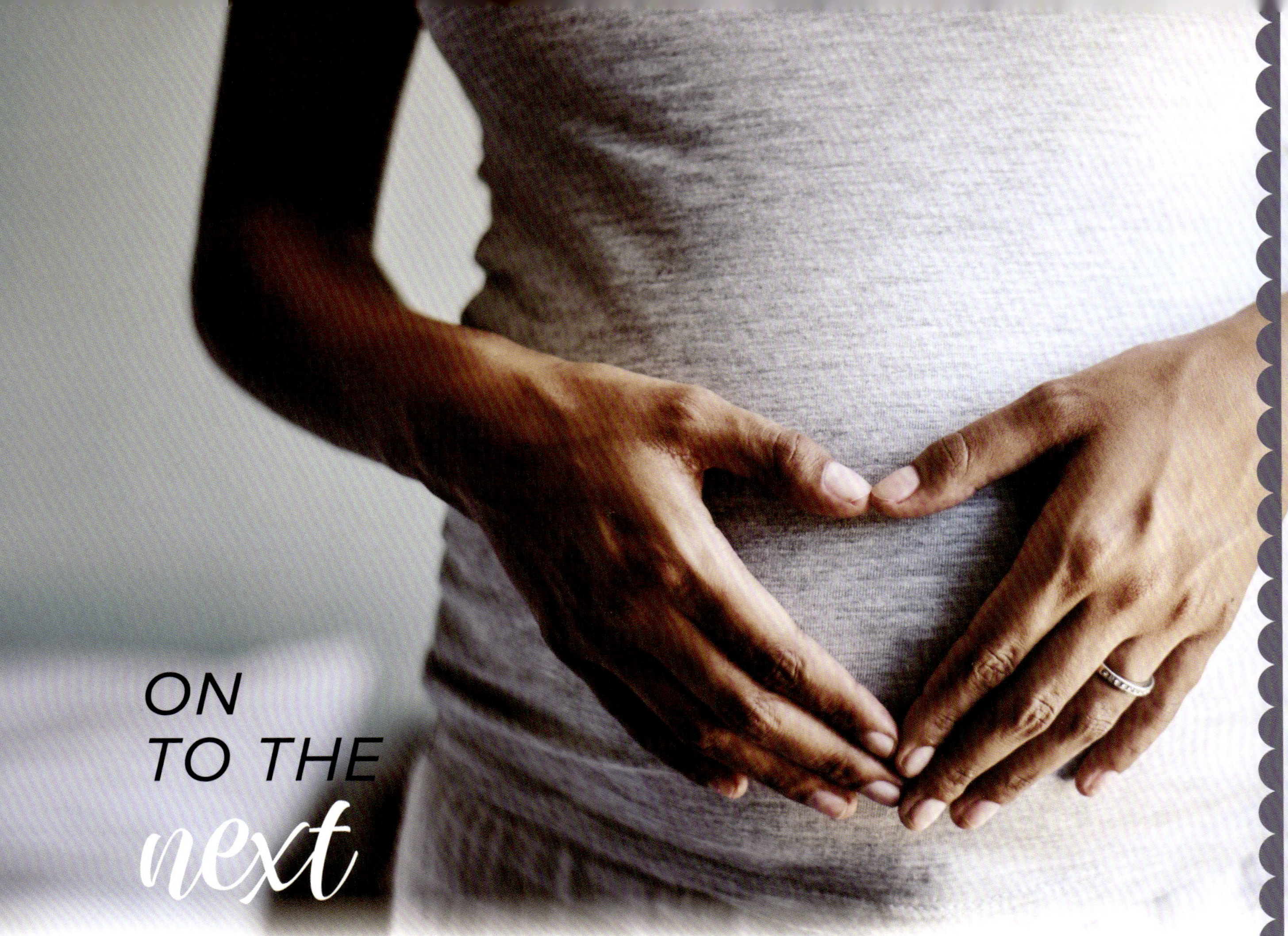

ON TO THE *next*

MOST WOMEN are relieved at the end of the first trimester of their pregnancy — and happy to move on. Hopefully, by the time the fourth month rolls around, you'll be feeling less nauseated and tired, and your appetite will have improved. You may also have a bump starting to show. If you're still feeling terrible at times, hang in there! Keep up with the nutrition tips from Trimester 1 and try to take things easy.

In Trimester 2, it's normal to be either feeling very hungry with the urge to enjoy lots of delicious food, or not having much of an appetite. If you have cravings for any food, go for it. Enjoy the food you want to eat, and banish the guilt! But if you don't feel hungry or don't feel like eating — think liquid nutrition. A good choice is bone broth, which is rich in protein, calcium, and fat. Smoothies are great too. They provide the vitamins and minerals you need, and they taste delicious.

Liquid foods and nutrient-rich drinks are a good solution when you need to keep your blood sugar stable and eat more often, yet don't have the energy to cook or the desire to eat.

Staying Healthy

In addition to staying active, getting enough sleep, and managing stress, eating lots of real food can give you the nutrients and energy you need to feel your best. If you aim for the rainbow each day (choosing veggies and fruit that are red, orange, green, purple, and yellow) and include plants at every meal, you are giving your body lots of vitamin C and a variety of anti-inflammatory antioxidants, which can help your immune system function well. Also try to add fermented foods to your plate once a day — kimchee, kefir, sauerkraut, yogurt, or miso can support the health of your gut and microbiome, which is directly related to your immune system.

On the other hand, excess sugar, especially refined sugars and grains, and processed foods and oils can impact immunity negatively. They can trigger inflammation, reduce the body's nutrient supply, and disrupt normal body functions.

NATURAL REMEDIES

Cold and flu season can be tough during pregnancy. Pregnancy suppresses your immune system slightly, and pharmaceutical remedies are mostly off the table. Food can help you to stay healthy — and to cope if you get sick.

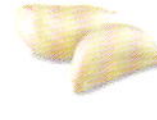

- **Garlic:** Smash a clove of garlic. Let it sit for 10 minutes, then swallow it down on a spoonful of honey.

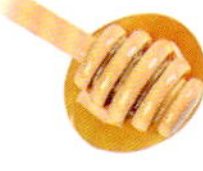

- **Honey:** Honey has antiviral properties and can suppress coughs. Have it straight off the spoon, or add it to ginger tea or an ice pop. Look for local honey.

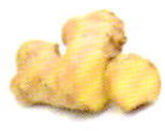

- **Ginger:** It helps! See pages 32 to 33 for three soothing and easy ginger remedies.

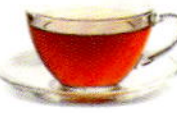

- **Fluids:** Keep drinking, and include bone broth and warming soups and stews for your meals.

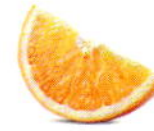

- **Vitamin C:** Keep up those rainbow veggies and fruit as much as you can!

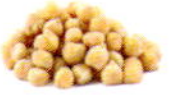

- **Zinc:** Zinc may help alleviate cold symptoms. Zinc is found in red meat, poultry, oats, nuts and seeds, and beans.

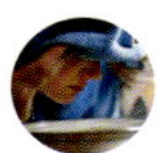

- **Rest and steam:** Steam can do wonders for congestion, and rest is best!

Talk to your healthcare professional about supplements such as vitamin C, vitamin D, and a probiotic — these can help to reduce the likelihood of getting and staying sick. Remember to always consult your health professional if you're sick and need medical advice.

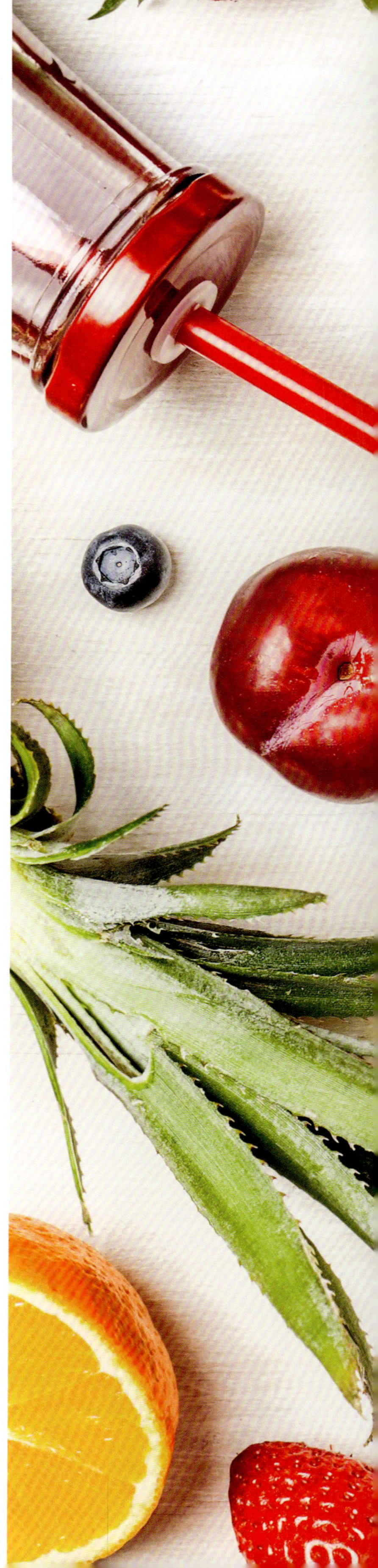

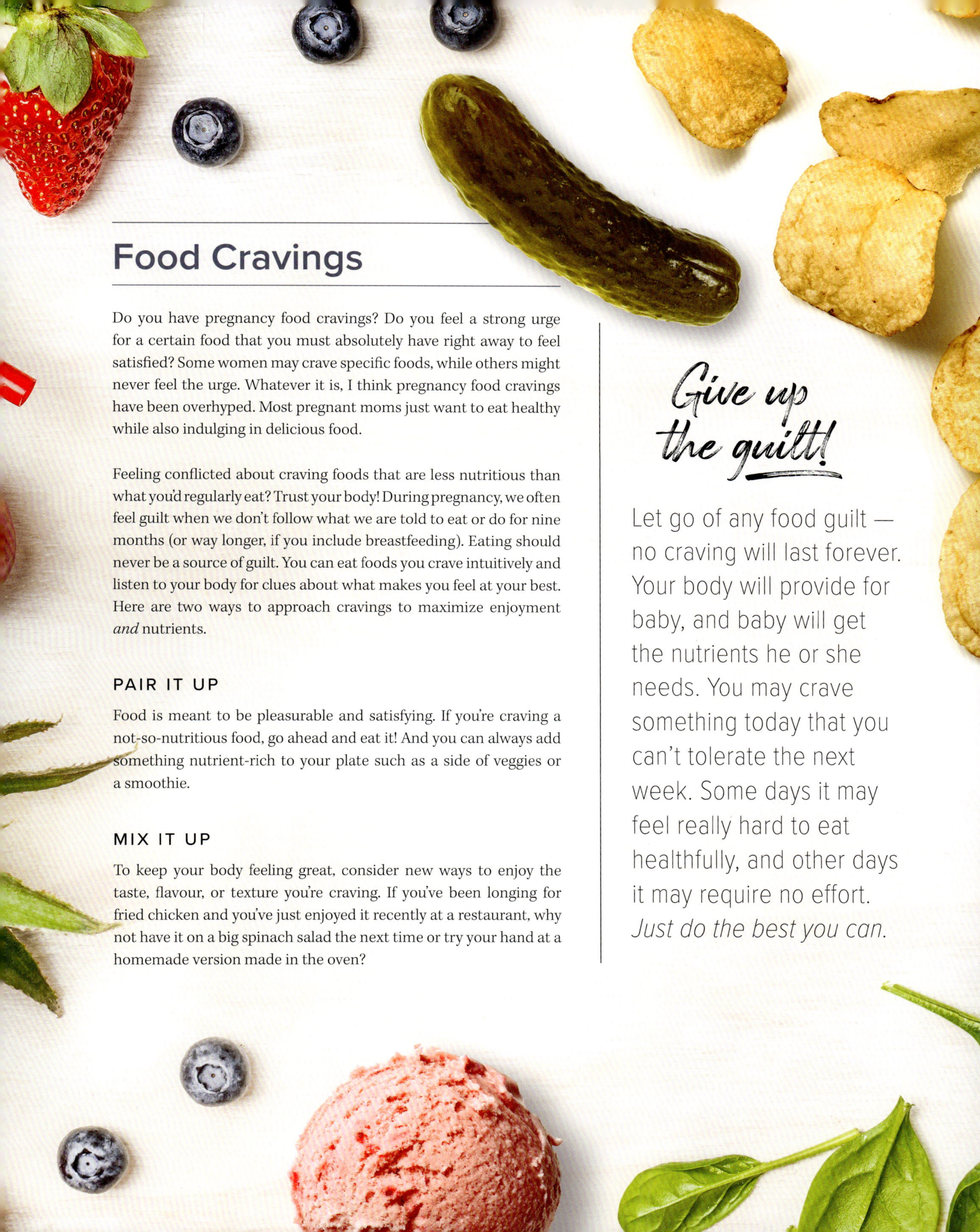

Food Cravings

Do you have pregnancy food cravings? Do you feel a strong urge for a certain food that you must absolutely have right away to feel satisfied? Some women may crave specific foods, while others might never feel the urge. Whatever it is, I think pregnancy food cravings have been overhyped. Most pregnant moms just want to eat healthy while also indulging in delicious food.

Feeling conflicted about craving foods that are less nutritious than what you'd regularly eat? Trust your body! During pregnancy, we often feel guilt when we don't follow what we are told to eat or do for nine months (or way longer, if you include breastfeeding). Eating should never be a source of guilt. You can eat foods you crave intuitively and listen to your body for clues about what makes you feel at your best. Here are two ways to approach cravings to maximize enjoyment *and* nutrients.

PAIR IT UP

Food is meant to be pleasurable and satisfying. If you're craving a not-so-nutritious food, go ahead and eat it! And you can always add something nutrient-rich to your plate such as a side of veggies or a smoothie.

MIX IT UP

To keep your body feeling great, consider new ways to enjoy the taste, flavour, or texture you're craving. If you've been longing for fried chicken and you've just enjoyed it recently at a restaurant, why not have it on a big spinach salad the next time or try your hand at a homemade version made in the oven?

Give up the guilt!

Let go of any food guilt — no craving will last forever. Your body will provide for baby, and baby will get the nutrients he or she needs. You may crave something today that you can't tolerate the next week. Some days it may feel really hard to eat healthfully, and other days it may require no effort. *Just do the best you can.*

Super Smoothies

Smoothies are a nutrient-dense snack or meal-on-the-go that can keep you feeling good and satiated. Why not have homemade smoothies throughout your pregnancy? Do it yourself — try out different options for a variety of tastes and flavours.

Follow the steps below to whip up super-nutritious green smoothies that are packed with protein, fat, and fibre. Don't care for green smoothies? Double up on the bonus veggies!

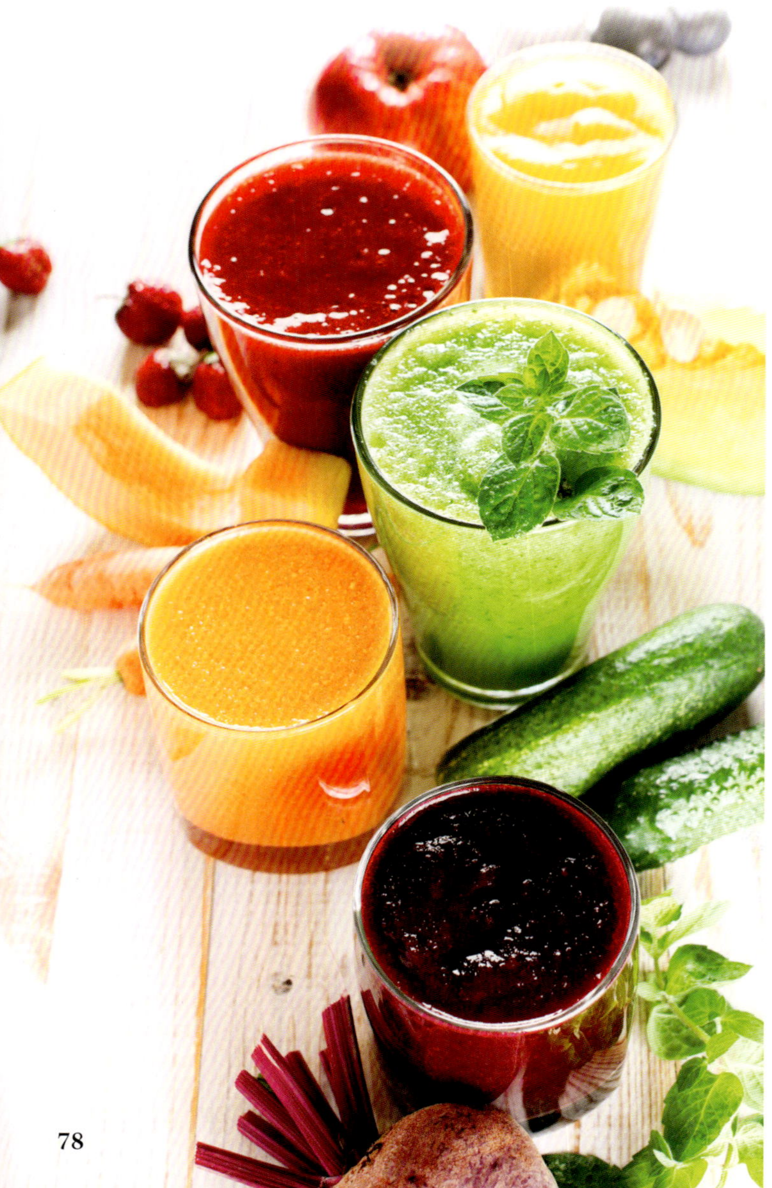

STEP 1

Start with the liquid, about 1½ to 2 cups.

Options: water, coconut water, cold herbal tea, or milk of choice

STEP 2

Add the greens, about 1½ to 2 cups.

Options: fresh kale, spinach, romaine lettuce, Swiss chard, or beet greens

STEP 3

Include the bonus veggies, about ½ cup.

Options: frozen cauliflower, zucchini, squash, sweet potato, beet, fresh cucumber, or parsley

STEP 4

Don't forget the fat, about 1 to 2 tablespoons.

Options: coconut oil, nut/seed butter, flax/pumpkin seed oil, avocado, or cashews

STEP 5

Follow up with the protein, about 2 tablespoons.

Options: hemp/chia/flax seeds, full-fat yogurt, lentils, collagen powder, or protein powder

STEP 6

Remember the fruit, about 1½ to 2 cups.

Options: mango, pineapple, peach, orange, berry, apple, pear, melon, plum, or banana

STEP 7 (OPTIONAL):

Punch up the flavour, about 1 tablespoon.

Options: lemon juice, sliced ginger, raw honey, coconut flakes, cacao powder, or mint

How cold?

If 1 or 2 of your items are frozen, you'll have an icy-cold smoothie. If not, add crushed ice to make the smoothie as cold as you like.

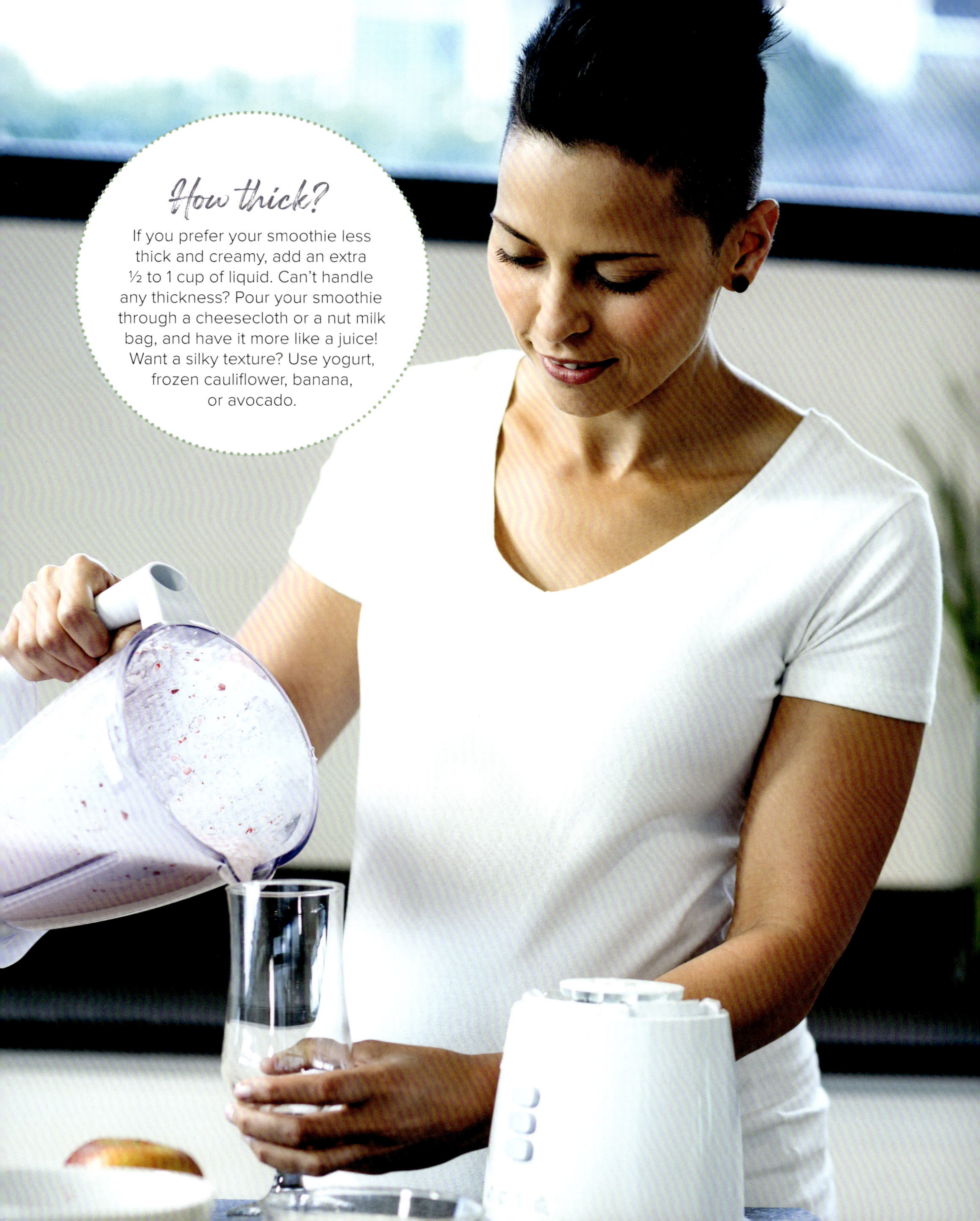

How thick?

If you prefer your smoothie less thick and creamy, add an extra ½ to 1 cup of liquid. Can't handle any thickness? Pour your smoothie through a cheesecloth or a nut milk bag, and have it more like a juice! Want a silky texture? Use yogurt, frozen cauliflower, banana, or avocado.

Cooking: Back in the Cards

If you're feeling more like your normal self in this trimester — that's wonderful! More interest in food means a rich nutrient intake for you and baby. If you feel okay to be around food and to get some meal planning and cooking done, try out my easy meal-planning guide below to get the healthy, wholesome nourishment you need at this stage of pregnancy.

MEAL PLANNING IN 3, 2, 1

Meal planning provides answers to these key questions: What am I having for dinner? How can I avoid cooking three meals each day? How can I easily pull together satisfying and healthy meals for me and my family throughout the week? Figuring these out means less stress, less time in the kitchen, less food waste (and therefore lower grocery bills), and more nutritious meals.

Meal planning assumes you have everyday go-to food items on your grocery list each week. Some essential stuff that will help you put together meals and snacks include fresh fruit and vegetables, bread and oats, nuts and seeds, flour, and eggs.

Meal planning in 3, 2, 1 is a guide to help you plan, in one sitting, what you'll have for dinner each night of the week and how you'll include your staples and leftovers to make up lunches and snacks. Here's what my meal planning looks like:

3

3 Dinners/Main Meals

Plan to cook three dinners or main meals a week. Make the components of each dinner last for three meals (two dinners and at least one lunch). Don't worry — you don't have to eat the same meal again and again!

2

2 Mix-and-Match Meal Makers

Stock up or prep two mix-and-match meal makers for the week. These meal makers will help you repurpose and transform your three main meals. Your goal is more variety and less cooking! I usually pick one protein and one base. See the next page for lots of examples!

1

1 Homemade Snack

Prep a homemade snack for the week — it could be muffins, trail mixes, granola bars, energy balls, or banana bread.

PLAN, PREP, PLATE

Pick a day during the week that works well for you, and write out your food plan for the week. Then use the 3Ps (Plan, Prep, Plate) to make it happen.

Plan

Start by writing down your three main meals. Next, think through how you might want to repurpose your main meals and decide on your two mix-and-match meal makers. The following are some examples:

Protein

Hardboiled eggs
Beans or lentils
Nuts or seeds
Crispy chickpeas
Fried eggs
Organic tofu
Ground almonds
Cheese (dairy or non-dairy)

Base

Broth
Large package of greens
Pot of quinoa, rice, millet, noodles, or pasta
Tortillas, flatbread, or crepes
Baked sweet potatoes
Pizza crust
Cauliflower rice or mash
Nori sheets

Write out your dinner plans for each night (including your main meals and repurposed meals), and jot down ideas for lunches and snacks for each day. Then make a grocery list of all the food items you will need (keep in mind that you'll have to cook more of each protein, grain, and veggie to provide for the additional meals).

Prep

Make a list of prep tasks that you can do in advance, either in one chunk of time or throughout the week. This will help to reduce stress when mealtimes come around. Here's what my prep tasks for a week might look like.

- Make muffins or another snack item.
- Cut up the veggies that I will use, either fresh or roasted.
- Make a pot of grains that I will use throughout the week.
- Make a breakfast item that can store well for several days, such as chia pudding, hardboiled eggs, baked egg cups, or pancakes.
- Make a salad dressing, dip, or spice mix.
- Roast the veggies or precook the meats to have them ready for my main meals.

Plate

Cook or assemble your meals at whatever time that works best for you. It could be 20 minutes after breakfast in the morning if this is the least stressful time of day for you. Simply reheat the food and finish up with the toppings later!

Repurpose Your Meals

Making the components of each dinner/main meal stretch out for other meals means scaling up on your cooking now in order to cook less later. Think about doubling your quantity of grains, salad dressings, roasted or chopped veggies, soups or stews, and meat. No point doing it again!

Repeating the same meals can be boring for most of us. Coming up with ideas for repurposing meals — using some or all of the meal components to create totally different meals — can give you a lot of satisfaction. It keeps you organized, saves you time, and rewards you with a variety of meals that you can whip up easily, providing wholesome eating for the whole family.

SAMPLE MAIN MEAL

After enjoying a main meal of baked chicken breast, roasted vegetables, and quinoa for dinner, I plan to use the same cooked and ready-to-go components along with some everyday staples and two mix-and-match items to make other meals. The results will be totally different yet appetizing and delicious meals that can be ready with little time and effort. Try any of the following:

- **Turn it into a soup**
  Sauté a few sliced veggies in a pot (onion, garlic, or carrot), add broth, and throw in some sliced leftover chicken and quinoa. Simmer, and done!

- **Turn it into a salad**
  Choose a favourite salad green. Add a scoop of leftover quinoa, chicken, and roasted veggies. Top it with a choice of extras (seeds, avocado, or cheese) and a dressing, and done!

- **Turn it into a taco, quesadilla, or wrap**
  Get a pack of tortillas, fill each with leftovers or extras (cherry tomatoes, black beans, salsa, avocado, or hot sauce), and done!

- **Turn it into a brunch platter**
  Reheat roasted veggies in a pan with olive oil, crack two eggs next to the veggies, and cover until cooked. Transfer them to a plate with leftover quinoa, add flavouring, and done!

- **Turn it into stuffed sweet potatoes or peppers**
  Prep and bake sweet potatoes or peppers. Mix leftover veggies, chicken, and quinoa together in a bowl with flavouring or spices, stuff, and done!

- **Turn it into a bowl**
  Arrange leftover chicken, roasted veggies, and quinoa in a bowl. Add extra flavouring (pink onions, sliced avocado, crumbled feta, sauce, or dressing), and done!

- **Turn it into a pasta bake**
  Cook a pot of pasta. Transfer cooked pasta to a baking dish of tomato sauce, leftover chicken, and roasted veggies. Bake it for 20 minutes, and done!

- **Turn it into a pizza**
  Spread sauce and cheese on a dough or crust. Add leftover chicken and roasted veggies, and done!

- **Turn it into a quiche or frittata**
  Create an egg mixture with eggs, cheese, and milk. Fold in leftover chicken and roasted veggies. Then bake, and done!

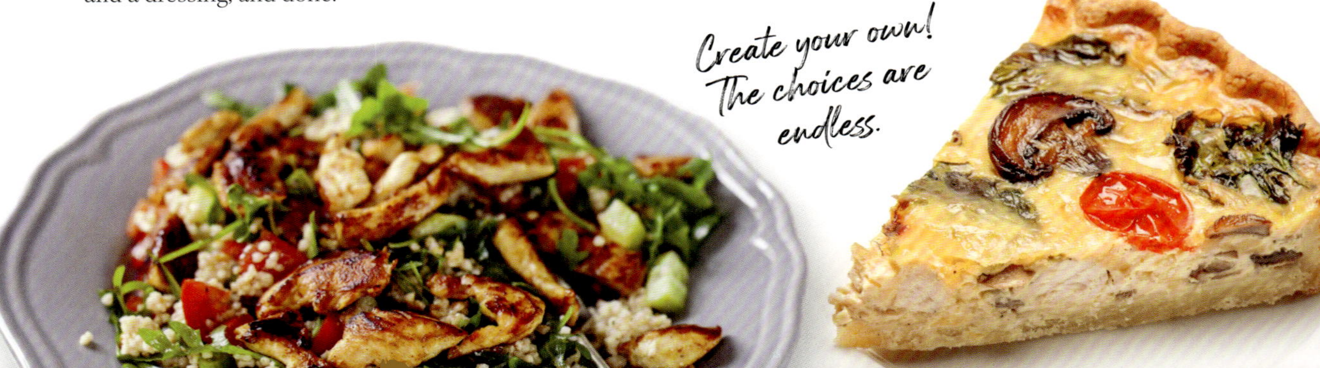

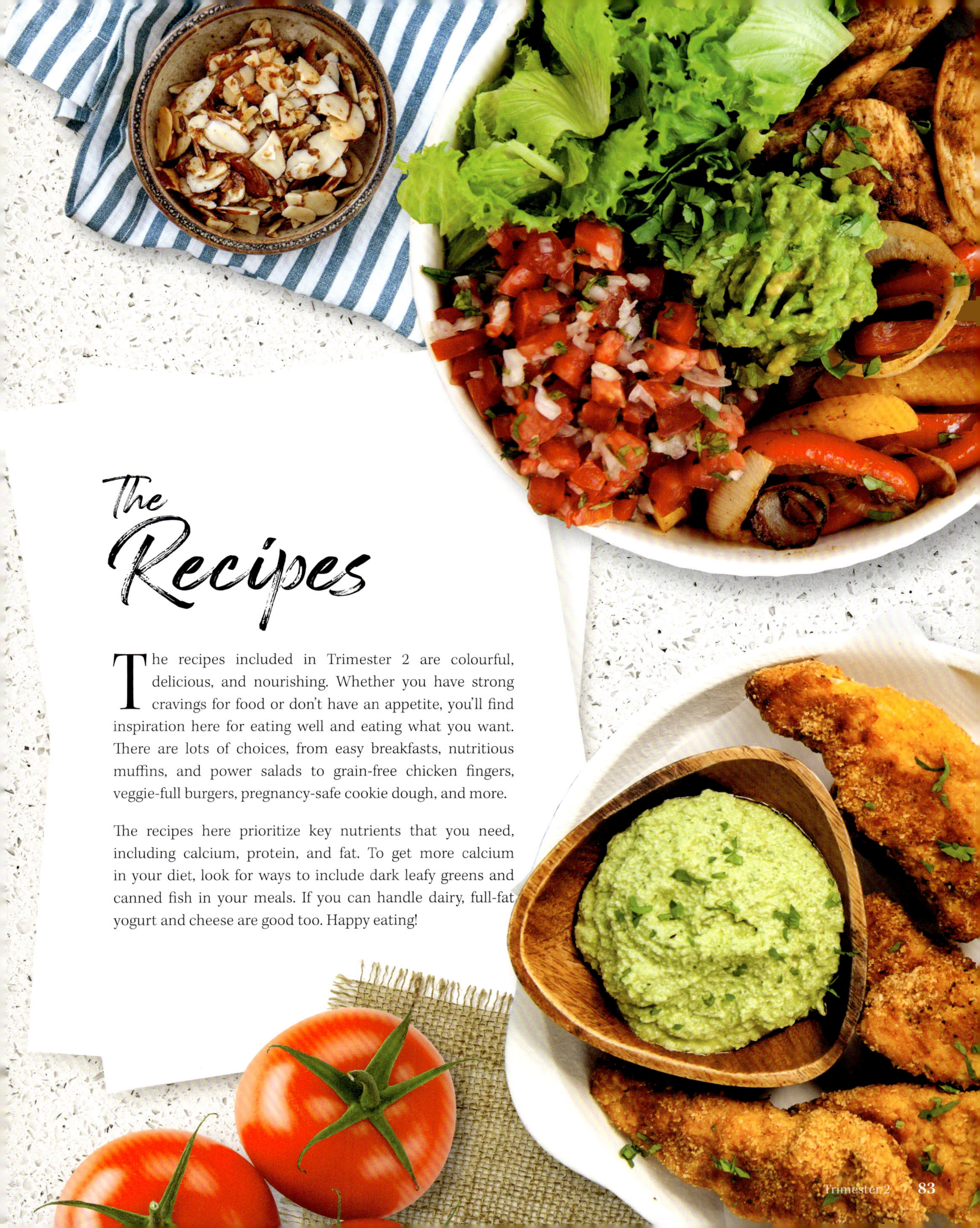

The Recipes

The recipes included in Trimester 2 are colourful, delicious, and nourishing. Whether you have strong cravings for food or don't have an appetite, you'll find inspiration here for eating well and eating what you want. There are lots of choices, from easy breakfasts, nutritious muffins, and power salads to grain-free chicken fingers, veggie-full burgers, pregnancy-safe cookie dough, and more.

The recipes here prioritize key nutrients that you need, including calcium, protein, and fat. To get more calcium in your diet, look for ways to include dark leafy greens and canned fish in your meals. If you can handle dairy, full-fat yogurt and cheese are good too. Happy eating!

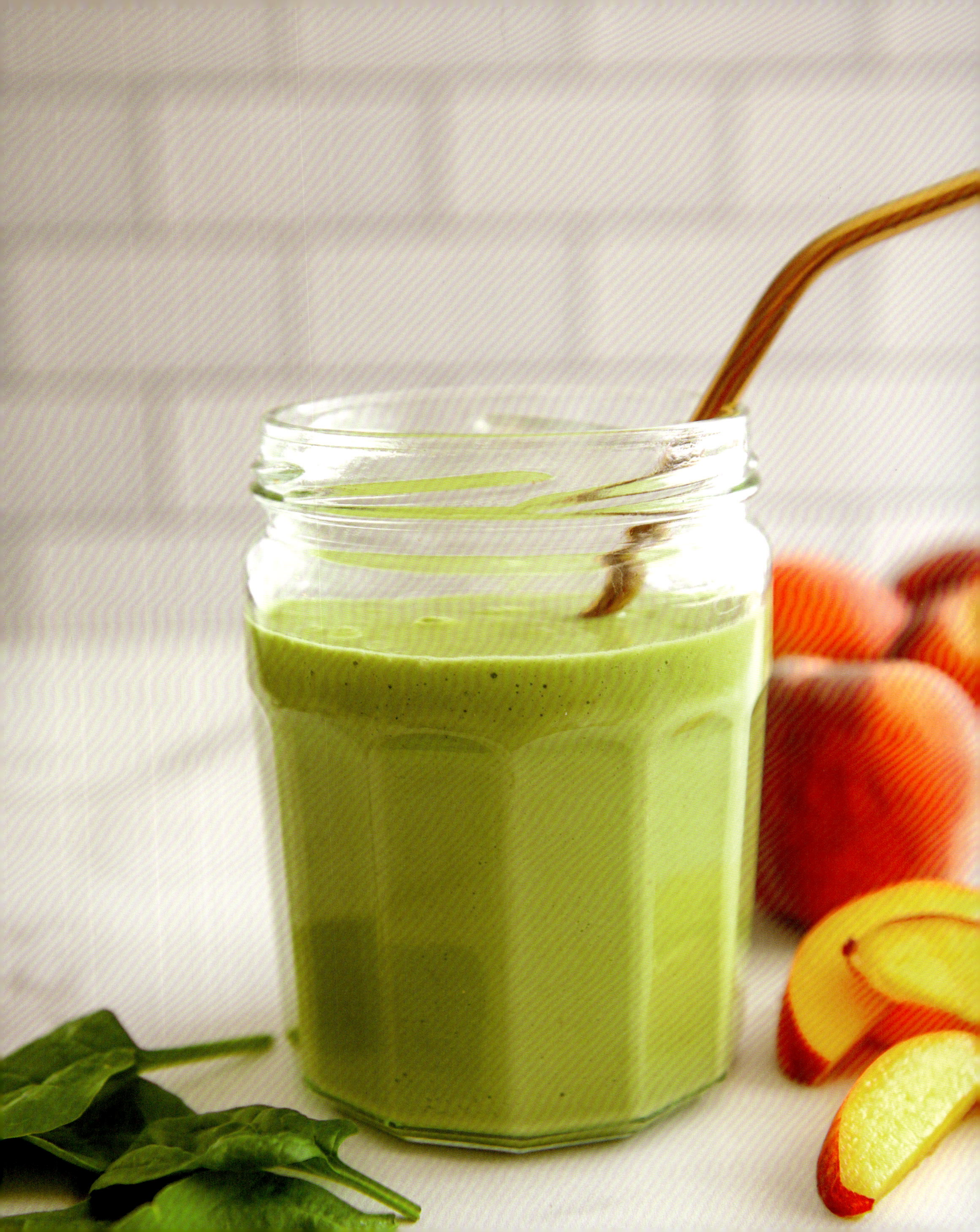

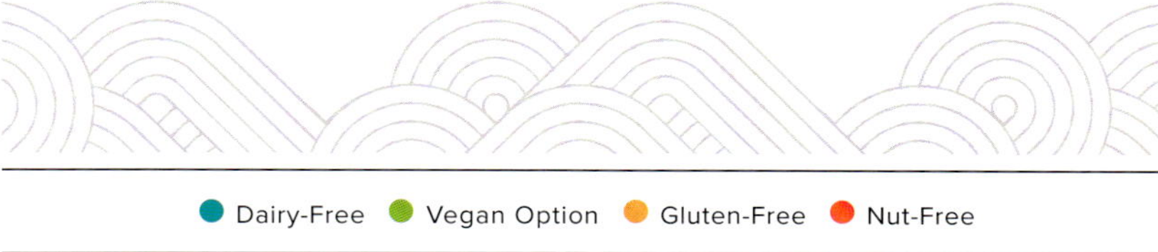

Dairy-Free · Vegan Option · Gluten-Free · Nut-Free

Peachy Green Smoothie

It's hard to resist taking a bite of a fresh, locally-grown peach in summer. It's sweet, juicy, and delicious! Extend peach season by freezing peach slices and enjoying them year-round in this peachy green smoothie. I like making this smoothie when I have coconut milk in the refrigerator or leftover from making another recipe, such as the Banana Coconut Nice Cream (page 99).

5 MINUTES PREPPING • 1 MINUTE BLENDING • MAKES 1 LARGE OR 2 SMALL SMOOTHIES

WHAT YOU NEED:	HOW TO MAKE IT:
2 cups (500 mL) coconut water or coconut milk (or water) 1 ½ cups (375 mL) frozen peaches 1 cup (250 mL) spinach, lightly packed ½ cup (125 mL) rolled oats 2 tbsp (30 mL) hemp hearts 1 tbsp (15 mL) lemon juice 1 ½ tsp (7.5 mL) honey (optional)	1. Add all ingredients to a high-powered blender. Blend until smooth, about 1 minute.

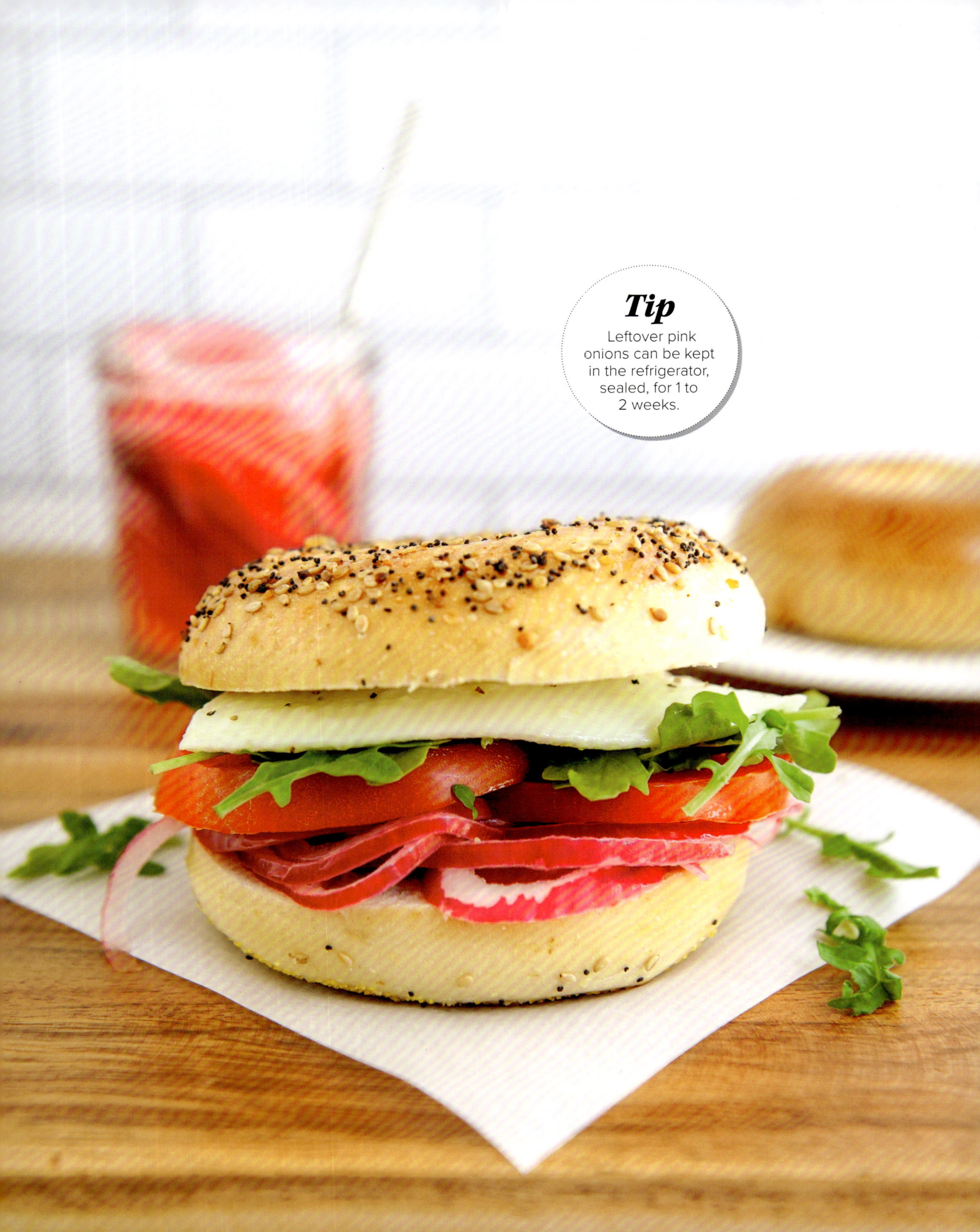

Tip

Leftover pink onions can be kept in the refrigerator, sealed, for 1 to 2 weeks.

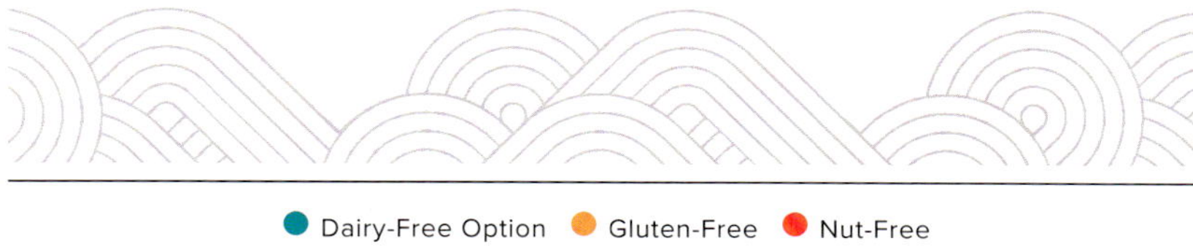

Dairy-Free Option · Gluten-Free · Nut-Free

Cravings Breakfast Sandwich

Sometimes you just need a good breakfast sandwich to start your day! You can easily scale up this recipe, depending on how many sandwiches you want to make. And don't skip the pink onions — you'll find the delicious flavour irresistible and will soon be adding pink onions to everything you eat.

10 MINUTES PREPPING (PLUS 30 MINUTES COOLING) • 5 MINUTES COOKING • MAKES 2 SERVINGS

WHAT YOU NEED:

For the sandwiches

1 tbsp (15 mL) butter or olive oil

2 gluten-free bagels (or substitute whole wheat for non-GF)

2 eggs

1 tomato, sliced

1 handful of arugula

Pink onions, as desired (see recipe below)

Salt and pepper, to taste

For the pink onions

1 large red onion

1 cup (250 mL) vinegar (white vinegar, apple cider vinegar, or a combination of the two)

1 tbsp (15 mL) honey

½ tsp (2 mL) sea salt

HOW TO MAKE IT:

1. Thinly slice the red onion, and place the slices in a wide-mouth jam jar or glass storage container.
2. Make the vinegar mixture: add the vinegar, honey, and sea salt to a small saucepan set to medium-high and heat until you start to see steam. Pour the hot vinegar mixture over the onions. Let cool for 30 minutes on your counter, then enjoy or keep them in the refrigerator until you're ready to eat.
3. Add butter/olive oil to a pan set to medium heat. When hot, crack your eggs into the pan and cover until cooked to your liking, about 4 to 5 minutes for a fully cooked yolk.
4. While eggs are cooking, toast your bagels. Top each toasted bagel with an egg, tomato slices, arugula, pink onions, and salt and pepper.

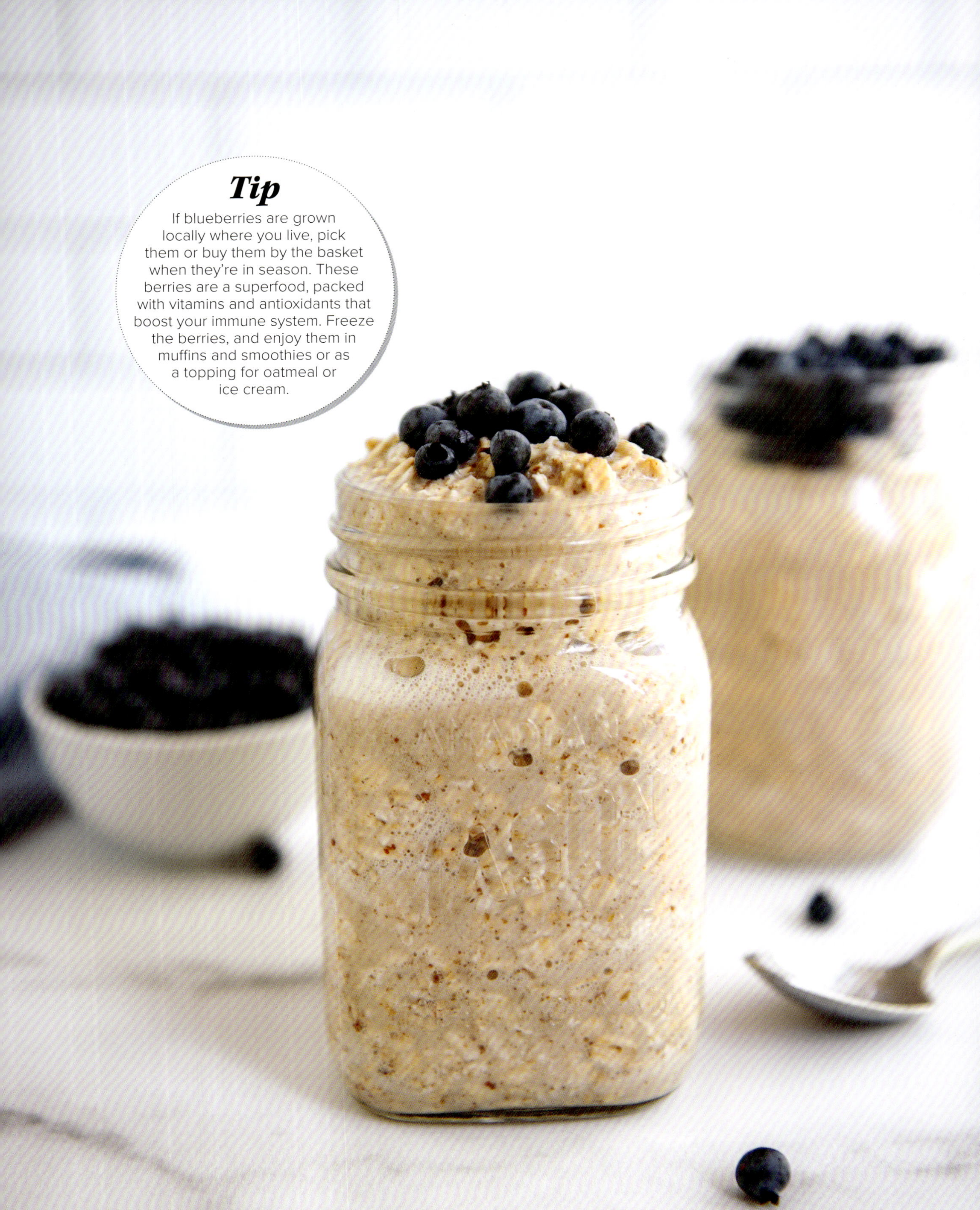

Tip

If blueberries are grown locally where you live, pick them or buy them by the basket when they're in season. These berries are a superfood, packed with vitamins and antioxidants that boost your immune system. Freeze the berries, and enjoy them in muffins and smoothies or as a topping for oatmeal or ice cream.

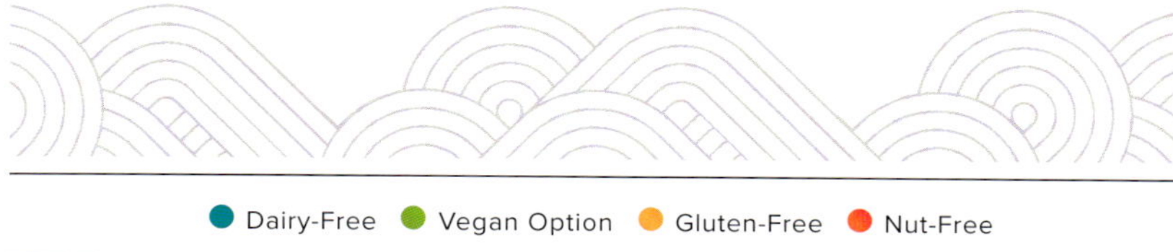

Dairy-Free · Vegan Option · Gluten-Free · Nut-Free

Wild Blueberry Overnight Oats

It feels wonderful to wake up to a breakfast that is already made and waiting to energize you! Do the prep the night before, and leave the oatmeal mixture to soften and combine overnight. In the morning, enjoy this nutritious breakfast cold, or heat it up. Have it the way you like it.

5 MINUTES PREPPING • OVERNIGHT CHILLING • MAKES 2 SERVINGS

WHAT YOU NEED:	HOW TO MAKE IT:
1 ½ cups (375 mL) non-dairy milk of choice 1 ¼ cups (310 mL) rolled oats ½ cup (125 mL) wild blueberries (or fruit of choice) 1 tbsp (15 mL) ground flaxseed 2 tsp (10 mL) honey or maple syrup ¼ tsp (1 mL) vanilla extract ⅛ tsp (0.5 mL) cinnamon Pinch of sea salt	1. Stir all the ingredients (except blueberries) together in a medium-sized bowl, storage container, or glass jar. Cover and let it sit overnight in the refrigerator. When ready to eat, top with the blueberries, and enjoy!

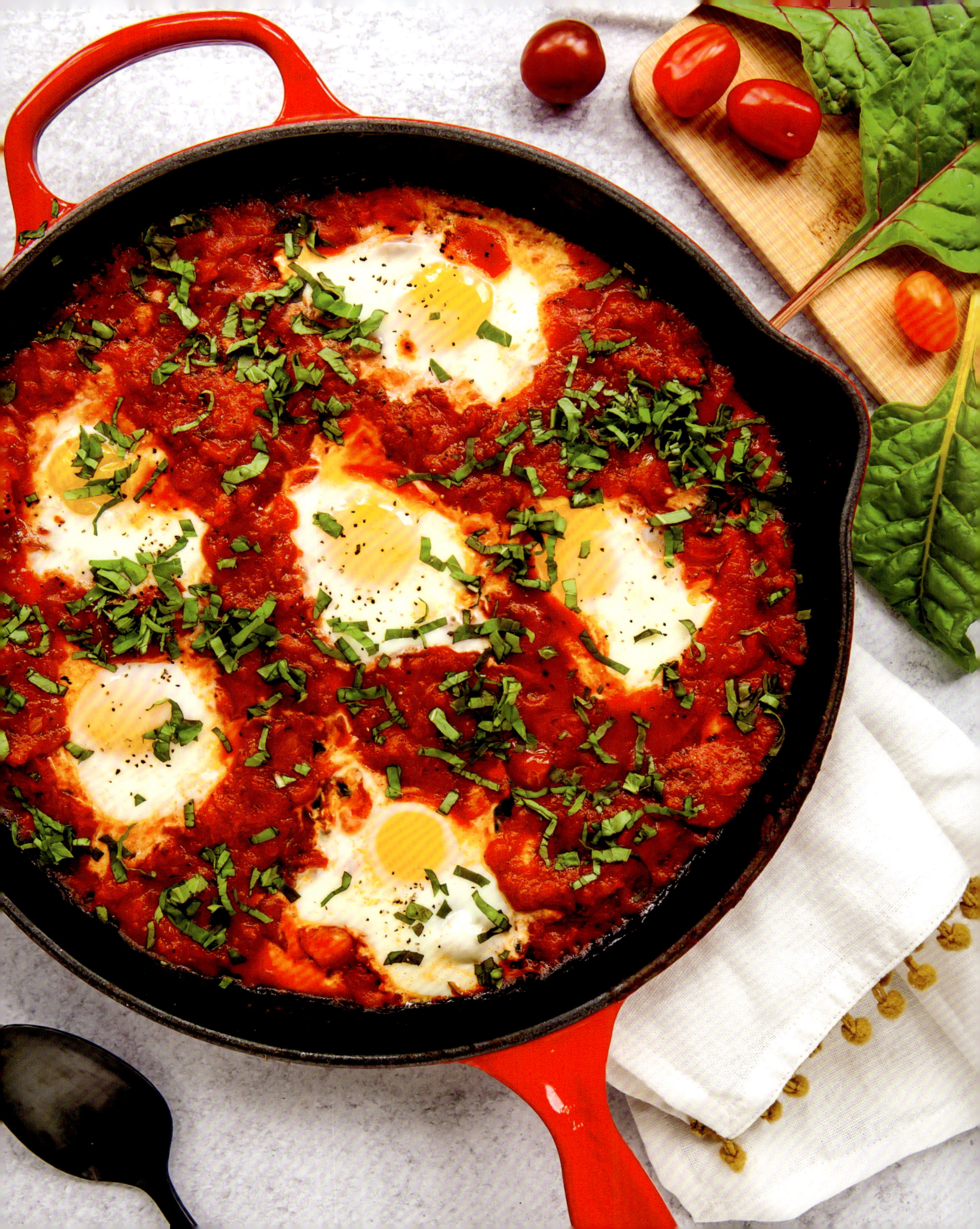

Dairy-Free • Gluten-Free • Grain-Free • Nut-Free

Shakshuka with Swiss Chard + Cherry Tomatoes

Here's a speedy take on an appetizing meal with its origins in North Africa. This dish is delicious with the Goodness Me Tomato Sauce (page 61), which is packed with tomatoes and grilled peppers. You can eat this on its own (for breakfast, lunch, or dinner) or serve with tortillas or crusty bread for dipping. I often scale down this recipe, using a small pan and 2 eggs if I'm cooking this just for myself.

5 MINUTES PREPPING • 20 MINUTES COOKING • MAKES 3 SERVINGS

WHAT YOU NEED:

1 tbsp (15 mL) olive oil

1 shallot, finely chopped

1 cup (250 mL) Swiss chard, chopped (or use kale)

1 cup (250 mL) cherry tomatoes

3 cups (750 mL) Goodness Me Tomato Sauce (page 61) or store-bought

4 to 6 eggs

¼ tsp (1 mL) pepper

Sea salt, to taste

Optional Toppings

Fresh basil (or use cilantro, parsley, or green onions)

Hot sauce, if you like it spicy

HOW TO MAKE IT:

1. Preheat your oven to 375°F (190°C).
2. In a large oven-safe skillet over medium heat, add olive oil. When oil is hot, add the shallots and cook, about 3 minutes. Next, add the cherry tomatoes and Swiss chard, and cook for 3 more minutes.
3. Add the sauce and heat until you see steam. Then one at a time, clear a little well in the sauce and crack an egg into it, gently spooning sauce over the edges of the egg whites to contain them.
4. Transfer your skillet to the oven and cook, about 10 to 12 minutes if you like eggs that are cooked through.
5. Top with salt, pepper, fresh basil, and hot sauce (if using). Leftovers can be kept in the refrigerator and enjoyed the next day.

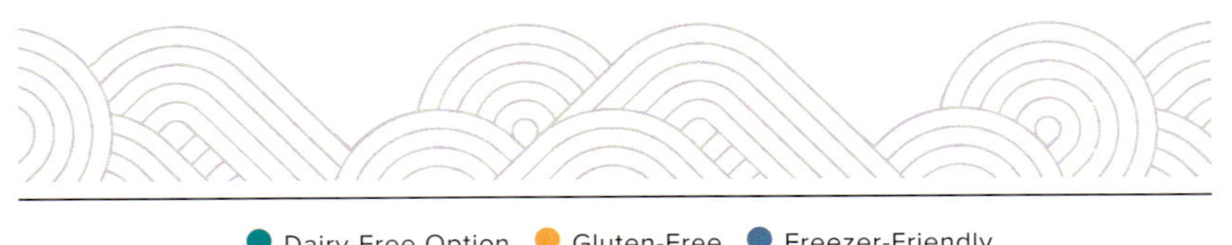

Dairy-Free Option • Gluten-Free • Freezer-Friendly

Blueberry Zucchini Muffins

Zucchini is a wonderful ingredient in baking — it doesn't have a strong vegetable flavour, and it adds moisture, softness, and nutrients such as fibre to baked goods. Everyone's favourite blueberry muffins are more nutritious, thanks to this green veggie!

15 MINUTES PREPPING • 20 MINUTES COOKING • MAKES 12 MUFFINS

WHAT YOU NEED:

Dry ingredients

2 cups (500 mL) gluten-free flour blend (or substitute whole wheat flour for non-GF)

½ cup (125 mL) almond flour

½ cup (125 mL) coconut sugar

1 tsp (5 mL) baking powder

1 tsp (5 mL) baking soda

½ tsp (2 mL) cinnamon

½ tsp (2 mL) sea salt

Wet ingredients

1 cup (250 mL) non-dairy milk of choice

¼ cup (60 mL) butter or coconut oil, melted and cooled

¼ cup (60 mL) apple sauce

1 egg

1 tbsp (15 mL) lemon juice

1 tbsp (15 mL) lemon zest (from half a lemon)

1 ½ tsp (7.5 mL) vanilla extract

Mix-in

1 cup (250 mL) zucchini, grated and squeezed of excess moisture (from 1 medium zucchini)

1 cup (250 mL) frozen wild blueberries

HOW TO MAKE IT:

1. Preheat oven to 350°F (180°C), and grease or line muffin pan with parchment paper liners.
2. In a large bowl, whisk together the dry ingredients.
3. In a medium bowl, whisk together the wet ingredients, then pour them into the dry ingredients. Add zucchini and blueberries to the bowl, and mix until just combined.
4. Spoon batter into the prepared muffin pan and bake, 18 to 22 minutes, until a toothpick inserted into the middle of a muffin comes out clean. Let cool in the pan for 5 minutes, then move to a cooling rack.

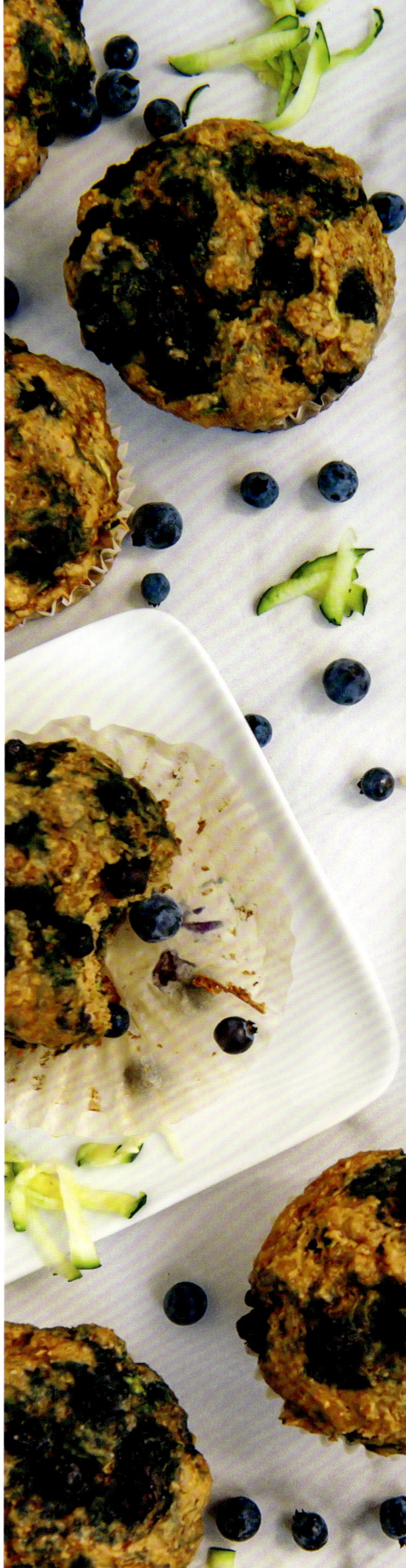

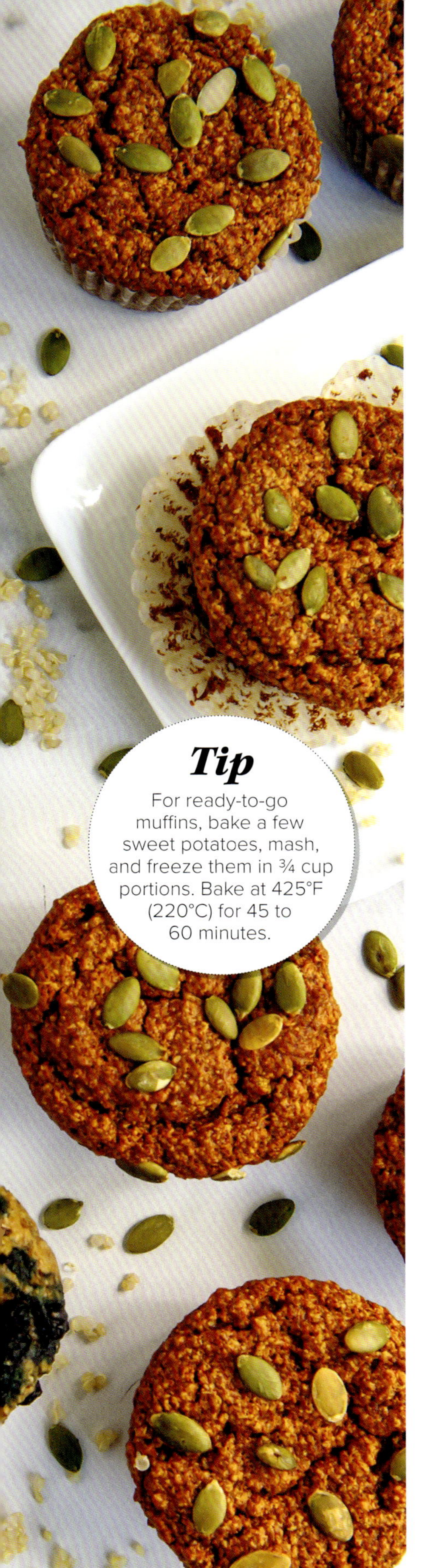

Tip

For ready-to-go muffins, bake a few sweet potatoes, mash, and freeze them in ¾ cup portions. Bake at 425°F (220°C) for 45 to 60 minutes.

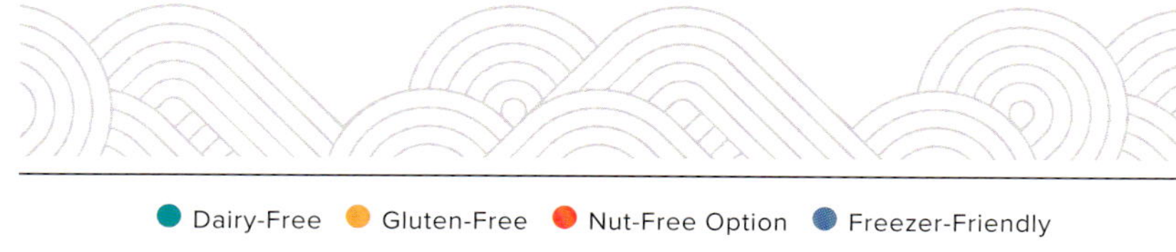

Dairy-Free • Gluten-Free • Nut-Free Option • Freezer-Friendly

Spiced Sweet Potato + Quinoa Muffins

Yes, these muffins have sweet potato and quinoa in them! They are packed with protein and fibre, which means they'll keep you full and feeling good too. And they are delicious — these muffins are perfect for breakfast or as a snack.

15 MINUTES PREPPING • 25 MINUTES COOKING • MAKES 12 MUFFINS

WHAT YOU NEED:

Dry ingredients

1 cup (250 mL) oat flour (or use whole wheat for non-GF)

¼ cup (60 mL) almond flour (or substitute whole wheat flour or oat flour for nut-free)

1 tbsp (15 mL) arrowroot starch (or use cornstarch)

1 tsp (5 mL) baking soda

1 tsp (5 mL) baking powder

1 ½ tsp (7.5 mL) cinnamon

1 tsp (5 mL) ground ginger

½ tsp (2 mL) sea salt

¼ tsp (1 mL) ground nutmeg

Wet ingredients

¾ cup (175 mL) sweet potato, cooked and mashed (from about 1 sweet potato)

½ cup (125 mL) maple syrup

¼ cup (60 mL) coconut oil, melted

1 egg

1 tbsp (15 mL) apple cider vinegar

1 tsp (5 mL) vanilla

Mix-in

¾ cup (175 mL) quinoa, cooked and cooled

Pumpkin seeds for topping (optional)

HOW TO MAKE IT:

1. Preheat oven to 350°F (180°C), and grease or line a muffin pan.
2. Whisk dry ingredients together in a large bowl.
3. Blend wet ingredients together in a high-powered blender, then pour into the dry ingredients. Add quinoa to the bowl, and mix the ingredients together until just combined.
4. Scoop into the muffin pan, top with the pumpkin seeds (if using), and bake for 20 to 25 minutes, or until a toothpick inserted into the centre of a muffin comes out clean. Cool for 5 minutes in the pan, then move to a cooling rack.

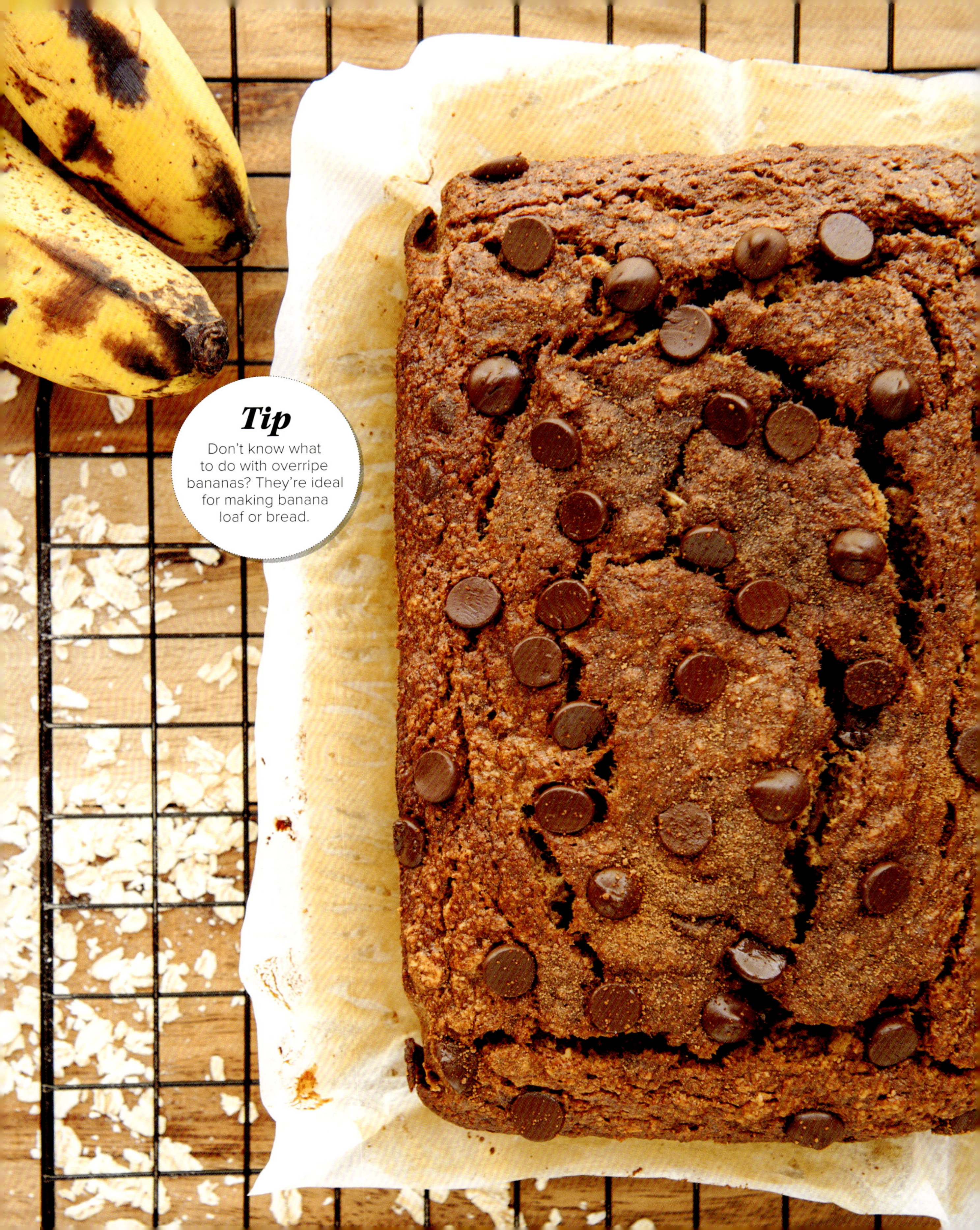

Tip

Don't know what to do with overripe bananas? They're ideal for making banana loaf or bread.

● Dairy-Free Option ● Gluten-Free ● Nut-Free ● Freezer-Friendly

Cinnamon Chocolate Banana Loaf

Banana bread is a favourite in most households — it's delicious, comforting, makes the house smell amazing, and often includes chocolate. This recipe is cinnamon-packed and sweetened by maple syrup (and bananas). Plus, it freezes perfectly.

15 MINUTES PREPPING • 45 MINUTES COOKING • MAKES ONE 8 × 5-INCH LOAF

WHAT YOU NEED:

Dry ingredients

1 ½ cups (375 mL) oat flour (or substitute whole wheat for non-GF)

1 cup (250 mL) rolled oats

1 tbsp (15 mL) cinnamon

1 tsp (5 mL) baking powder

1 tsp (5 mL) baking soda

½ tsp (2 mL) fine sea salt

Wet ingredients

3 to 4 very ripe bananas (about 1 ½ cups/375 mL), puréed in a blender

2 eggs

½ cup (125 mL) maple syrup

¼ cup (60 mL) coconut oil, melted

1 tbsp (15 mL) vanilla extract

Mix-in

½ cup (125 mL) chocolate chips (dairy-free or regular)

Optional toppings

Cinnamon sugar sprinkle: 1 tsp (5 mL) coconut sugar mixed with ¼ tsp (1 mL) cinnamon

Extra chocolate chips

HOW TO MAKE IT:

1. Preheat oven to 350°F (180°C), and line a 8 x 5-inch loaf pan with parchment paper.
2. Whisk together the dry ingredients in a large bowl.
3. Mix together the wet ingredients, either in a blender or a medium-sized bowl, until smooth.
4. Pour the wet ingredients into the dry bowl and mix until combined. Fold in the chocolate chips.
5. Pour the mixture into the prepared loaf pan, and top it with cinnamon sugar sprinkle and extra chocolate chips, if using.
6. Bake for about 45 minutes, or until the centre is cooked. Remove from the oven and cool for 10 minutes in the pan, then move to a cooling rack.

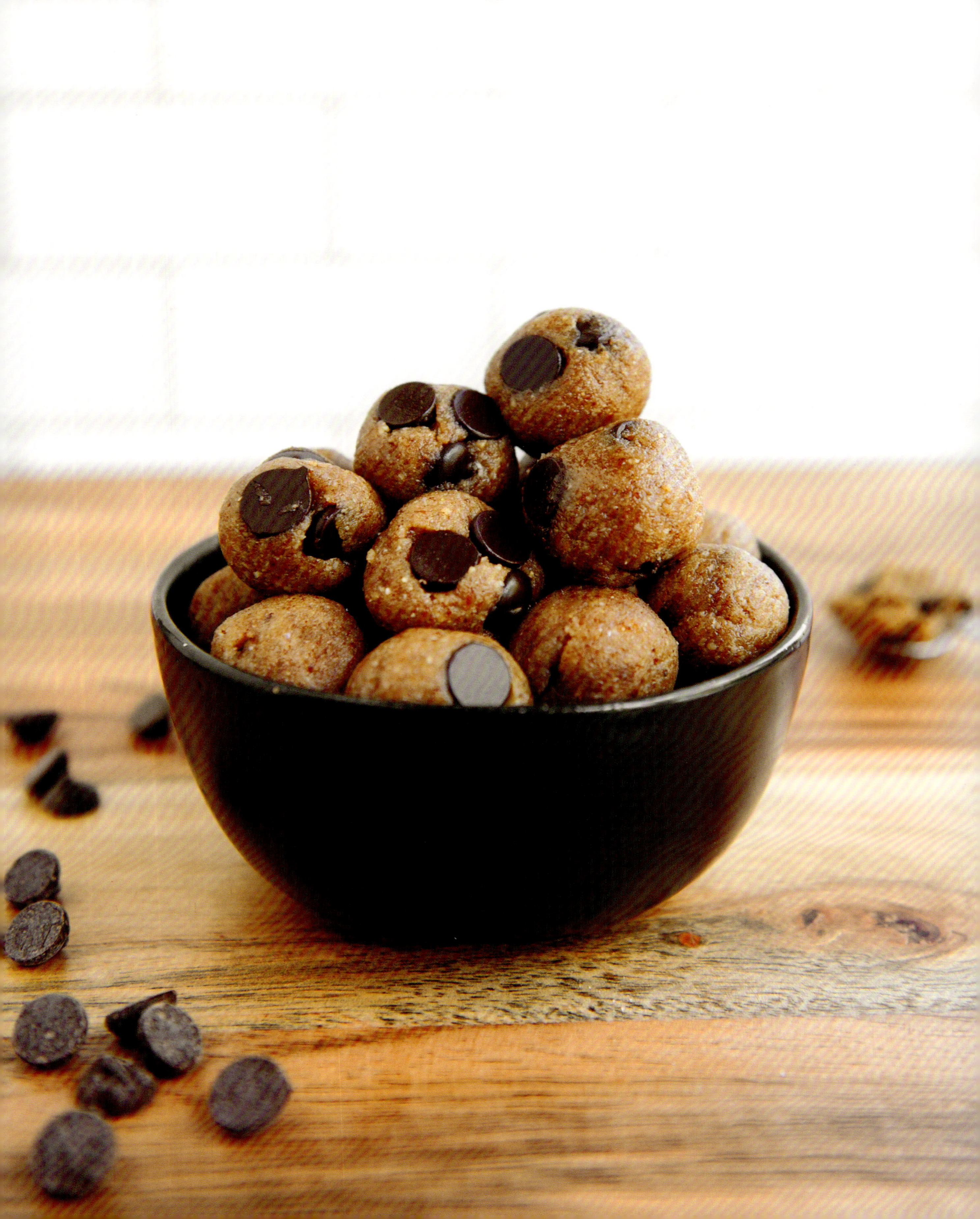

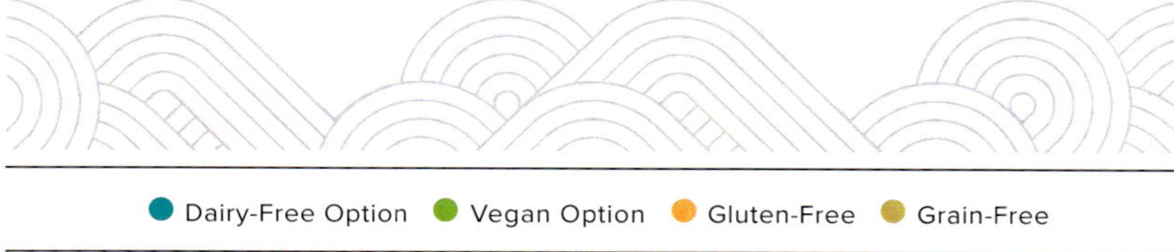

Dairy-Free Option · Vegan Option · Gluten-Free · Grain-Free

Cookie Dough Bites

With this recipe, you can have all the softness and richness of cookie dough without the worry of eating raw eggs! There's no baking involved too.

5 MINUTES PREPPING • 5 MINUTES ROLLING • MAKES 22 BITES

WHAT YOU NEED:	HOW TO MAKE IT:
1 cup (250 mL) almond flour ¼ cup (60 mL) ground flaxseed ¼ cup (60 mL) maple syrup ¼ cup (60 mL) chocolate chips (dairy-free or regular) 3 tbsp (45 mL) almond butter 1 tsp (5 mL) vanilla extract ⅛ tsp (0.5 mL) sea salt	**1.** Combine all the ingredients in a large bowl with a spatula. Then, using a ½ tbsp (7 mL) scoop for size, roll the cookie dough into small bite-sized balls with your hands. **2.** Once rolled, the cookie dough bites can be kept in a storage container in the refrigerator for about a week.

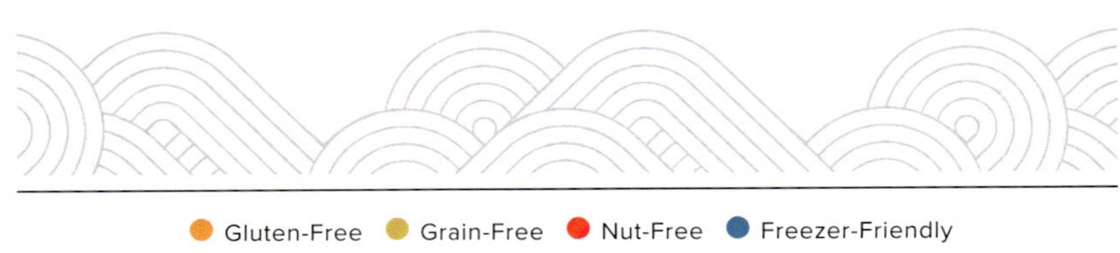

Gluten-Free · Grain-Free · Nut-Free · Freezer-Friendly

Chickpea Flour Ginger Cookies

If you're experimenting with gluten-free or grain-free flours, chickpea flour is a great place to start. It packs in the protein (the 1 ½ cups in this recipe has more than 30 g of protein!) and fibre, and it contains an impressive range of micronutrients, including iron and folate. These ginger cookies will easily become your favourite snack — they're a perfect treat with a cup of tea!

10 MINUTES PREPPING (PLUS 2 HOURS CHILLING) • 10 MINUTES COOKING • MAKES 1 DOZEN

WHAT YOU NEED:

Wet ingredients

½ cup (125 mL) butter, softened

½ cup (125 mL) coconut sugar

1 egg

1 tsp (5 mL) vanilla extract

Dry ingredients

1 ½ cups (375 mL) chickpea flour

1 tbsp (15 mL) ground ginger

1 tsp (5 mL) cinnamon

½ tsp (2 mL) baking soda

¼ tsp (1 mL) nutmeg

¼ tsp (1 mL) sea salt

HOW TO MAKE IT:

1. In a large bowl, cream together the softened butter and the coconut sugar, using a hand mixer or spatula. Then add the egg and vanilla, and mix well.
2. In another bowl, whisk to combine the dry ingredients. Pour this mixture over the wet ingredients and mix until just combined. Transfer the dough to the refrigerator, covered, for 1 to 2 hours (or overnight).
3. Preheat the oven to 350°F (180°C), and remove the dough from the refrigerator. On a cookie sheet lined with parchment paper, portion out the cookie dough into 1-inch (2.5-cm) balls. Bake, about 10 to 12 minutes. Let cool for a few minutes, then transfer to a cooling rack.

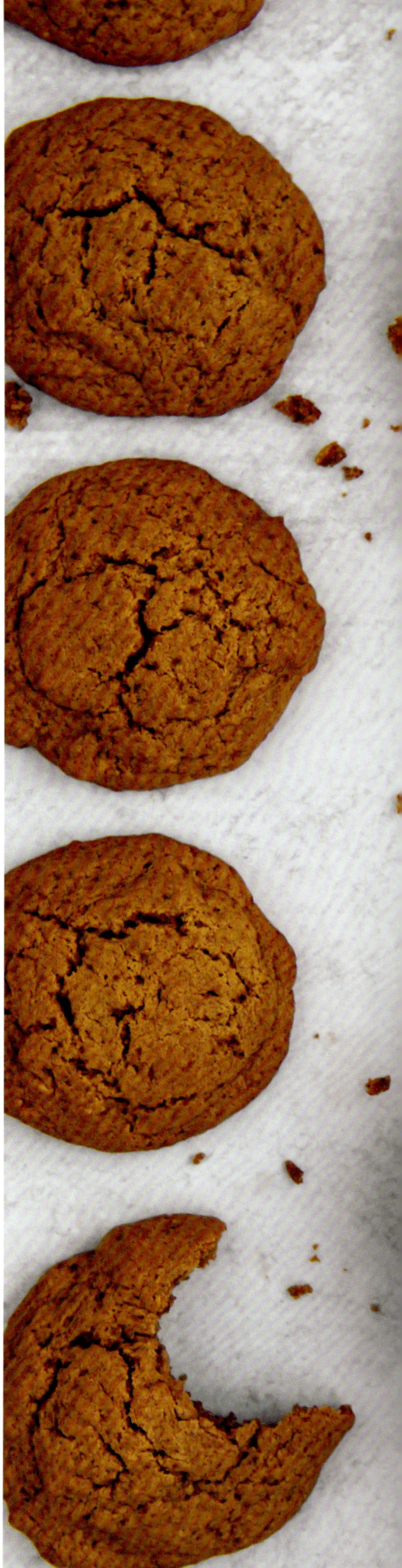

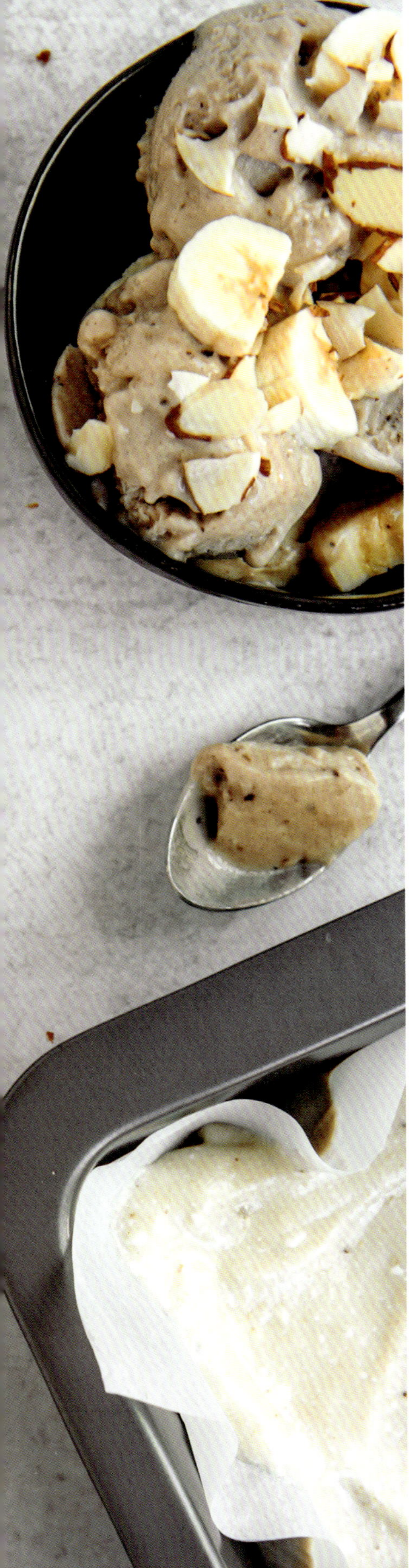

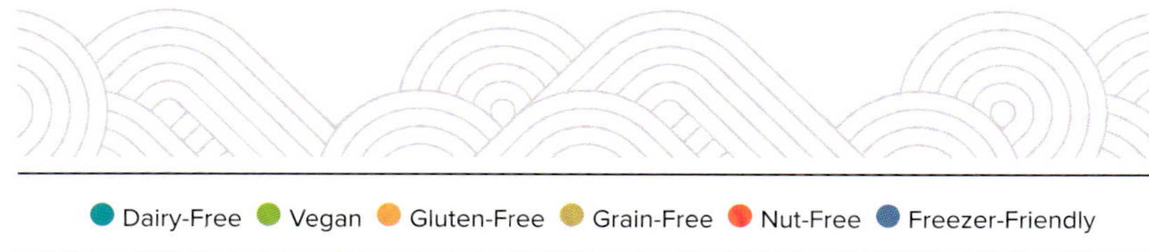

Dairy-Free • Vegan • Gluten-Free • Grain-Free • Nut-Free • Freezer-Friendly

Banana Coconut Nice Cream

"Nice Cream" is a dairy-free soft-serve frozen dessert made almost entirely of bananas! It is free of refined sugar and is a healthy and delicious treat for the whole family. You can customize this treat any way you like it. Add peanut butter, frozen berries, cacao powder, or anything you fancy — and make it your own.

5 MINUTES PREPPING • 3 MINUTES BLENDING • MAKES 4 SERVINGS

WHAT YOU NEED:

4 ripe, frozen bananas, sliced (see Note below)

½ cup (125 mL) coconut cream (scooped off the top of a can of coconut milk)

½ tsp (2 mL) vanilla extract

Optional toppings

Toasted coconut, chocolate chips, or berries

HOW TO MAKE IT:

1. Add your frozen, sliced bananas to a high-powered food processor or blender. Top up the bananas with the coconut cream and vanilla extract. Blend until smooth, scraping the sides or pressing down with your tamper, as necessary.
2. Enjoy immediately as soft-serve ice cream in a bowl, or freeze it to scoop out later, like traditional ice cream. (Be warned — you'll need to let it sit out of the freezer for a good 15 minutes before it's soft enough to scoop!)

NOTE

To make it easier to get smooth "Nice Cream," it's best to use frozen sliced bananas. If you have whole bananas in your freezer, take them out and slice them into pieces. If you are using fresh, ripe bananas, first slice them into rounds and freeze them on a parchment-lined baking tray until they are frozen.

Link-up

Use the coconut water that remains in the can of coconut milk as the liquid for the **Peachy Green Smoothie** (page 85).

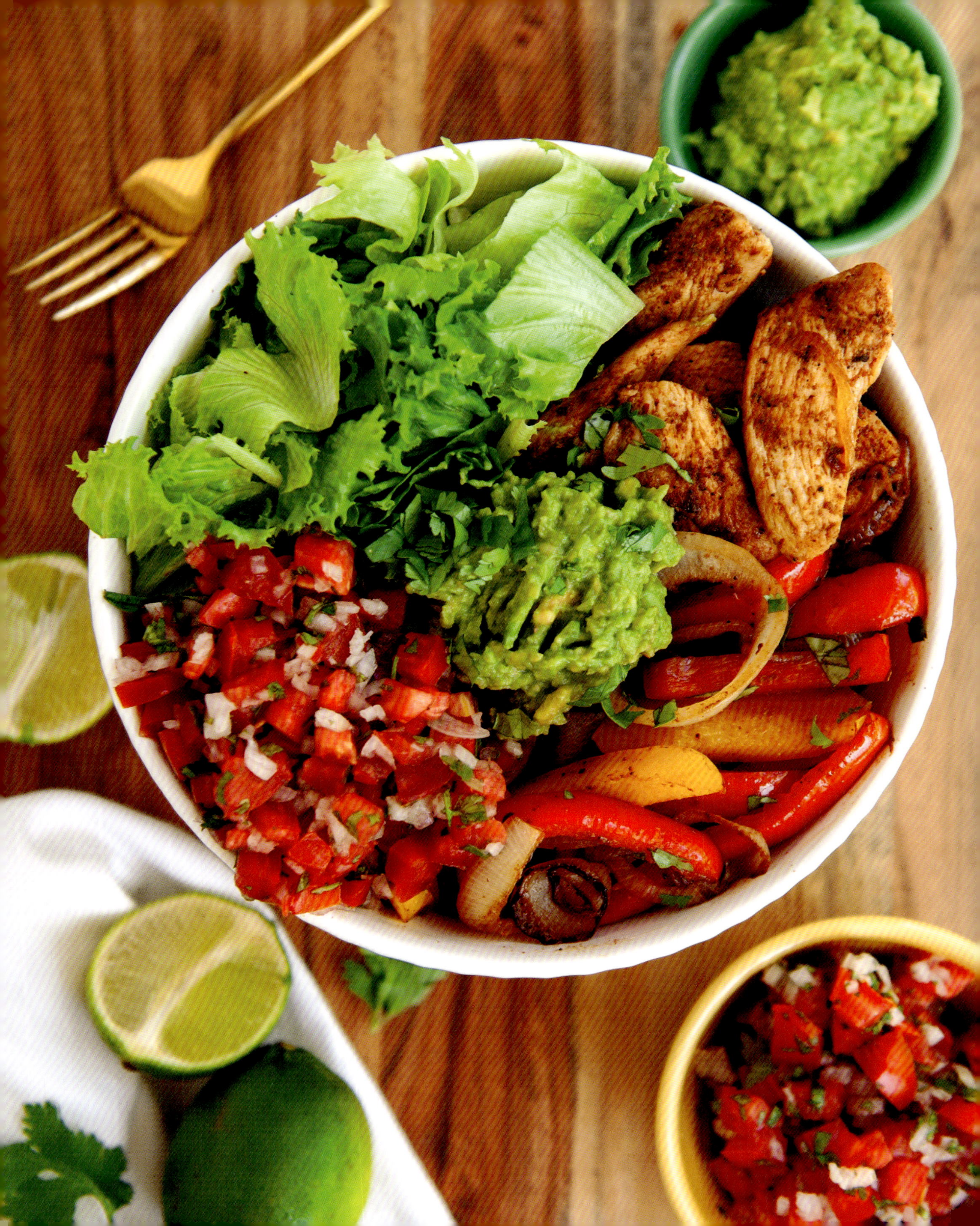

● Dairy-Free ● Gluten-Free Option ● Nut-Free

Fajita Bump Bowl

Fajitas are a weeknight staple in my house, and these bowls are one of my favourite ways to enjoy fajitas. They're fresh, bright, and full of Mexican flavour. If I have leftovers from the Slow Cooker Chicken Fajitas (page 71) or the Paprika + Cinnamon Pulled Pork (page 217), I'll make this meal the next day. I go straight to step 3, and have my dinner ready in no time.

10 MINUTES PREPPING • 15 MINUTES COOKING • MAKES 3 TO 4 SERVINGS

WHAT YOU NEED:

For the bowls

2 tbsp (30 mL) olive oil, divided

1 lb (450 g) boneless chicken breast, sliced into thin strips

1 ½ tbsp (22 mL) fajita spice mix (page 71)

2 bell peppers, sliced

1 onion, thinly sliced

8 cups (2 L) romaine lettuce, chopped

1 large avocado, sliced or smashed

Pico de gallo (see recipe below or store-bought)

2 limes, halved

Homemade Tortilla Chips (page 137) or store-bought (optional)

For the pico de gallo

4 ripe plum tomatoes, chopped into small pieces

½ cup (125 mL) onion, finely chopped

¼ cup (60 mL) fresh cilantro, finely chopped

1 garlic clove, minced

2 tbsp (30 mL) lime juice

¼ to ½ tsp (1 to 2 mL) fine sea salt

½ to 1 jalapeno pepper, finely chopped (optional)

HOW TO MAKE IT:

1. Heat 1 tbsp (15 mL) of the olive oil over medium heat in a big skillet. Add the chicken strips and the fajita spice mix, and cook about 5 minutes, or until the chicken is cooked through. Remove the chicken to a plate.
2. Heat the remaining 1 tbsp (15 mL) of olive oil in the skillet, and add the peppers and onions, stirring to coat with any spices remaining in the pan. Cook until the mixture is softened, about 8 minutes.
3. Assemble your bowls. Split up the chicken and veggie mixture, lettuce, avocado, and pico de gallo in the bowls, then finish each bowl with the juice of half a lime and a handful of tortilla chips. (I like to crush mine up!)

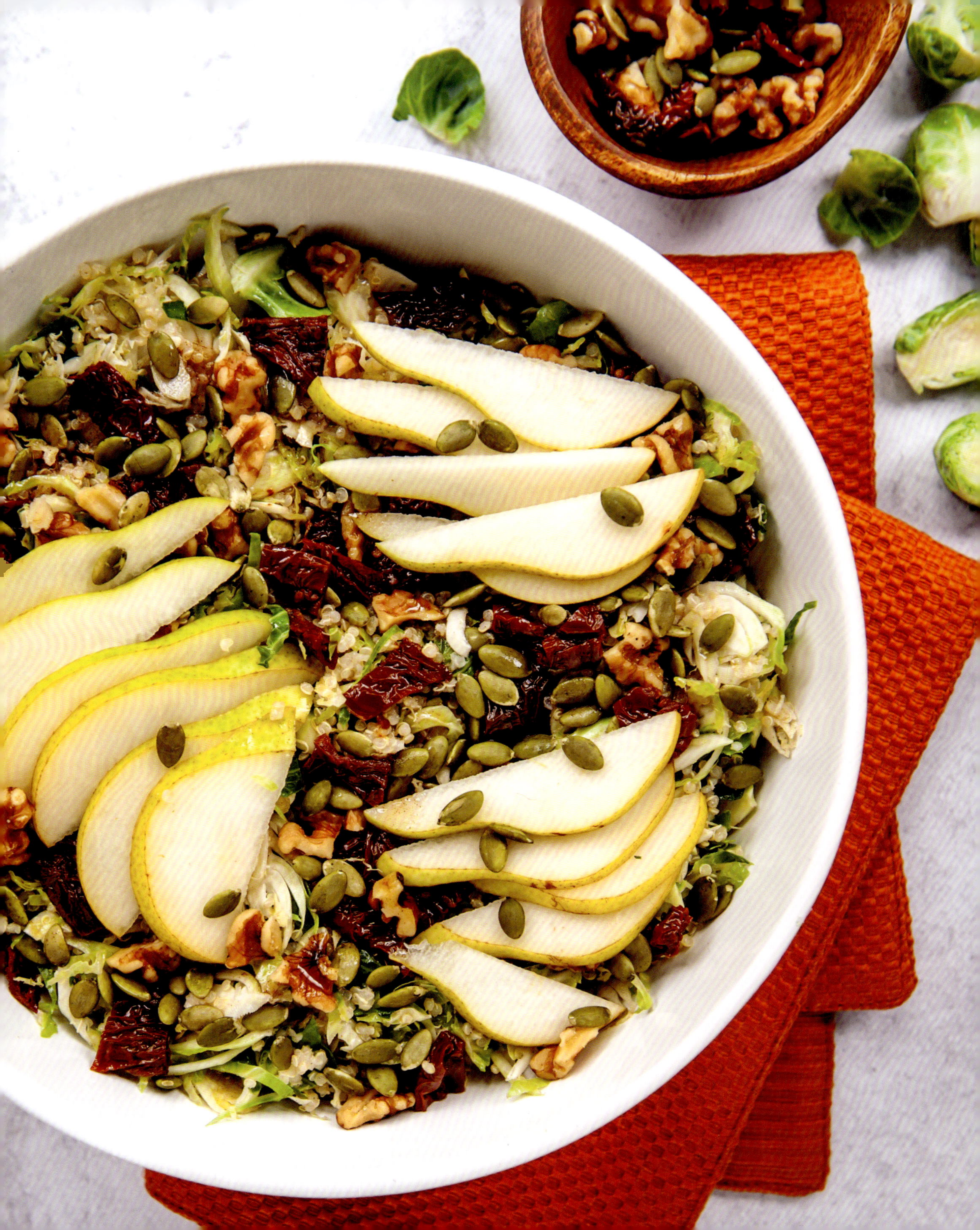

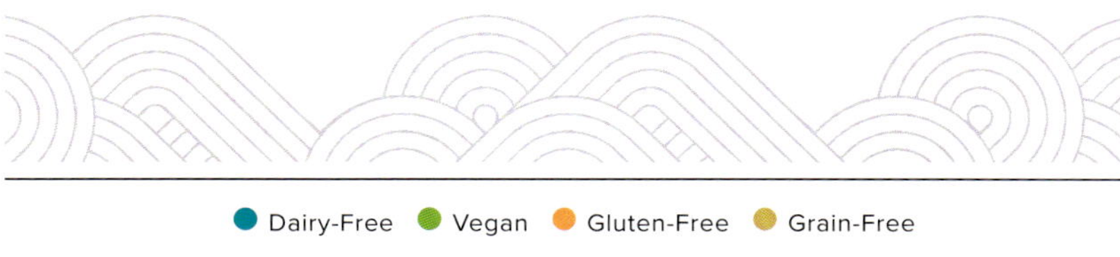

Dairy-Free · Vegan · Gluten-Free · Grain-Free

Brussels Sprout + Pear Salad with Quinoa

Fall is a wonderful season and a great time to be pregnant — the weather is sunny with a cool breeze, and ideal for layered clothing and light, comfortable boots. The food is delicious too — from an abundant fall harvest of hardy vegetables and crisp fruit to the warming spices that we love in food and drinks. This recipe is a fall salad through and through, right down to the maple cinnamon vinaigrette!

15 MINUTES PREPPING • 0 MINUTES COOKING • MAKES 4 TO 6 SERVINGS

WHAT YOU NEED:

For the salad

1 lb (450 g) Brussels sprouts

2 cups (500 mL) cooked quinoa

½ cup (125 mL) oil-packed sun-dried tomatoes, chopped

⅓ cup (75 mL) walnuts, chopped

¼ cup (60 mL) pumpkin seeds (pepitas)

1 pear, thinly sliced

1 shallot, finely chopped

For the maple cinnamon vinaigrette

⅓ cup plus 1 tbsp (90 mL) olive oil

3 tbsp (45 mL) apple cider vinegar

1 tbsp (15 mL) maple syrup

½ tsp (2 mL) cinnamon

¼ tsp (1 mL) sea salt

HOW TO MAKE IT:

1. Make the vinaigrette by combining all the ingredients in a jar or bowl.
2. Shred the Brussels sprouts. The easiest and quickest way to do this is by using the blade attachment of a food processor. Otherwise, slice the Brussels sprouts thinly by hand.
3. In a large bowl, combine the Brussels sprouts, quinoa, sun-dried tomatoes, walnuts, pumpkin seeds, pear, and shallots. Then add the dressing, toss the salad, and enjoy. Keep leftovers in the refrigerator for 2 days.

Link-up

Double up on the dressing and use it for the **Warm Golden Cauliflower + Carrot Salad** (page 205). That's another fall favourite meal!

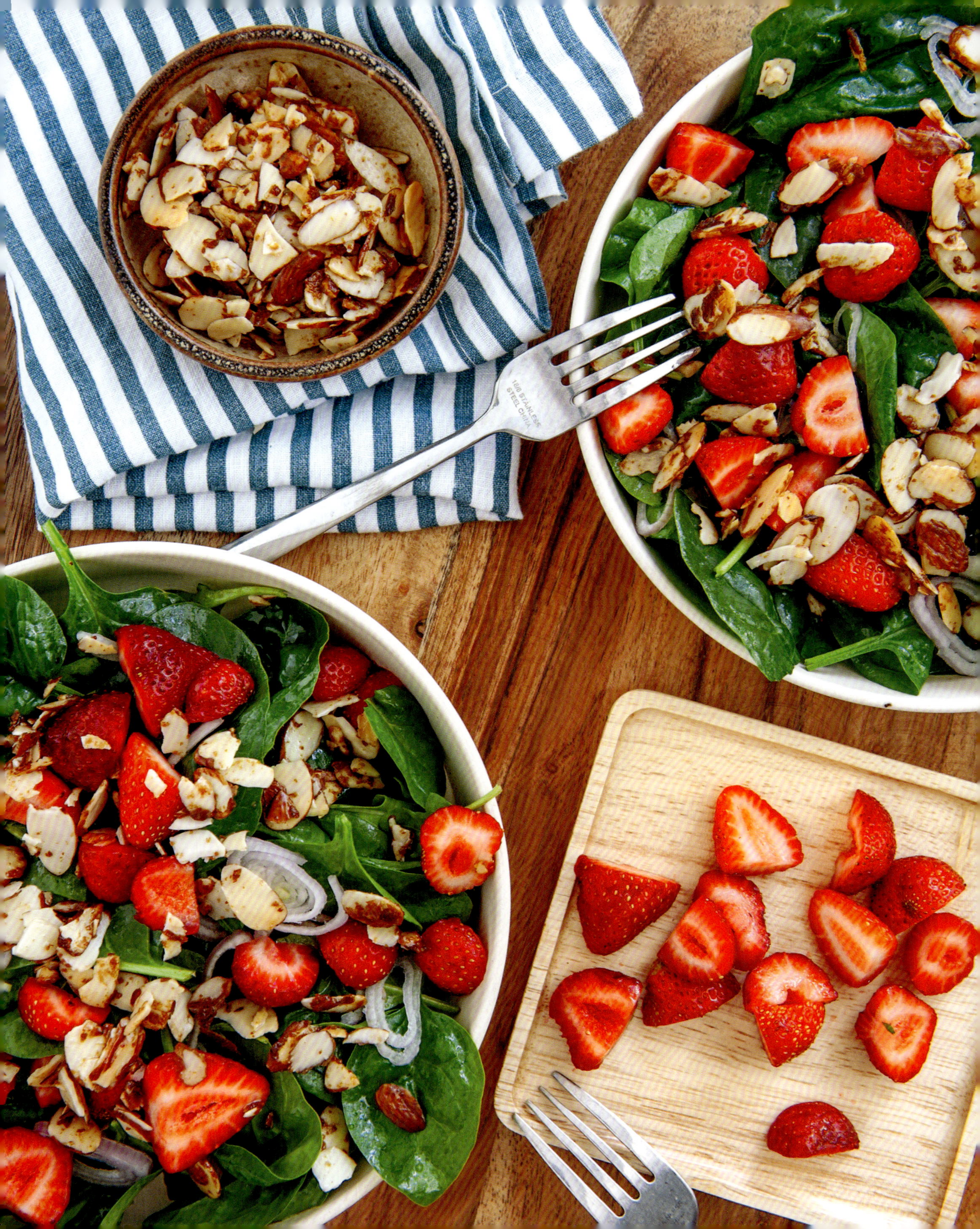

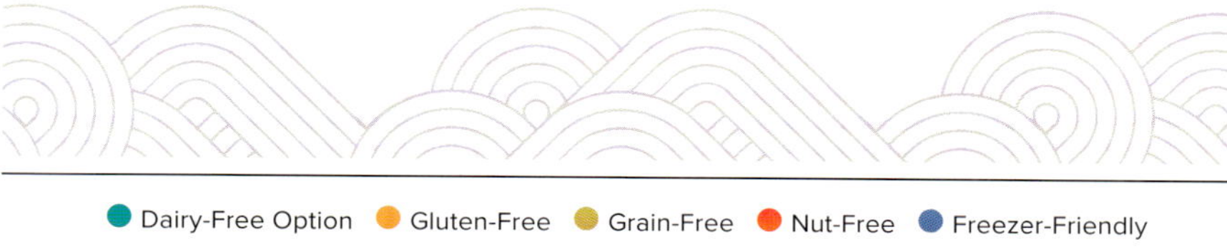

● Dairy-Free Option ● Gluten-Free ● Grain-Free ● Nut-Free ● Freezer-Friendly

Hidden Greens Meatballs

These meatballs are gluten-free and dairy-free, and they're full of the flavour that you'd expect in a meatball. They're versatile too — enjoy them hot in spaghetti, or try them cold tucked into a pita with crunchy veggies and a zesty dip. If you take the pasta route — why not have more veggies? Mix your favourite pasta with sweet potato, carrot, zucchini, or squash noodles.

15 MINUTES PREPPING • 30 MINUTES COOKING • MAKES 20 LARGE MEATBALLS

WHAT YOU NEED:

- 1 lb (450 g) ground beef (ideally grass-fed)
- 1 lb (450 g) ground pork (or use ground beef)
- 1 cup (250 mL) spinach, lightly packed
- ¼ cup (60 mL) fresh parsley, lightly packed
- ¼ cup (60 mL) non-dairy milk
- ¼ cup (60 mL) oat flour
- 1 small onion, roughly cut into chunks
- 2 garlic cloves
- 1 egg
- 2 to 3 heaping tbsp (40 to 60 mL) nutritional yeast (or Parmesan cheese)
- 1 tsp (5 mL) salt
- ½ tsp (2 mL) pepper

HOW TO MAKE IT:

1. Preheat the oven to 400°F (205°C), and line a 13 x 9-inch baking dish with parchment paper.
2. In a food processor, pulse together the veggies (spinach, parsley, onion, and garlic), until they are finely chopped. Or chop the veggies by hand.
3. In a large bowl, mix together all ingredients, using your hands until just combined. Gently portion into balls. (A soft pat to shape is enough; there's no need to pack or form perfect circles.)
4. As each meatball is finished, place it on the baking dish. Then transfer it to the oven and bake for about 30 minutes, or until cooked through.
5. If using sauce, add meatballs to the sauce and simmer until ready to eat.

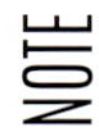

You can freeze these meatballs at any stage in the cooking process: raw, baked, or in sauce. With the cooked meatballs, first wait for them to cool before placing them on a parchment-lined baking sheet in the freezer. Once frozen, move them to a freezer-safe bag or container.

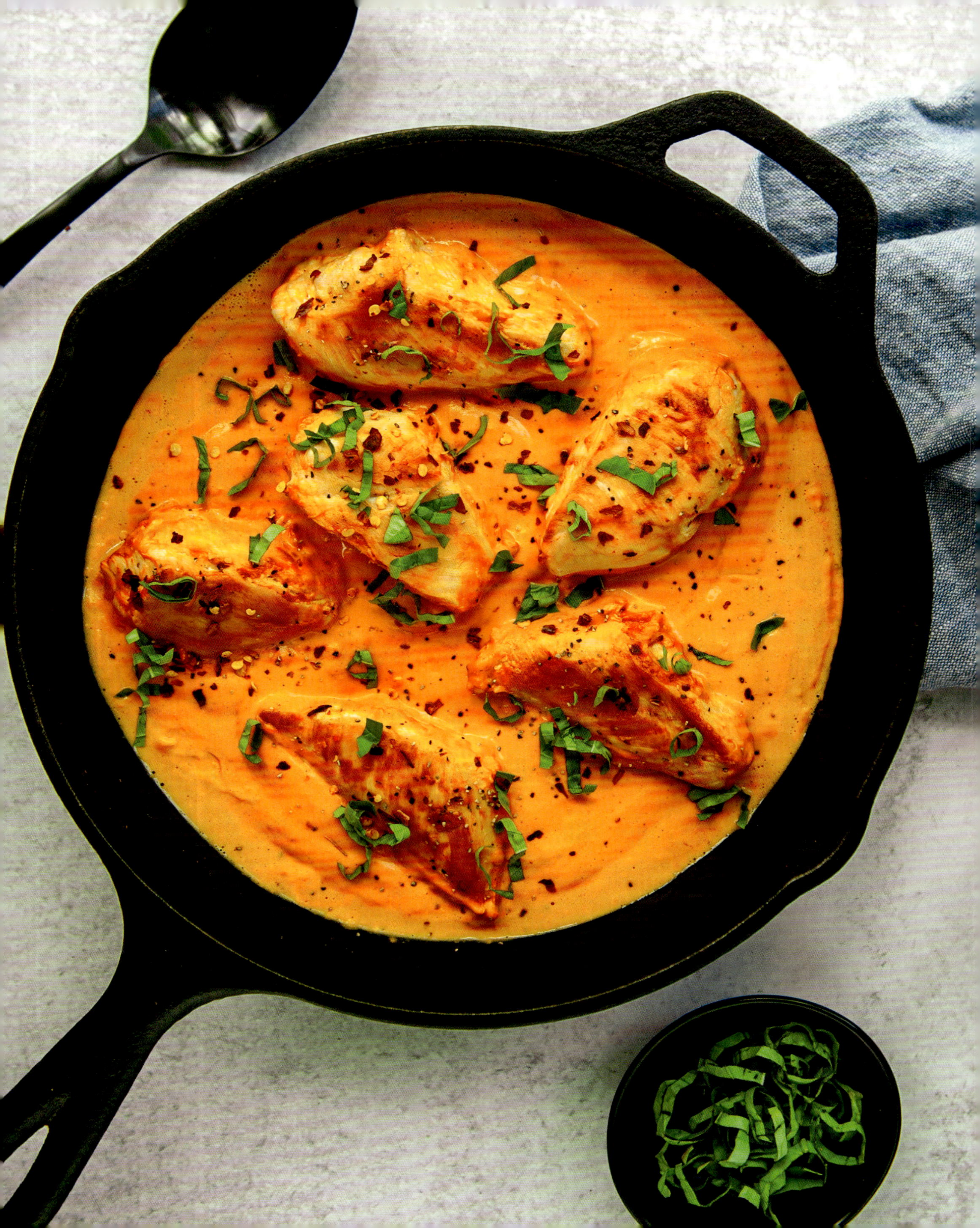

Dairy-Free • Gluten-Free • Grain-Free

One-Pan Chicken in Red Pepper Cashew Sauce

This one-pan chicken dish is super tasty and comes together in no time. You'll love the blended roasted red pepper cashew sauce — you can make it in advance or while you're cooking the chicken.

10 MINUTES PREPPING (PLUS 2 HOURS SOAKING) • 20 MINUTES COOKING • MAKES 3 TO 4 SERVINGS

WHAT YOU NEED:

For the sauce

1 cup (250 mL) cashews, soaked overnight or in boiling water, 1 to 2 hours

¾ cup (175 mL) warm water

3 roasted red peppers

3 cloves garlic

3 tbsp (45 mL) olive oil

¾ tsp (4 mL) sea salt

½ tsp (2 mL) dried oregano

½ tsp (2 mL) dried thyme

¼ tsp (1 mL) crushed red pepper flakes

¼ tsp (1 mL) pepper

For the chicken

2 lbs (900 g) boneless chicken breasts, cut into equal-sized large pieces (3 pieces per breast)

2 tbsp (30 mL) olive oil

Salt and pepper

For serving (optional)

Handful of fresh basil, finely chopped

HOW TO MAKE IT:

1. Combine all sauce ingredients in a high-powered blender or food processor. Pulse the ingredients until smooth.
2. Heat the olive oil in a large pan over medium heat. While the oil is heating, season both sides of the chicken pieces with the salt and pepper. Then place the chicken in the pan and cook, about 4 to 6 minutes per side, or until golden brown and cooked through. Transfer the chicken to a plate.
3. Add the sauce to the pan and stir, about 2 minutes, or until it is warm. Bring the chicken pieces back to the pan, tossing them in the sauce to coat evenly. Turn off heat, garnish with basil (if using), and serve immediately.

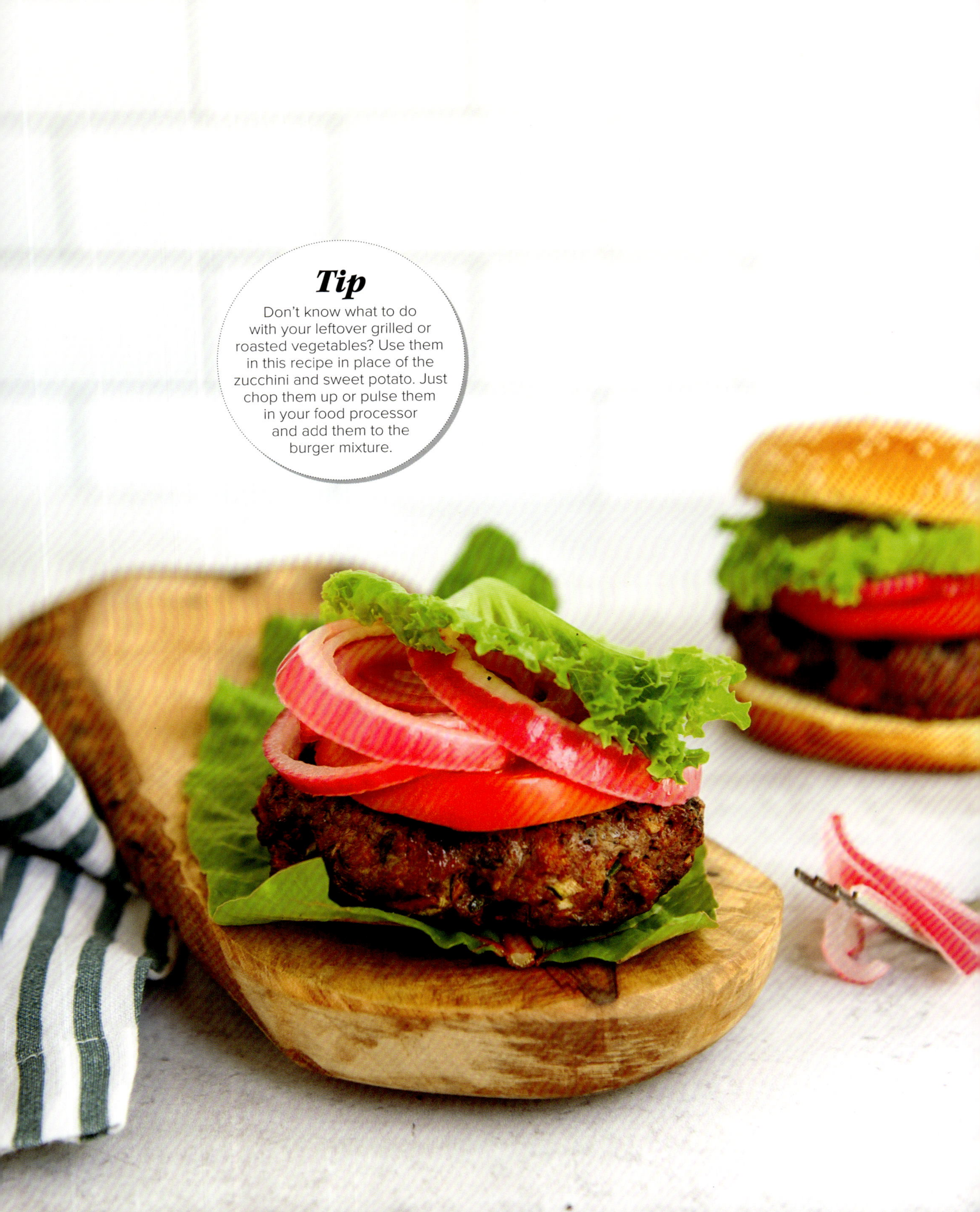
Tip
Don't know what to do with your leftover grilled or roasted vegetables? Use them in this recipe in place of the zucchini and sweet potato. Just chop them up or pulse them in your food processor and add them to the burger mixture.

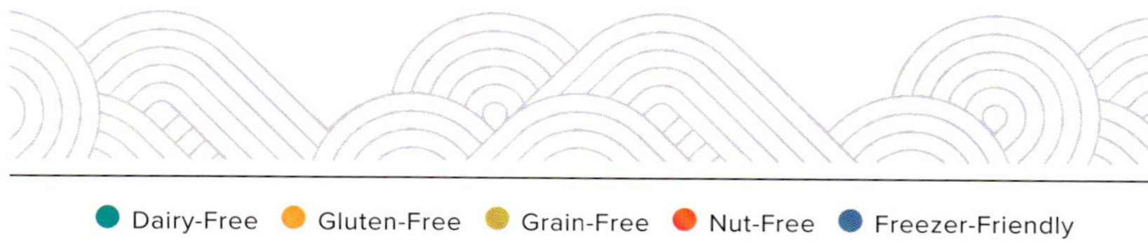

Dairy-Free · Gluten-Free · Grain-Free · Nut-Free · Freezer-Friendly

Veggie-Full Burgers

Have your burger, and lots of veggies too! If you have any reluctant veggie eaters in the family who may not like visible veggies in their burgers, here's a solution. Chop the veggies roughly, then pulse them in a food processor — they'll be virtually unrecognizable.

15 MINUTES PREPPING • 10 MINUTES COOKING • MAKES 8 BURGERS

WHAT YOU NEED:

- 2 lbs (900 g) ground beef (ideally grass-fed)
- 1 medium zucchini, grated and squeezed of excess moisture
- 1 small sweet potato, grated
- 1 small red onion, finely chopped
- 3 cloves garlic, minced
- 2 eggs
- 1 tbsp (15 mL) balsamic vinegar
- 1 tsp (5 mL) salt
- ½ tsp (2 mL) pepper

HOW TO MAKE IT:

1. Preheat the grill to high heat.
2. Add the ground beef, veggies, eggs, balsamic vinegar, salt, and pepper to a large bowl. Use your hands to gently combine the ingredients. Divide into patties about 1-inch (2.5-cm) thick and 4-inches (10-cm) across. Transfer the patties to the refrigerator until they're ready to cook.
3. When the grill is heated, transfer the patties to cook, about 10 minutes, or until cooked through, flipping as needed for even cooking.
4. Enjoy the burgers with your favourite toppings!

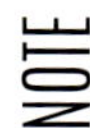

To freeze these burgers, line a baking tray with parchment paper and fill it with uncooked patties. Transfer the tray to the freezer until the patties are frozen, then store them in a freezer-safe container or bag.

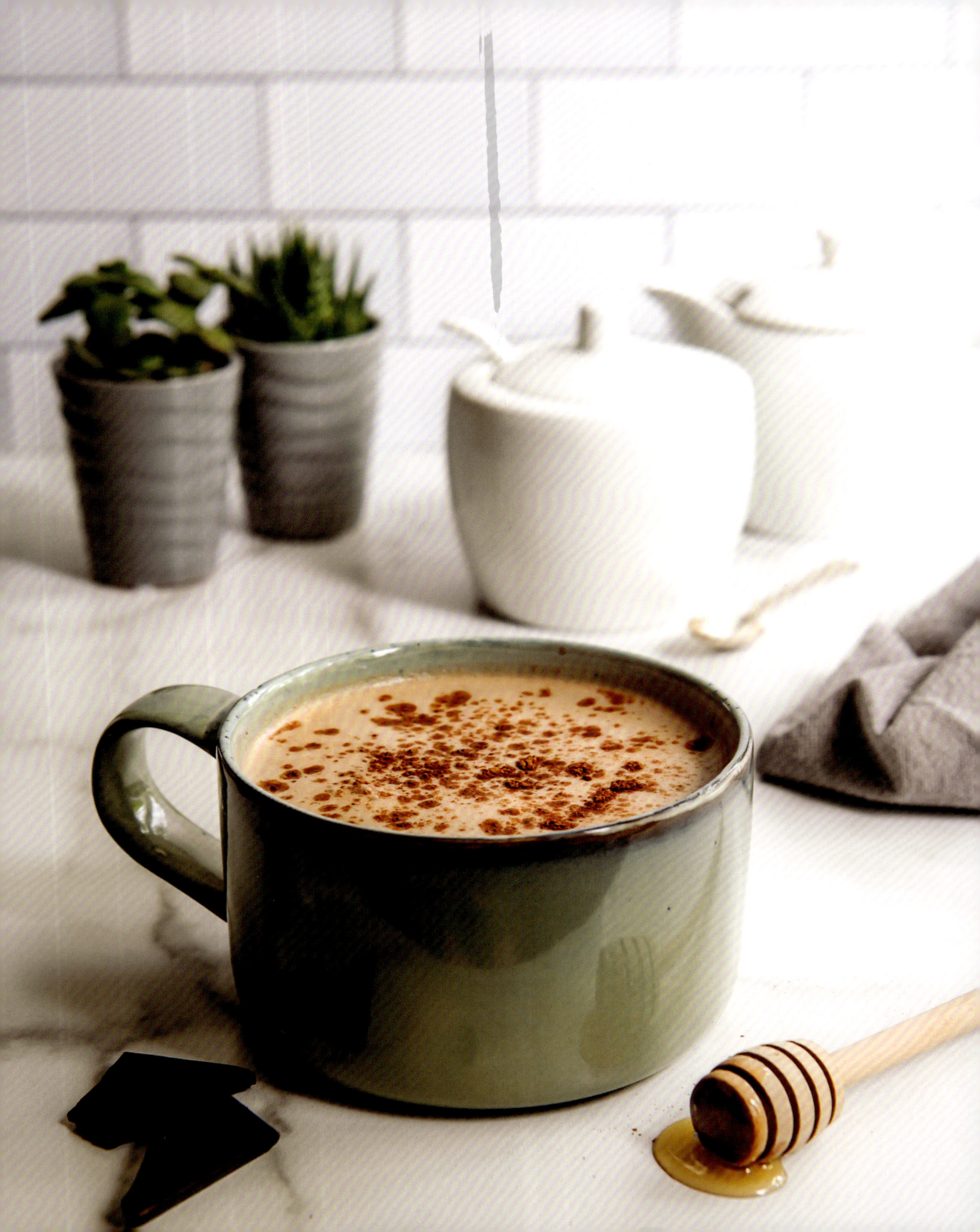

Dairy-Free Option · Gluten-Free · Grain-Free · Nut-Free

Heavenly Hot Chocolate

Rich and frothy, this is perfect on a cold day or when you're in need of a soothing hot drink in the evening. Who can resist hot chocolate?

5 MINUTES PREPPING • 5 MINUTES COOKING • MAKES 1 SERVING

WHAT YOU NEED:

½ to 1 tbsp (7 to 15 mL) cacao butter (or use coconut butter/oil or ghee)

2 cups (500 mL) milk of choice

1 ½ tbsp (22 mL) cacao powder

1 tbsp (15 mL) honey

HOW TO MAKE IT:

1. In a small pot, heat the cacao butter over medium heat. Meanwhile, combine the milk, cacao powder, and honey in a blender. Blend on low speed, about 30 seconds.
2. Once the cacao butter has melted, pour the mixture from the blender into the pot, and heat until hot and steaming but not boiling, about 3 minutes.

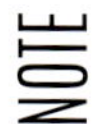

The cacao butter is optional, but it's highly recommended for its flavour and aroma.

TRIMESTER 3

(WEEKS 29–40)

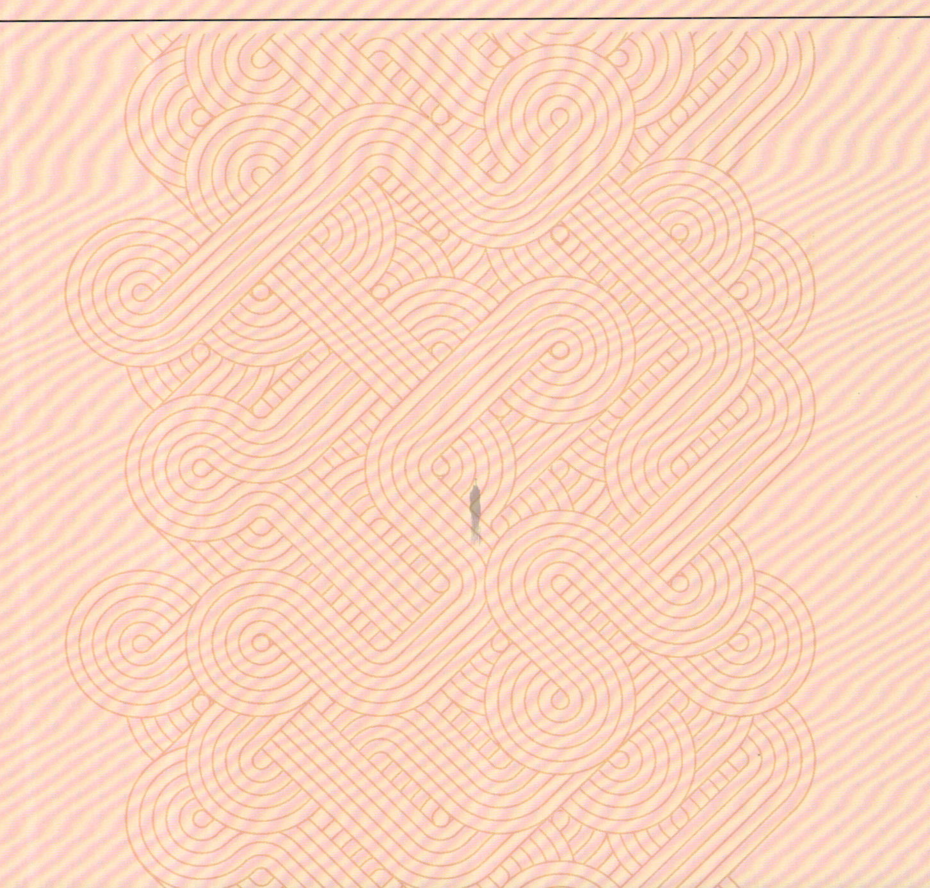

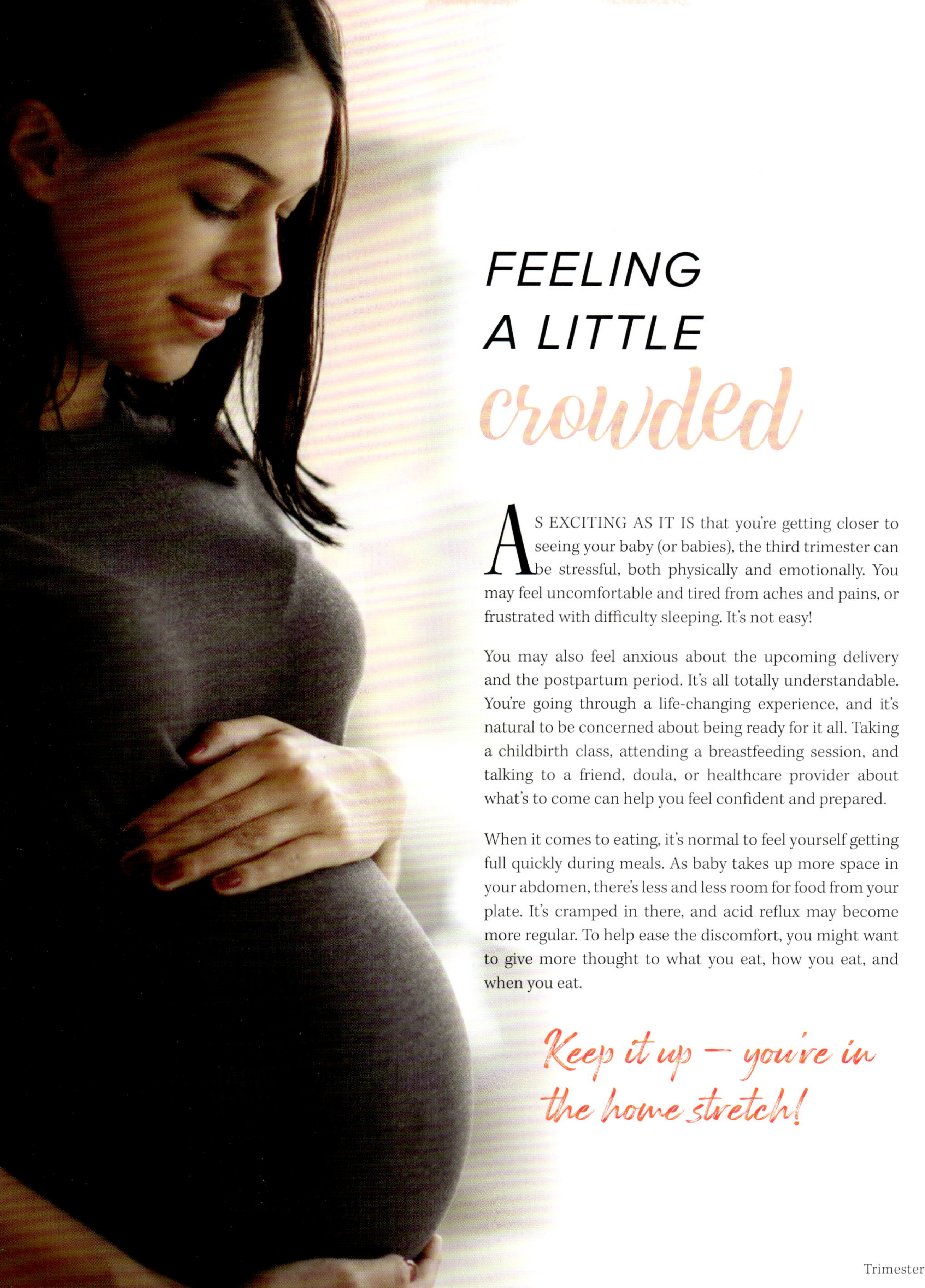

FEELING A LITTLE crowded

AS EXCITING AS IT IS that you're getting closer to seeing your baby (or babies), the third trimester can be stressful, both physically and emotionally. You may feel uncomfortable and tired from aches and pains, or frustrated with difficulty sleeping. It's not easy!

You may also feel anxious about the upcoming delivery and the postpartum period. It's all totally understandable. You're going through a life-changing experience, and it's natural to be concerned about being ready for it all. Taking a childbirth class, attending a breastfeeding session, and talking to a friend, doula, or healthcare provider about what's to come can help you feel confident and prepared.

When it comes to eating, it's normal to feel yourself getting full quickly during meals. As baby takes up more space in your abdomen, there's less and less room for food from your plate. It's cramped in there, and acid reflux may become more regular. To help ease the discomfort, you might want to give more thought to what you eat, how you eat, and when you eat.

Keep it up — you're in the home stretch!

Eating for the Third Trimester

WHAT TO EAT

Consider fuelling up on less filling, but still nutrient-rich meals and snacks. This might mean eating fewer grains — switch to a burger on a lettuce bun, a stir-fry with a side of cauliflower rice, and everything fresh such as big green salads, fruit salads, and smoothies. Not getting too full on grains means you'll have room for the good fats and proteins that your body needs right now.

For a grain-free meal plan, try out these recipes: Overnight Flax + Chia Pudding (page 135) for breakfast; Romaine Calm Lettuce Wraps (page 163) for lunch; and Greek Chicken Skewers (page 150) and Greek Garlic Kale Salad (page 151) for dinner. If you feel like having a refreshing snack, reach out for a fruit salad. The Pineapple + Lime Fruit Salad (page 144) or Mango Mint Salad (page 145) are delicious choices.

If reflux is becoming more constant, try eating less spicy, greasy, and acidic food. And go one step further by thinking about not just what you eat, but *how* and *when*.

HOW TO EAT

When you chew your food slowly and thoroughly, you make it easier for your body to digest the food and absorb its nutrients. It's the reason that well-cooked, soft food is recommended in the early weeks postpartum. Food that is already broken down is easier on your gut and less likely to give you digestive problems.

WHEN TO EAT

Smaller, more frequent meals might work best if you're getting full too quickly and dealing with acid reflux. You might consider going back to the No-More Nausea Meal Schedule on page 26 to break each of the three main meals for the day into two parts.

Eating smaller, more frequent meals also supports your digestive system, which tends to slow down in the third trimester because of the added pressure of your uterus taking up more space. You may experience constipation as a result. Here are some tips to help you feel better:

- Make up a batch of Overnight Flax + Chia Pudding (page 135) and enjoy this on its own, or heap a tablespoon or two of the pudding on a smoothie, fruit salad, or oatmeal.
- Add an extra serving of fresh fruit and vegetables to your usual intake each day.
- Add 1 tbsp of fermented food to your meals each day. Try kefir, sauerkraut, kimchee, yogurt, miso, or kombucha.
- Have a slow, short walk every hour or two. It keeps your system moving and helps to relieve aches, pains, and swelling.

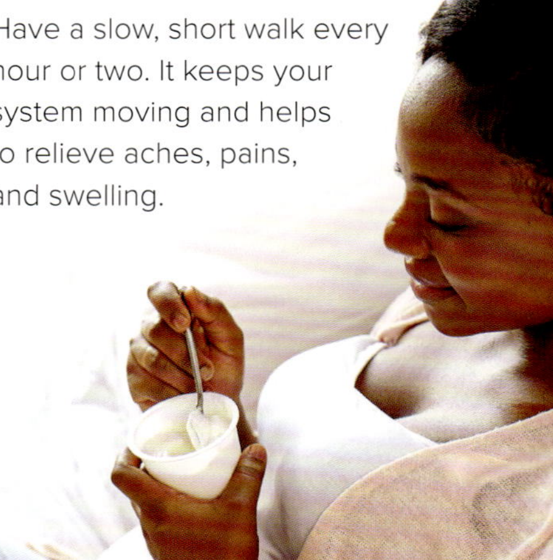

WATER WORKS

Water is essential right now. It helps your digestive system to function well; it enables your uterus to maintain proper blood flow and fluid levels; it is crucial for keeping amniotic fluid levels stable; and it's important to help you stay hydrated. Dehydration can cause cramping and contractions that feel like preterm labour, causing undue stress or even a visit to the hospital.

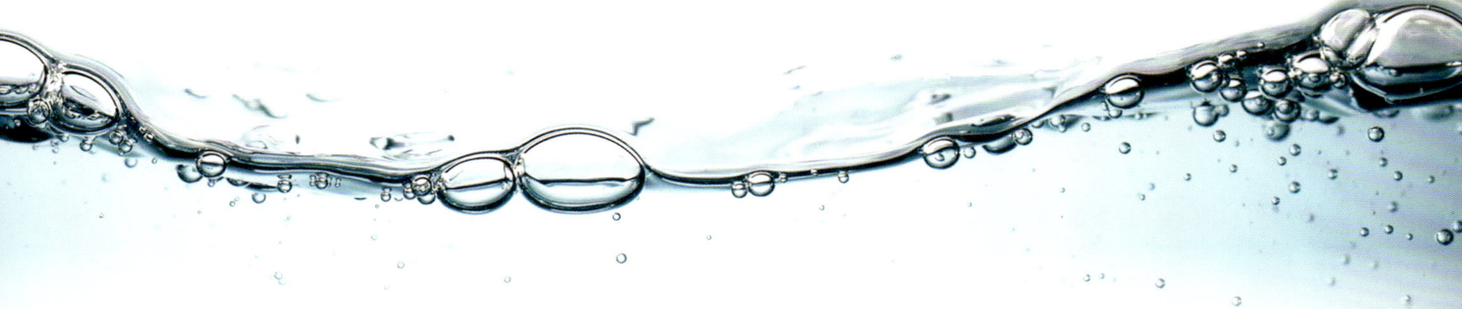

If you find it difficult to drink enough water (2.5–3 L daily), try these strategies:

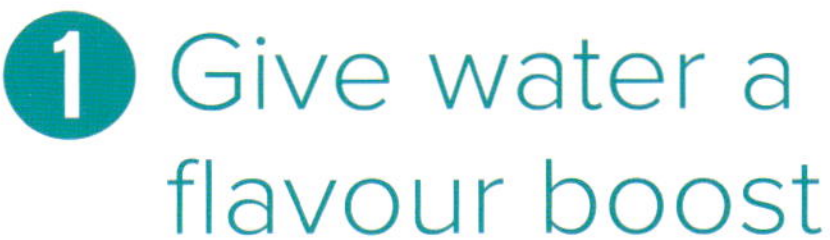

1 Give water a flavour boost

- Drink **flavour-infused water**. Add citrus, frozen berries, or slices of cucumber to water for taste and flavour.
- Enjoy fruity **ice cubes**. Mash into ice-cube trays pieces of cut-up watermelon, berries, or mangoes, add water, and freeze.

2 Consider a variety of sources

Water is also in broths, tea, and **smoothies**. It adds up. Here's what 3 L of water a day could look like:

6 cups water + 3 cups broth + 1 cup smoothie + 2 cups tea

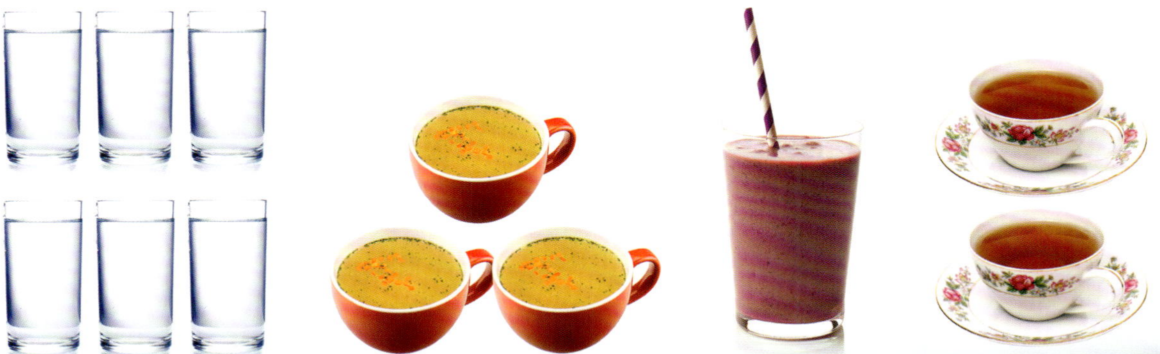

Baby's Growth Spurt

The third trimester is your baby's major growth spurt — this is the time baby puts on weight to prepare for birth. Many nutrients, vitamins, and minerals are important right now, including fat, iron, calcium, and protein. Don't worry too much about specific nutrients, however. Eating a variety of real food and selecting nourishing meals most of the time will ensure you're getting in what you need.

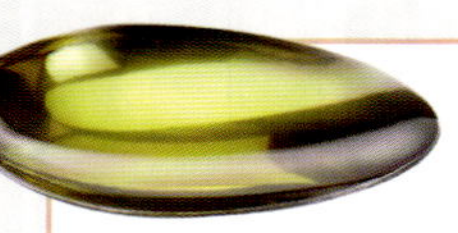

Fat

It helps baby with brain development and weight gain (that's baby's job right now!) and it's the most important component of healthy breast milk. So load up on healthy fats such as **olive oil**, **avocado oil**, **coconut oil**, **grass-fed butter**, and **ghee**, and include **eggs**, **nuts** and **seeds**, **animal products**, **avocado**, and **fish** in your diet.

Omega-3 fatty acids, especially **DHA**, help with the healthy development of baby's central nervous system. Getting in lots of DHA may lower the risk of preterm birth and low birthweight as well as your risk of perinatal mood disorders. Cold-water fish such as **salmon**, **sardines**, **mackerel**, and **herring** are the best choices.

Iron

It's common for women to become iron-deficient or anemic by the third trimester. This has been associated with higher risks of preterm birth, low birthweight, and babies born smaller than normal for their gestational age. Babies born to moms with higher iron levels have shown higher scores on alertness and social interaction as infants. To raise your iron level, consider **meat** and **fish**, or get iron from plant-based food such as **beans**, **lentils**, **seeds**, **greens**, and **dark chocolate**. Pair iron-rich food with colourful produce high in vitamin C for best absorption (see page 30).

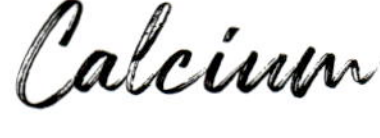

Calcium

Your calcium needs and the amount you absorb from food kick into high gear in this trimester as your body fuels the development of baby's bones and teeth. A diet full of **fruit** and **vegetables** and a steady dose of calcium may also help protect you against pre-eclampsia and other hypertensive disorders of pregnancy. Include **kefir**, **bone broth**, and **dark leafy greens** in your meals.

Protein

Your protein needs are at their highest level now to support baby's growth spurt. The protein sources you choose should be what you feel like eating. The following recipes feature a variety of protein choices that cater to different dietary requirements:

Eggs: Breakfast Bowlritto (page 133)
Meat: Arugula + Quinoa Steak Salad (page 149)
Poultry: One-Pan Chicken + Golden Rice (page 161)
Peas and Beans: Everyday Hummus (page 139)
Lentils: Sheet Pan Roasted Lentil Bowl (page 147)
Nuts and Seeds: Overnight Flax + Chia Pudding (page 135)

Planning for Postpartum

Some women experience "the nesting instinct" toward the end of pregnancy. You may get the urge to prepare the nest for baby's arrival, to make sure everything is in order, and to be ready to welcome baby. One of the best ways to plan for nesting postpartum is to have a freezer full of nutritious pre-made meals, so that you can focus on recovering, resting, and bonding with baby.

Toward the end of the third trimester, prepping for postpartum meals can be a big stress reliever, particularly for new parents who don't have family or friends around to help out after baby is born. Pick a weekend to focus on postpartum meal prep — enlist a helper if you can. If you happen to have friends at the same stage of pregnancy as you, do it together! Make more and share, split up the work, and save time.

TIPS FOR POSTPARTUM MEAL PREP

- Decide on a weekend when you don't have lots going on so you can focus and do all the cooking in the morning, leaving time to rest later. Select a date not too close to your due date just in case baby comes early, and not too far away either (so that food stays fresh and delicious when enjoyed postpartum). Sometime in the seventh month of pregnancy is ideal.
- Set aside time to make your grocery list and to prep in advance for your weekend cooking. Chop up vegetables for the meals and store them in separate containers, whip up spice mixes, and so on.
- Have food containers ready: stock up on various sizes of freezer-safe glass containers suitable for individual servings and full entrees. Prepare a label for each meal you prep with its recipe name, date of cooking, as well as defrosting and reheating instructions.
- Make sure everything is clean and ready: counter tops, stove, cookware, and cooking/baking essentials.
- Write down a list of all meals and snacks you have in the freezer (stick the list on the fridge door or somewhere visible so that a postpartum helper can easily see it).

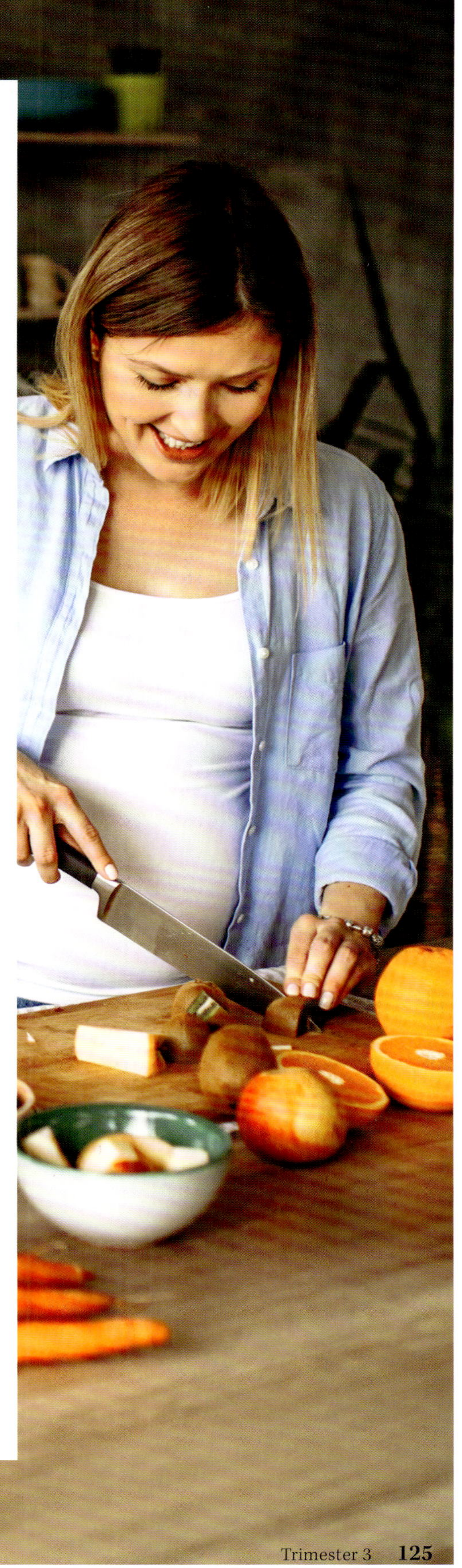

POSTPARTUM Meal Prep GUIDE

ALL MEALS IN THIS MEAL PREP GUIDE are dairy-free, gluten-free, and of course, freezer-friendly. This guide provides steps for two days of meal prep during a weekend. If it works better for you to do two days of prep further apart, look out for the notes below about additional freezing.

DAY ONE (4 HOURS)

Meals and Snacks to Make: Paprika + Cinnamon Pulled Pork, Simplest Roast Chicken, Everyday Bone Broth, Hidden Greens Meatballs (×2), Mama's Freezer Fudge (×2), and Apple Pie Oat Bars or Almond Chocolate Oat Bars (×2).

Step 1: Make the Paprika + Cinnamon Pulled Pork (page 217) in a slow cooker and set the timer for eight hours.

Step 2: Follow the Simplest Roast Chicken recipe (page 210) and get the chicken in the oven.

Step 3: While chicken bakes, make Mama's Freezer Fudge (page 197), then prepare your two trays of meatballs. When chicken is done, let it sit until cool to the touch, and transfer meatballs to the oven.

Step 4: Move on to the double batch of either the Apple Pie Oat Bars (page 196) or Almond Chocolate Oat Bars (page 49). By the time your batter is ready, your meatballs should be done, and can be left to cool.

Step 5: Shred your chicken, transferring the bones to a large pot. *Move shredded chicken to the fridge for use on Day 2 or freezer if you will not be doing Day 2 for more than three days.*

Step 6: Transfer meatballs to two freezer-safe containers or bags and move to the fridge. Then, score the bars and transfer them to freezer-safe containers, separating each layer with parchment paper to prevent sticking.

Step 7: Following the recipe for Everyday Bone Broth (page 181), get the broth going on the stove (letting it simmer until the end of the day or overnight in a slow cooker for use on Day 2). *If you are not doing Day 2 for more than three days, transfer lukewarm broth to the fridge, and freeze when it's cold. Defrost in the fridge two days before you need it.*

Step 8: Transfer the cooled oat bars to the freezer. Well done! The fudge is freezing, the meatballs are cooling, the shredded chicken is in the fridge, and the broth and pulled pork are softly simmering away.

Step 9: When the 8-hour timer for the pulled pork rings, remove the pork and let it sit on the cutting board for 10 minutes. Move on to do something else: Move your cooled meatballs to the freezer, then remove the fudge from the freezer (if frozen!), slice it into small squares with a serrated knife, and transfer them to a freezer-safe container and back to the freezer. Then shred the pork, transferring meat and juice to one or two large freezer-safe containers. Cool in the fridge overnight before freezing.

DEFROSTING INSTRUCTIONS ON LABELS

Pulled Pork: Defrost in the fridge overnight; transfer to a parchment-lined baking sheet, and broil for 10 minutes (flip with tongs after 5 minutes).

Bone Broth: Defrost individual containers in the fridge overnight.

Meatballs: Defrost in the fridge overnight. Then reheat in sauce or use in another dish.

Freezer Fudge: Grab a square, and let it sit for about 5 minutes before you have your sweet pick-me-up.

Apple Pie or Almond Chocolate Oat Bars: Remove squares from the freezer, individually or by batch. Keep them on counter (in sealed container) for a couple of days or in the fridge for a week.

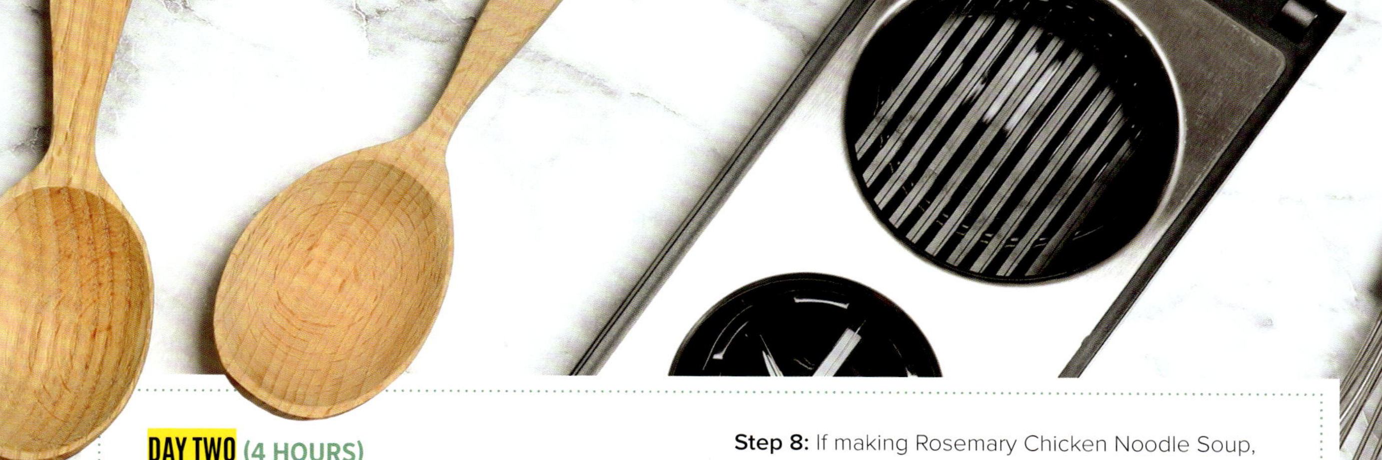

DAY TWO (4 HOURS)

Meals and Snacks to Make: Golden Mama Healing Stew, Slow Cooker Chicken Fajitas (×2), Sheet Pan Pumpkin Pancakes (×2), Rosemary Chicken Noodle Soup or Chicken + Spinach Enchiladas, and Little Lactation Cookies (×2).

Step 1: Finish up Day One's meals. Transfer shredded pulled pork to the freezer and finish up the bone broth, following recipe steps 3 and 4 (page 181). No need to wash the pot, as you'll be using it right away.

Step 2: Make the Golden Mama Healing Stew (page 203) in the soup pot.

Step 3: While the soup is simmering, prep everything you need to make two batches of the Slow Cooker Chicken Fajitas (page 71). Transfer all ingredients, raw, into two freezer bags or containers, and store in the freezer (optionally, keep bell peppers separate in a smaller bag).

Step 4: Transfer the stew to individual freezer-safe jars or large containers and let cool on the counter, then move to the fridge. If you're making the Rosemary Chicken Noodle Soup, just give the pot a rinse.

Step 5: Preheat oven and make a double batch of Sheet Pan Pumpkin Pancakes (page 187), letting them cool on the counter when done.

Step 6: When the pancakes are in the oven, use the shredded chicken you prepared on Day One to make either the Rosemary Chicken Noodle Soup (page 213, follow all steps) or Chicken + Spinach Enchiladas (page 218, follow steps 1 to 3).

Step 7: When pancakes are cooled, slice them into squares, and transfer them to a freezer-safe bag or container, separating each layer with a sheet of parchment paper. Then move to the freezer.

Step 8: If making Rosemary Chicken Noodle Soup, transfer soup to freezer-safe jars or containers and allow to cool on counter until lukewarm, then move to the fridge. If making Chicken + Spinach Enchiladas, transfer the chicken and veggie mixture and remaining Lazy Enchilada Sauce to separate freezer-safe containers, and keep them in the fridge when cool.

Step 9: While the meals are cooling, make a double batch of Little Lactation Cookies. Leave some cookies to celebrate a job well done, and move the rest to a freezer-safe jar or container. Finally, when the stew and soup and enchilada mix have cooled completely in the fridge, move them to the freezer, along with the cookies.

DEFROSTING INSTRUCTIONS ON LABELS

Golden Mama Healing Stew: Defrost in the fridge, then reheat it on the stove until hot.

Chicken Fajitas: Defrost in the fridge overnight, then cook in a slow cooker according to recipe directions (page 71).

Pumpkin Pancakes: Defrost a slice or a batch in the fridge or on the counter.

Rosemary Chicken Noodle Soup: Defrost overnight in the fridge, then heat it on the stove until hot.

Chicken + Spinach Enchiladas: Defrost the enchilada mix and sauce in the fridge overnight, then proceed with the recipe (follow steps 4 to 7).

Little Lactation Cookies: Defrost a single cookie or a batch on the counter.

Approaching Labour

If you're heading to the hospital for baby's birth, consider packing snacks in your hospital bag to support your energy needs. Choose snacks that will be okay out of the fridge for at least a few hours; are easy to eat with one hand; and provide long-lasting energy. For drinks, bring a large reusable water bottle or consider other options such as coconut water, cold-pressed juices, or cooled teas. If you are birthing at home, you may want to have a couple of the following snack and hydration choices in your fridge.

- **Apple Pie Oat Bars** (page 196)
- **Sunflower Flax Energy Balls** (page 199)
- **Raspberry Date Labour Prep Smoothie** (page 131)
- **Iced or Warm Raspberry Leaf Tea** (page 130)

You may have heard that eating and drinking during labour is prohibited due to concerns over complications if general anaesthetic becomes necessary. Recent research has shown, however, that this concern is unfounded, and that women should be free to decide if and when they want to eat or drink to support their energy needs during childbirth. In fact, having this choice has been shown to decrease stress and the length of labour!

The majority of hospitals in Canada no longer have policies preventing women from eating or drinking, so talk to your healthcare professional and follow what feels right for you. Maybe you will want to eat to keep up your energy, or maybe you just feel like taking sips of water or another drink. It is likely that your desire to eat will fade as labour progresses — let your body guide you.

Excitement awaits — *get ready to welcome your baby!*

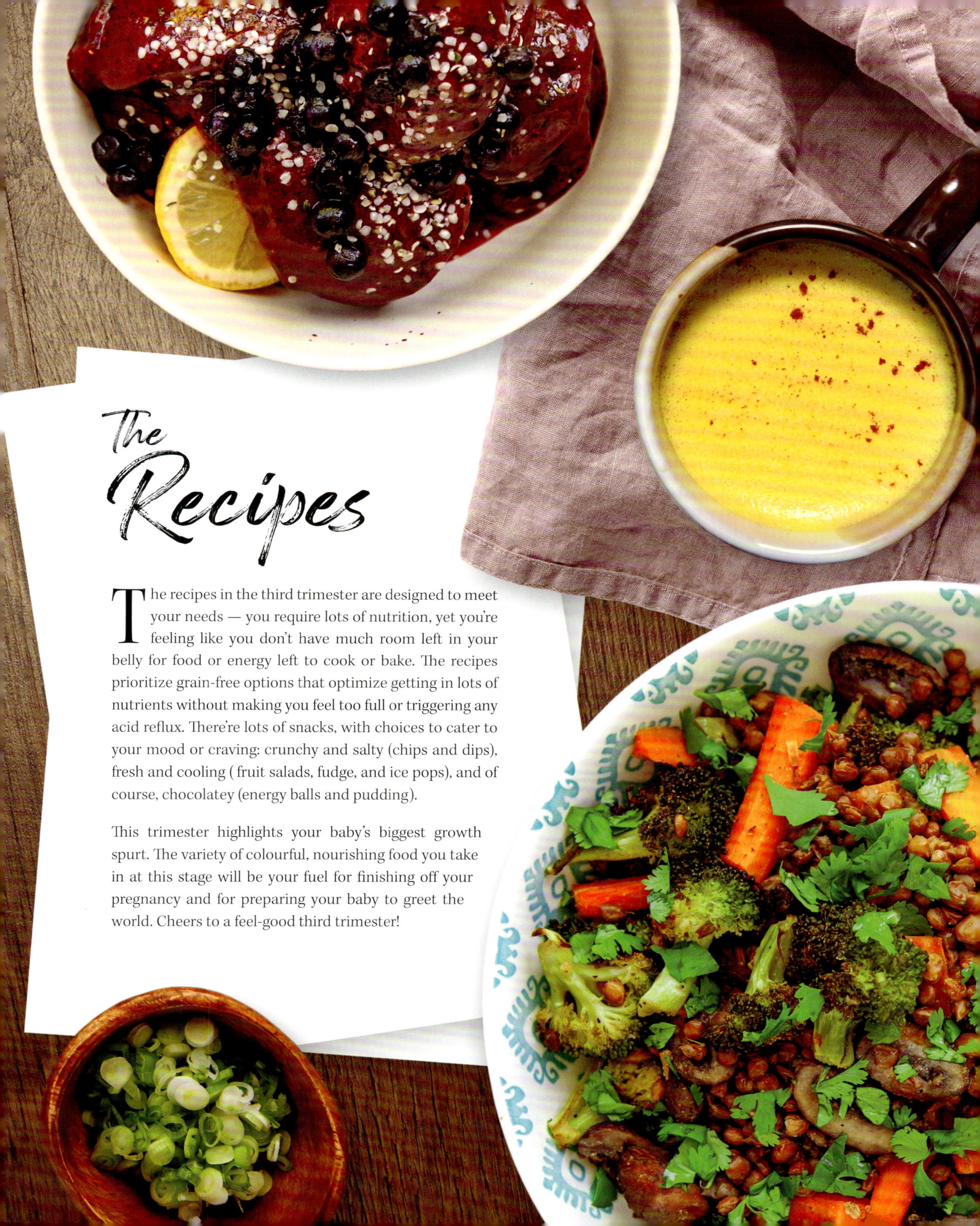

The Recipes

The recipes in the third trimester are designed to meet your needs — you require lots of nutrition, yet you're feeling like you don't have much room left in your belly for food or energy left to cook or bake. The recipes prioritize grain-free options that optimize getting in lots of nutrients without making you feel too full or triggering any acid reflux. There're lots of snacks, with choices to cater to your mood or craving: crunchy and salty (chips and dips), fresh and cooling (fruit salads, fudge, and ice pops), and of course, chocolatey (energy balls and pudding).

This trimester highlights your baby's biggest growth spurt. The variety of colourful, nourishing food you take in at this stage will be your fuel for finishing off your pregnancy and for preparing your baby to greet the world. Cheers to a feel-good third trimester!

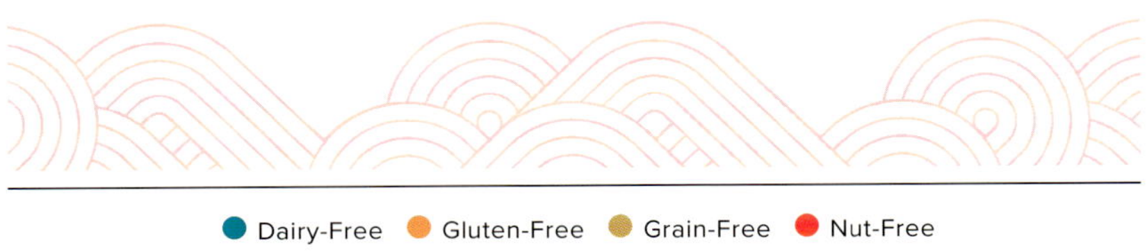

Dairy-Free • Gluten-Free • Grain-Free • Nut-Free

Iced Raspberry Leaf Tea

Red raspberry leaf has long been used as a medicinal herb, especially toward the end of pregnancy, thanks to its reputation as a labour support. We need more research to know if and how this herb can contribute to an easier or faster labour. Regardless, this herb is rich in vitamins and minerals, and it is delicious and refreshing as a homemade iced tea!

5 MINUTES PREPPING • 15 MINUTES COOKING • MAKES 4 CUPS (1 L)

WHAT YOU NEED:

4 red raspberry leaf tea bags

4 cups (1 L) water

Juice of 1 lemon

1 tbsp (15 mL) honey

Ice, as desired

HOW TO MAKE IT:

1. Bring the water to a boil and pour into a large glass jar along with the 4 tea bags. Let it steep about 15 minutes. Then remove tea bags.
2. Stir in the lemon juice and honey, and let it cool.
3. Serve over ice, keeping leftovers in the refrigerator for several days.

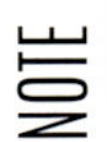

As with any herb, it's best to consult with a healthcare professional prior to incorporating red raspberry leaf into your third trimester diet.

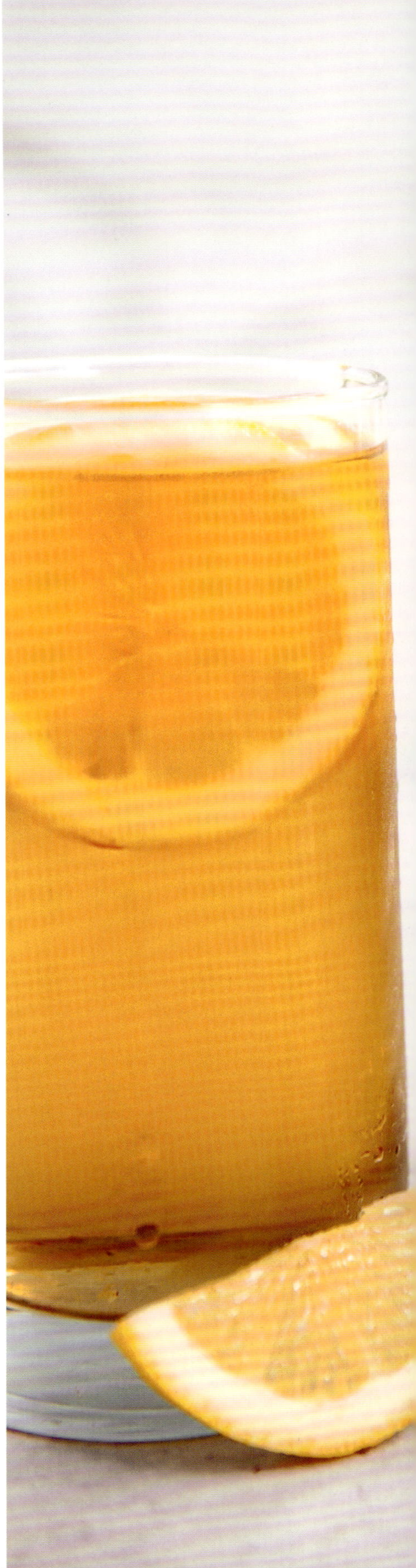

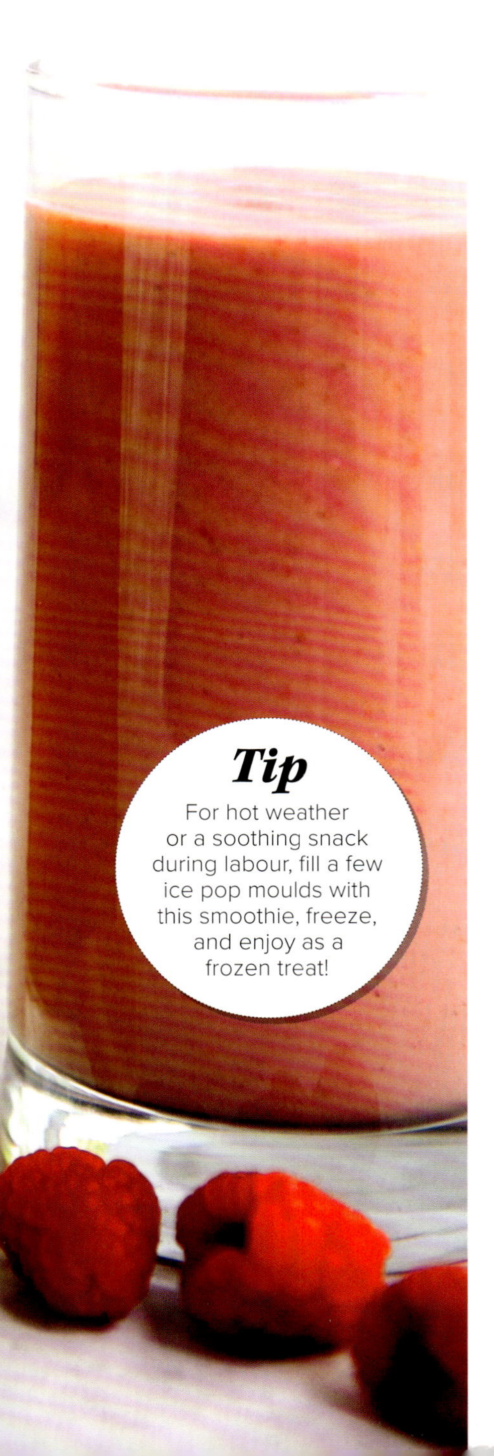

Tip

For hot weather or a soothing snack during labour, fill a few ice pop moulds with this smoothie, freeze, and enjoy as a frozen treat!

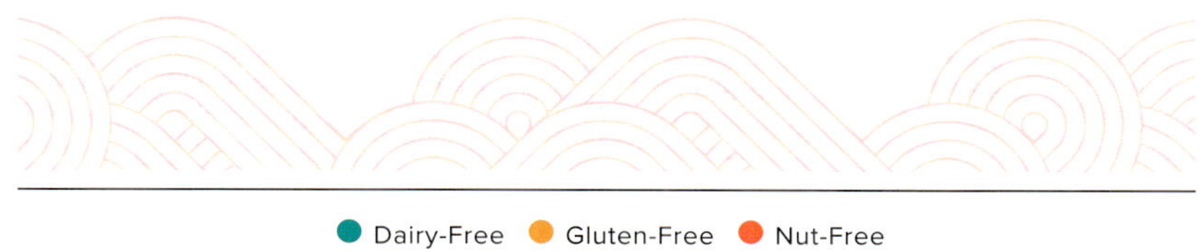

Dairy-Free • Gluten-Free • Nut-Free

Raspberry Date Labour Prep Smoothie

This pretty pink smoothie is perfect for the last stage of pregnancy since it's a combo of red raspberry leaf tea and dates, two foods thought to support labour when consumed regularly at the end of pregnancy. To balance the natural sweetness from the raspberries and dates, the oats, avocado, flax, and collagen add ample fat, protein, and fibre to fill you up and keep you feeling good!

5 MINUTES PREPPING • 1 MINUTE BLENDING • MAKES 1 LARGE SMOOTHIE

WHAT YOU NEED:

- 2 cups (500 mL) iced raspberry leaf tea (page 130)
- 1 cup (250 mL) frozen raspberries
- ¼ cup (60 mL) rolled oats
- ¼ cup (60 mL) frozen avocado chunks (or use 1 tbsp/15 mL coconut oil)
- 3 medjool dates
- 2 tbsp (30 mL) collagen powder (optional)
- 1 tbsp (15 mL) ground flaxseed
- 1 tbsp (15 mL) lemon juice

HOW TO MAKE IT:

1. Add all ingredients to your high-powered blender, and blend at high speed for 1 minute, or until smooth.

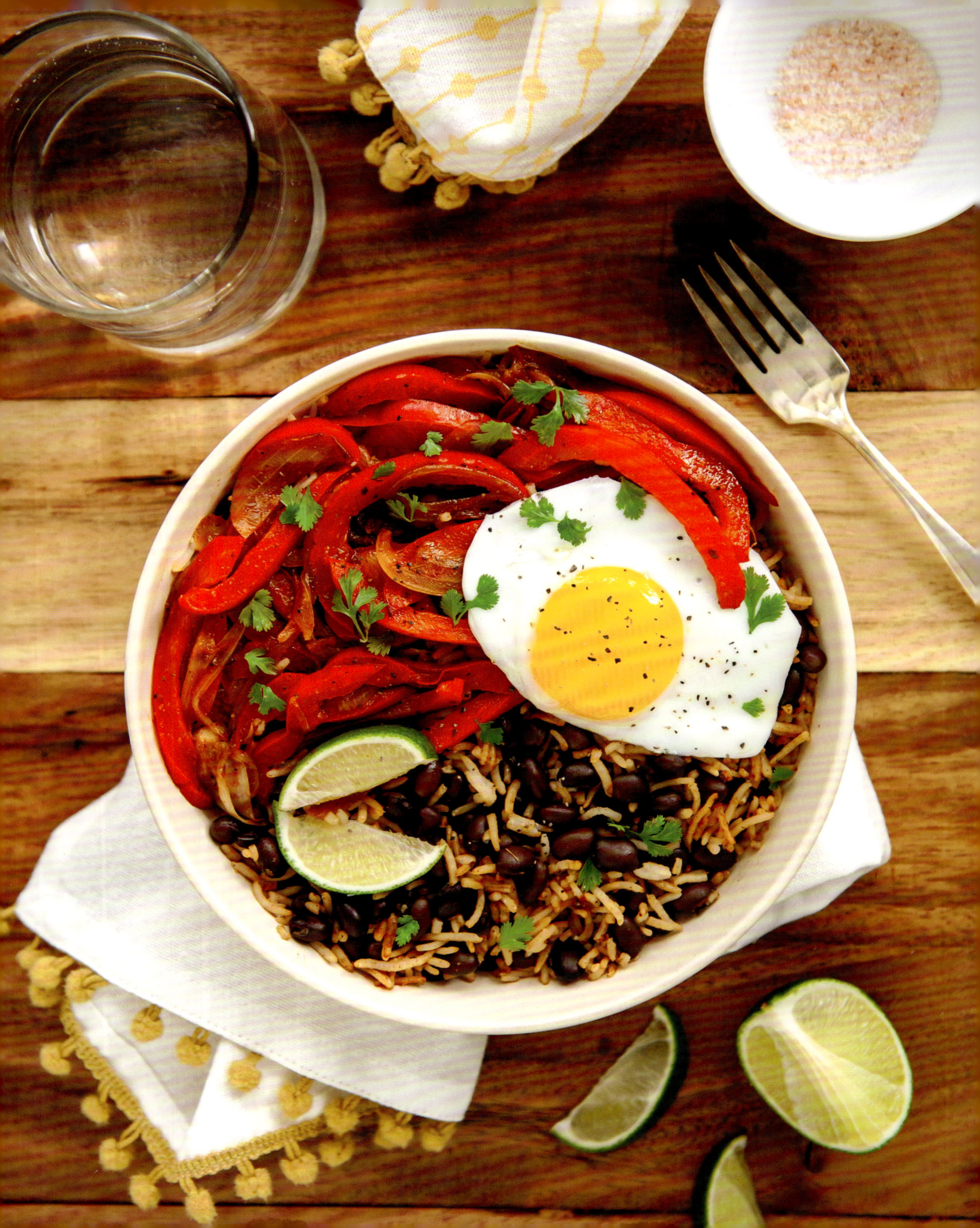

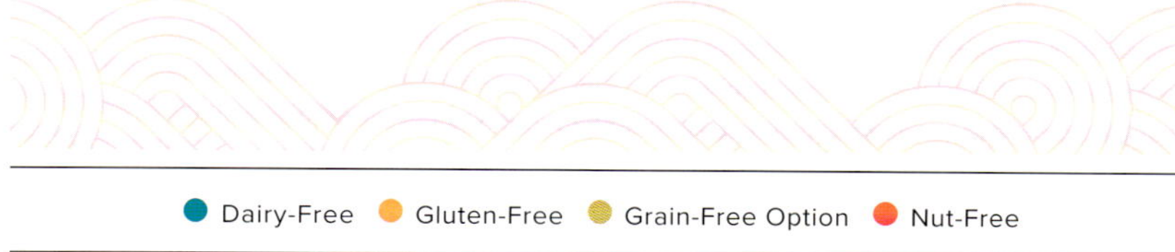

● Dairy-Free ● Gluten-Free ● Grain-Free Option ● Nut-Free

Breakfast Bowlritto

A big boost for all-morning energy has never tasted so good. This bowl is perfect for early morning or brunch. You can easily double or triple this recipe as long as you have a large pan. Don't have leftover quinoa or rice in the fridge? Simply omit it, and heap everything onto a piece of toast or enjoy it on a bed of greens.

5 MINUTES PREPPING • 10 MINUTES COOKING • MAKES 1 SERVING

WHAT YOU NEED:

2 tbsp (30 mL) olive oil, divided

⅔ cup (150 mL) red bell pepper, thinly sliced

⅓ cup (75 mL) onion, thinly sliced

1 tsp (5 mL) fajita spice mix (page 71)

½ cup (125 mL) cooked rice, quinoa, or cauliflower rice (optional)

½ cup (125 mL) black beans, rinsed

1 egg

Optional toppings

Chopped cherry tomatoes, cilantro, lime, hot sauce, or avocado

HOW TO MAKE IT:

1. In a pan set to medium-high heat, add 1 tbsp (15 mL) of the olive oil, and cook the pepper and onion with the fajita spice mix for 5 minutes, or until onion is translucent and starting to turn golden.
2. Take the pan off the heat for a moment, remove the pepper and onion mix, and transfer to a bowl.
3. Turn heat down to low, and add the remaining 1 tbsp (15 mL) olive oil. Stir in the rice/quinoa and black beans. Add the pepper and onion mix, and give it a quick stir to soak up the spices. Then move the mixture to one side of the pan. Crack the egg on the other side of the pan, cover for 3 to 5 minutes, or until the egg is done to your liking.
4. Transfer everything to a bowl, add optional toppings, and enjoy!

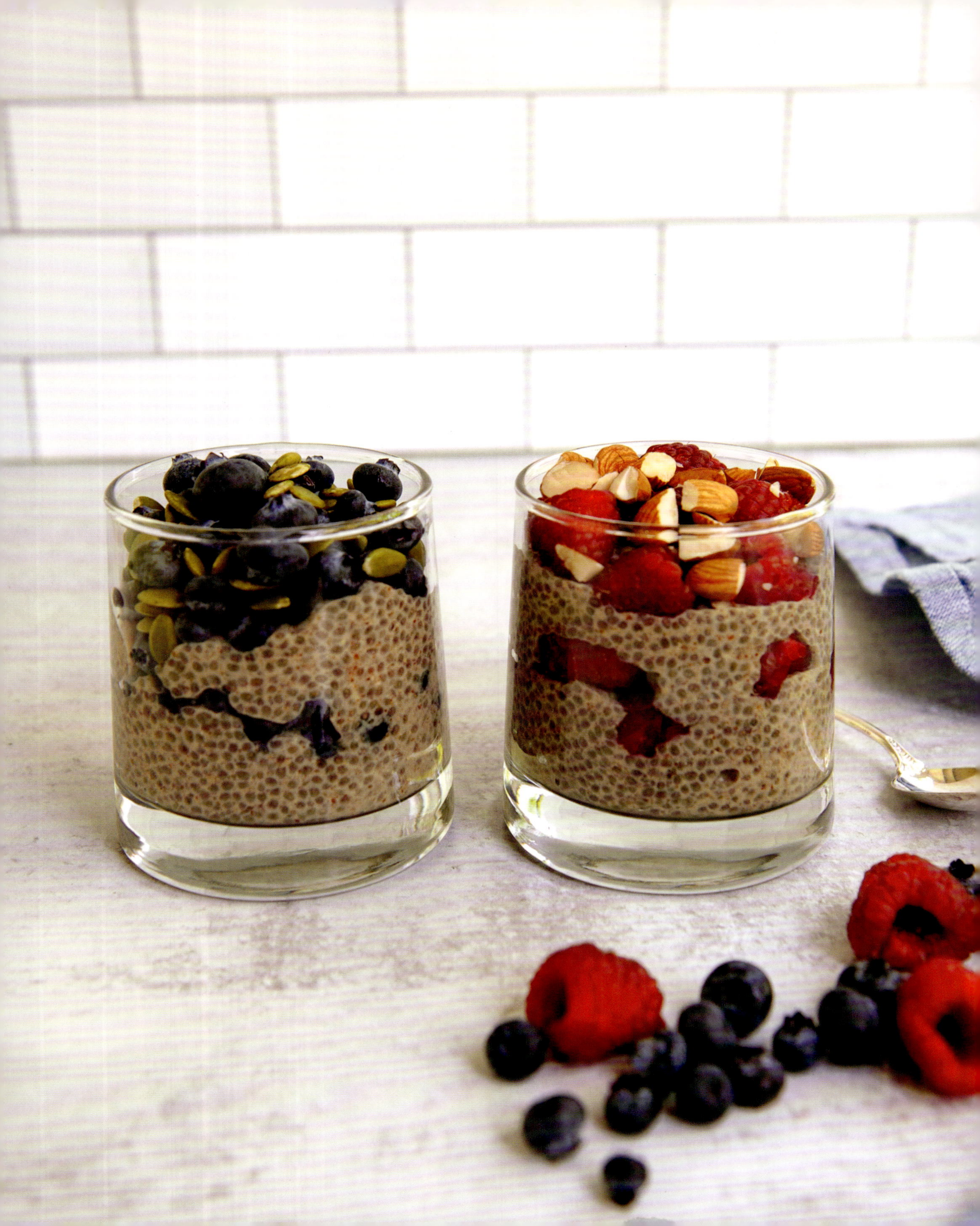

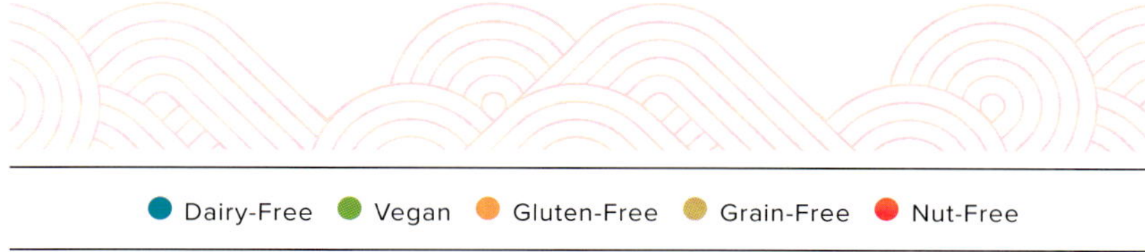

Dairy-Free · Vegan · Gluten-Free · Grain-Free · Nut-Free

Overnight Flax + Chia Pudding

Fuelling, filling, portable, and full of omega-3 fats and fibre, this grain-free pudding makes a perfect breakfast or morning snack. It can also double up as a digestion aid, thanks to the fibre content and gel-like texture of chia seeds. Have extra? Add a heaping scoop to your smoothies for a protein and fat boost!

5 MINUTES PREPPING • OVERNIGHT CHILLING • MAKES 2 TO 3 SERVINGS

WHAT YOU NEED:

1 ½ cups (375 mL) dairy-free milk of choice

¼ cup (60 mL) chia seeds

2 tbsp (30 mL) ground flaxseed

1 to 2 tsp (5 to 10 mL) maple syrup

1 tsp (5 mL) vanilla

Optional flavour

¼ tsp (1 mL) cinnamon, ½ tsp (2 mL) cacao powder, or a small handful of shredded coconut

Optional toppings

Berries, nuts, seeds, coconut flakes, cacao nibs, banana, mango, or pineapple

HOW TO MAKE IT:

1. In a small bowl, stir or whisk together all ingredients for a few minutes until pudding has slightly thickened in texture and chia seeds are dispersed throughout.
2. Transfer pudding to a storage container (one or several, split up by servings), and allow it to thicken overnight. Keeps in refrigerator for 3 days.

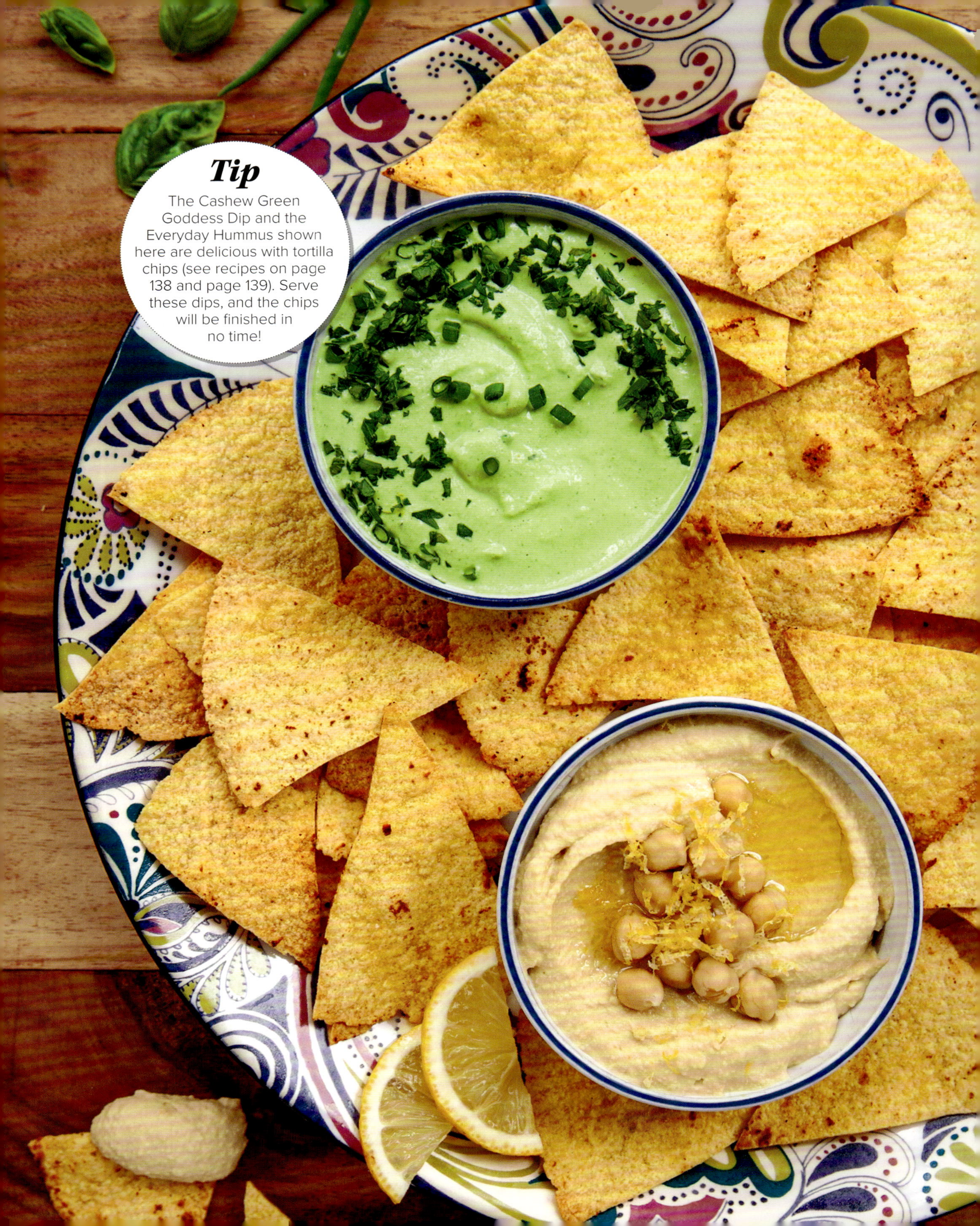

Tip
The Cashew Green Goddess Dip and the Everyday Hummus shown here are delicious with tortilla chips (see recipes on page 138 and page 139). Serve these dips, and the chips will be finished in no time!

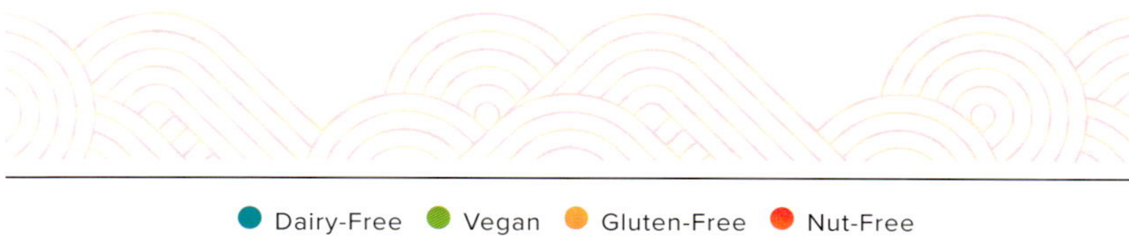

Dairy-Free • Vegan • Gluten-Free • Nut-Free

Homemade Tortilla Chips

It's so fast and easy to make your own tortilla chips, and you get to control the flavour and ingredient list! These tortilla chips have a Tex-Mex flavour — perfect for enjoying them with dips, salsa, or guacamole.

5 MINUTES PREPPING • 15 MINUTES COOKING • MAKES 4 TO 6 SERVINGS

WHAT YOU NEED:

- 10 (7-in) corn tortillas (or use wheat tortillas)
- 1 ½ tbsp (22 mL) olive oil
- 1 tbsp (15 mL) lime juice
- 1 tbsp (15 mL) lime zest
- 1 tsp (5 mL) garlic powder
- ½ tsp (2 mL) salt
- ½ tsp (2 mL) cumin

HOW TO MAKE IT:

1. Preheat oven to 350°F (180°C) and line 2 baking sheets with parchment paper.
2. Mix together oil, lime juice, lime zest, and spices in a bowl. Then brush the mixture on to both sides of each tortilla.
3. Arrange 5 of the tortillas on top of one another. Using kitchen shears, cut tortillas in half, then cut each half into 4 triangles. Repeat with remaining tortillas.
4. Scatter triangles in a single layer on the 2 prepared baking sheets and bake for 14 minutes. Rotate the baking sheets halfway, and watch closely for the final few minutes to prevent burning.

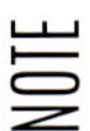

To keep chips crispy, store them in a container with the lid on top but not snapped closed.

Link-up

Use tortilla chips as a fun topping for the **Fajita Bump Bowl**, page 101.

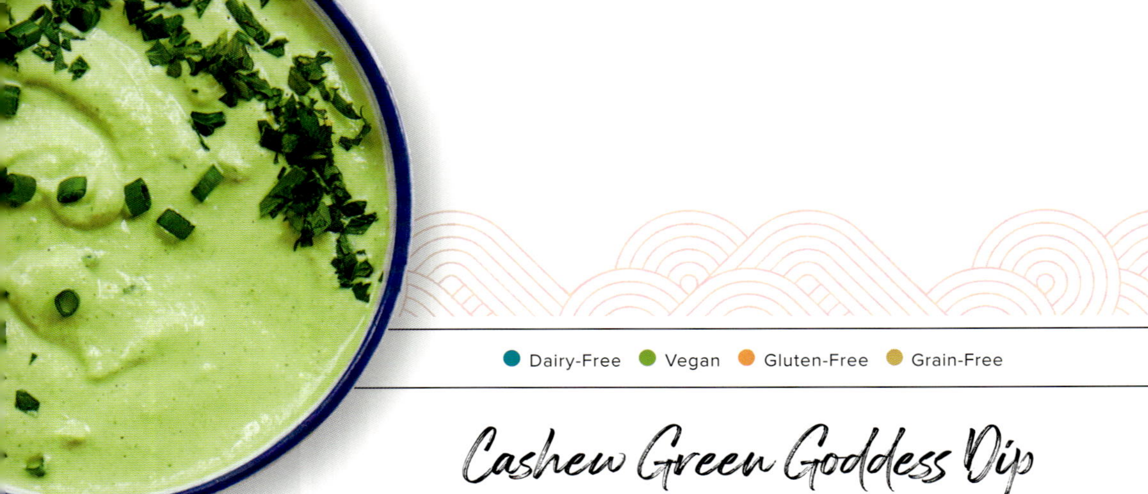

Dairy-Free · Vegan · Gluten-Free · Grain-Free

Cashew Green Goddess Dip

Fresh herbs take centre stage in this fresh, garlicky, and dairy-free dip. Herbs such as parsley, cilantro, and basil are much more than the occasional garnish. They are nutrient rich, with lots of vitamin K, folate, iron, vitamin C, and vitamin A. This is a delicious dip for tortilla chips, raw vegetables, and Grain-Free Chicken Fingers (page 106) — go ahead and try it!

10 MINUTES PREPPING (PLUS 1 TO 2 HOURS SOAKING) • 3 MINUTES BLENDING • MAKES 2 CUPS (500 ML)

WHAT YOU NEED:

- 1 ⅓ cups (325 mL) cashews, soaked in water overnight (or in boiling water for 1 to 2 hours) and rinsed
- 1 bunch (about 1 cup/250 mL, lightly packed) parsley (or use cilantro)
- 1 cup (250 mL) fresh basil, lightly packed
- 4 green onions
- 3 to 4 garlic cloves
- Juice of 2 lemons
- ¼ cup (60 mL) olive oil, plus another ¼ cup (60 mL) as needed
- ½ tsp (2 mL) sea salt

HOW TO MAKE IT:

1. Combine all ingredients in a high-powered blender or food processor, and blend until smooth. Transfer to a sealed storage container, and keep in the fridge for 3 to 4 days. Add extra olive oil as needed to thin the dip (it will thicken up as it sits in the refrigerator).

Link-up

This dip is a sure winner with the **Homemade Tortilla Chips** (page 137). It's also delicious with the **Grain-Free Chicken Fingers** (page 106).

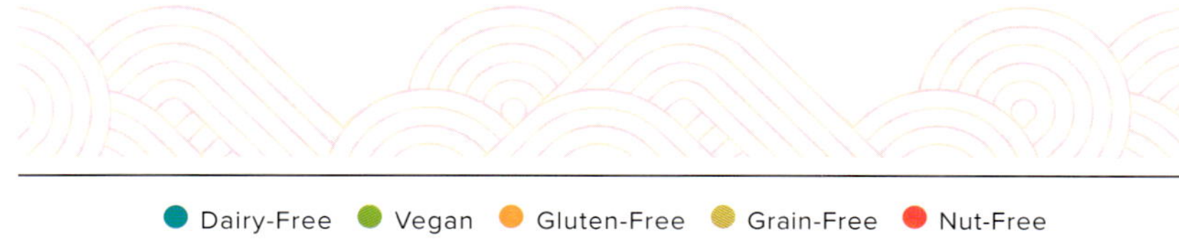

Dairy-Free • Vegan • Gluten-Free • Grain-Free • Nut-Free

Everyday Hummus

This recipe gives you a creamy, smooth, and mild hummus with a hint of lemon that can be customized to your taste! The optional nutritional yeast called for in this recipe lends a bit of a cheesy flavour, mellows the tahini, and provides a vegan dose of B vitamins, including folate, B6, and B12.

10 MINUTES PREPPING • 5 MINUTES BLENDING • MAKES 3 CUPS

WHAT YOU NEED:

- 2 (19 oz/540 mL) cans of chickpeas
- ¼ cup (60 mL) tahini
- ¼ cup (60 mL) olive oil, plus more for drizzling
- ¼ cup (60 mL) lemon juice
- 2 tsp (10 mL) lemon zest
- 2 garlic cloves
- 1 tsp (5 mL) sea salt
- 2 to 4 tbsp (30 to 60 mL) water to thin as necessary

Optional

- 1 to 2 heaping tbsp (15 to 30 mL) nutritional yeast

HOW TO MAKE IT:

1. Add all ingredients to a food processor or blender and purée until hummus is smooth, scraping the sides occasionally.
2. Customize it! Taste and adjust to your preference: you may want more salt, more tahini (for a nuttier flavour), more garlic (for zing), more lemon (for tartness), or more water (for a thinner consistency). Keep in the refrigerator in a sealed container for about a week.

Link-up

Enjoy your hummus with the **Sheet Pan Roasted Lentil Bowl**, page 147.

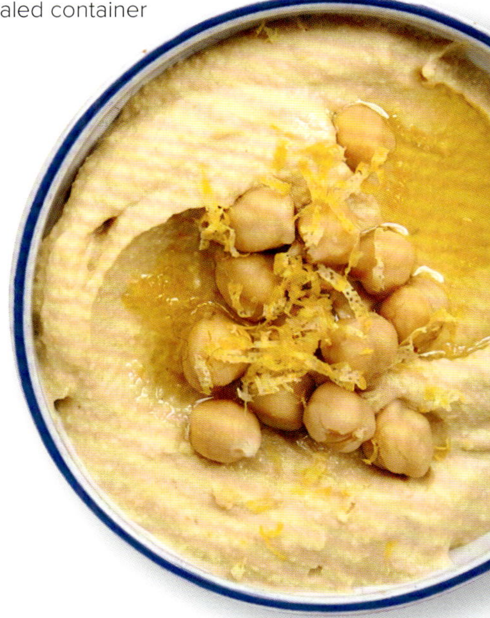

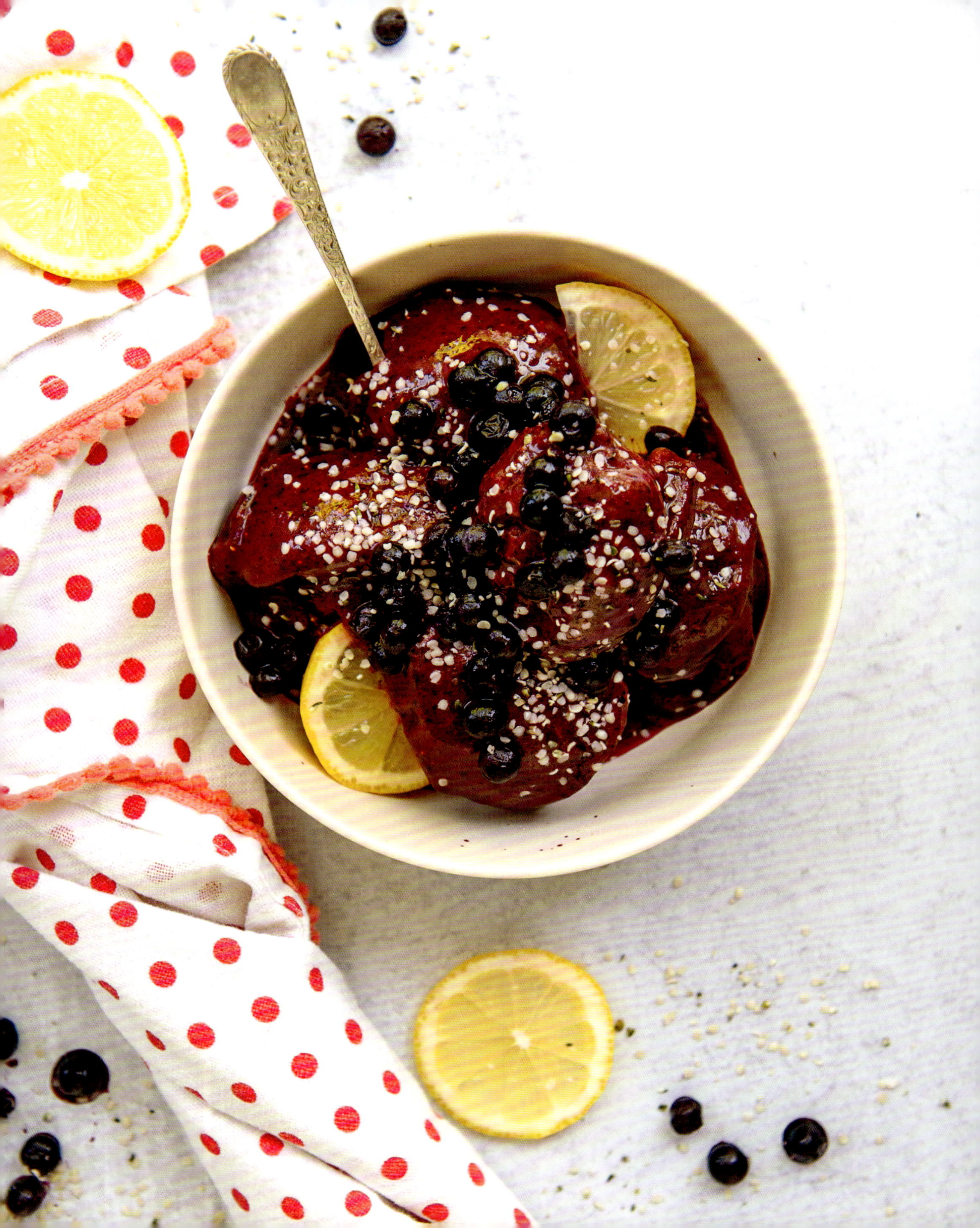

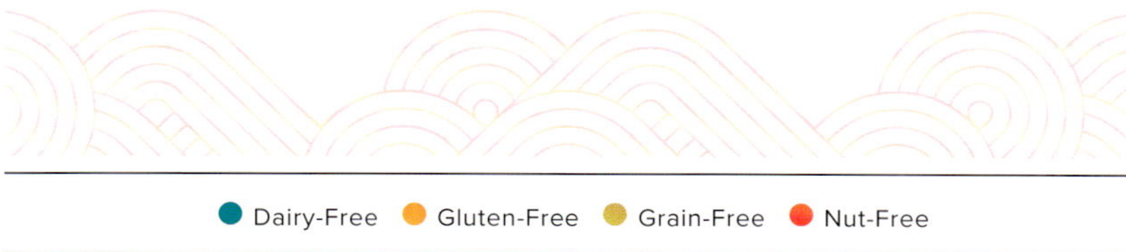

● Dairy-Free ● Gluten-Free ● Grain-Free ● Nut-Free

Berry Sorbet

Can you think of anything better to cool off with than a scoop of sorbet? Try out this recipe — you'll have a frozen treat free of refined sugars and artificial flavours, ready to enjoy in minutes! Use whatever combination of frozen fruit you have for a sweet surprise!

5 MINUTES PREPPING • 10 MINUTES BLENDING • MAKES 2 SERVINGS

WHAT YOU NEED:

¼ cup (60 mL) warm water, plus more if needed

Juice of 1 lemon

2 tbsp (30 mL) honey

1 ½ cups (375 mL) frozen strawberries

1 ½ cups (375 mL) frozen blueberries

1-inch (2.5-cm) piece of ginger, minced (about 1 tsp/5 mL)

For topping

Frozen blueberries, hemp hearts, or topping of choice

HOW TO MAKE IT:

1. Add all ingredients in the order listed to your high-powered blender.
2. Blend, starting slowly, then increasing speed as the consistency of your sorbet gets smoother. You may need to use a tamper or stir, in between pulses, a couple of times, adding more water (1 tbsp/15 mL at a time) as necessary.
3. Scoop mixture out of blender into bowl, add toppings as desired, and enjoy immediately.

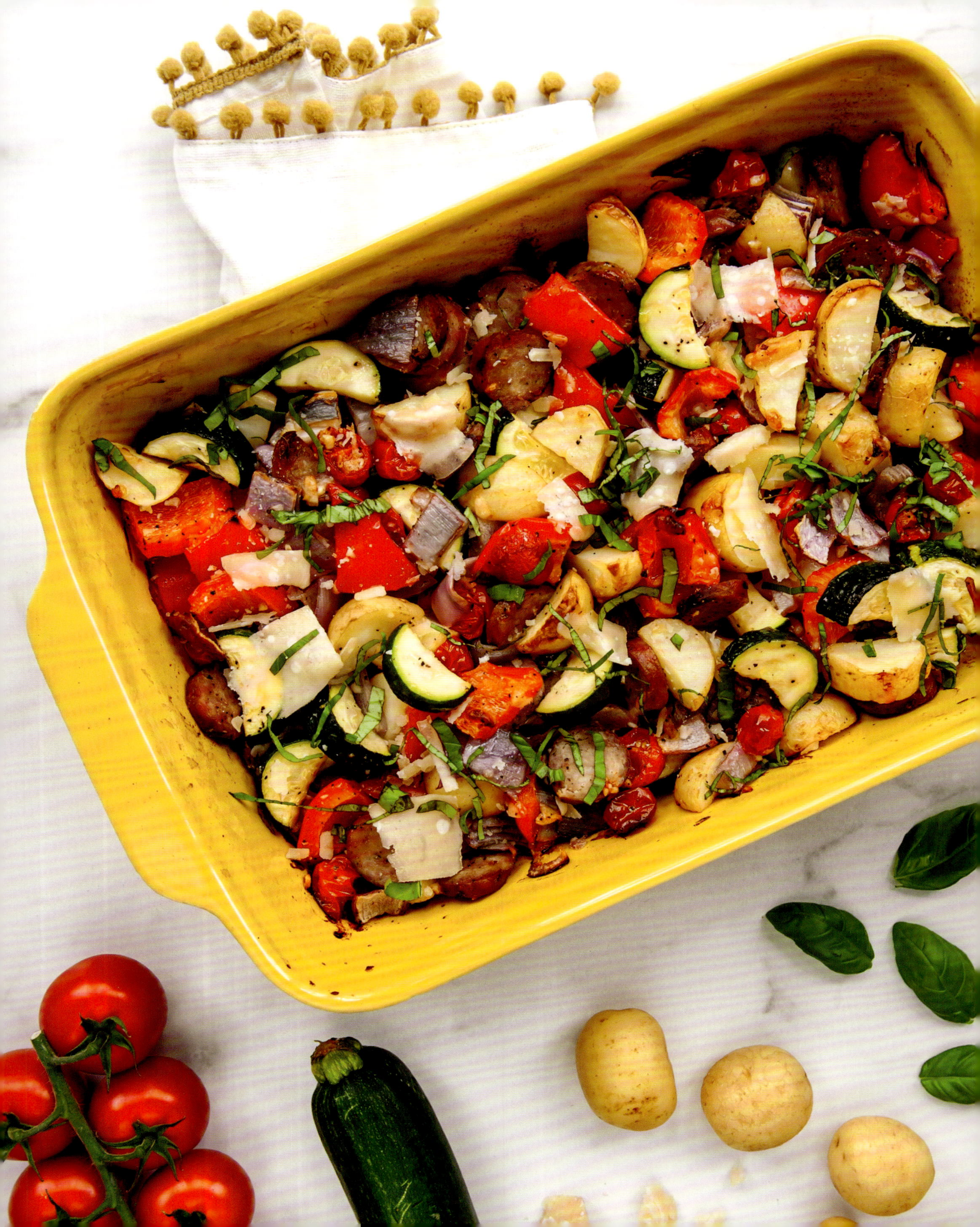

Gluten-Free Option • Grain-Free Option • Nut-Free

Rainbow Sausage Bake

A rustic, comforting meal that combines abundant summer produce and BBQ leftovers. It's equally delicious as dinner with a big green salad or as breakfast topped with a fried egg. No sausage? Try using meatballs instead!

10 MINUTES PREPPING • 45 MINUTES COOKING • MAKES 3 TO 4 SERVINGS

WHAT YOU NEED:

- 2 to 3 cooked sausage links, sliced (gluten-free or regular)
- 2 bell peppers (about 3 cups/ 750 mL) chopped into medium-sized pieces
- 1 to 2 zucchinis (about 2½ cups/ 625 mL), thick sliced and halved
- 1 ½ cups (375 mL) baby potatoes, halved or quartered (try to match size of zucchini)
- 1 ½ cups (375 mL) red onion, roughly chopped
- 1 ½ cups (375 mL) cherry or grape tomatoes
- 3 cloves garlic, minced
- 2½ tbsp (37 mL) olive oil
- 1 tsp (5 mL) sea salt
- ¼ tsp (1 mL) pepper
- 2 small handfuls Parmesan cheese, grated (about ¼ cup/60 mL), divided
- 3 tbsp (45 mL) fresh basil, chopped

HOW TO MAKE IT:

1. Preheat oven to 400°F (205°C) and have a 9 × 13-inch baking dish ready.
2. Add sausage and vegetables (zucchini through garlic) to your baking dish, and toss with olive oil, salt, pepper, and one small handful of Parmesan cheese.
3. Bake for about 45 minutes, giving a quick gentle stir halfway, or until potatoes are soft when pierced with a fork.
4. Stir in second small handful of Parmesan and fresh basil and enjoy!

Link-up

More basil on hand?
Enjoy it on the **Shakshuka with Swiss Chard + Cherry Tomatoes** (page 91) or **Mango Mint Salad** (page 145).

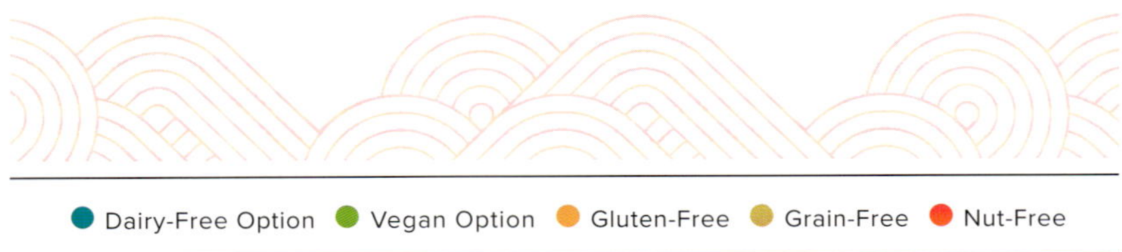

Dairy-Free Option · Vegan Option · Gluten-Free · Grain-Free · Nut-Free

Pineapple + Lime Fruit Salad with Poppy Seed Dressing

If you're craving fresh and juicy fruit, you'll enjoy this delicious tropical fruit salad. There is no scientific evidence that pineapple should be on the "do not eat" list during pregnancy. Dig into the pineapple — the rumour about not eating pineapple during pregnancy is just a myth!

15 MINUTES PREPPING • 0 MINUTES COOKING • SERVES 4

WHAT YOU NEED:

- 1 pineapple, cored and cubed (about 4 cups/1 L)
- 1 container strawberries (16 oz/454 g), halved
- 1 container blueberries (6 oz/170 g)
- Juice of 2 limes, zest of 1 lime
- 2 tsp (10 mL) honey or maple syrup
- 2 to 3 tsp (10 to 15 mL) poppy seeds
- ¼ tsp (1 mL) cinnamon
- Pinch of sea salt
- For dipping, consider full-fat yogurt, coconut cream, or kefir

HOW TO MAKE IT:

1. In a large bowl big enough to serve your fruit salad, mix together the lime juice, lime zest, honey, poppy seeds, cinnamon, and salt.
2. Add pineapple cubes, strawberries, and blueberries to the bowl and toss to coat fruit evenly.
3. Serve with yogurt, coconut cream, or kefir on the side for dipping. Keeps well in refrigerator for 2 days.

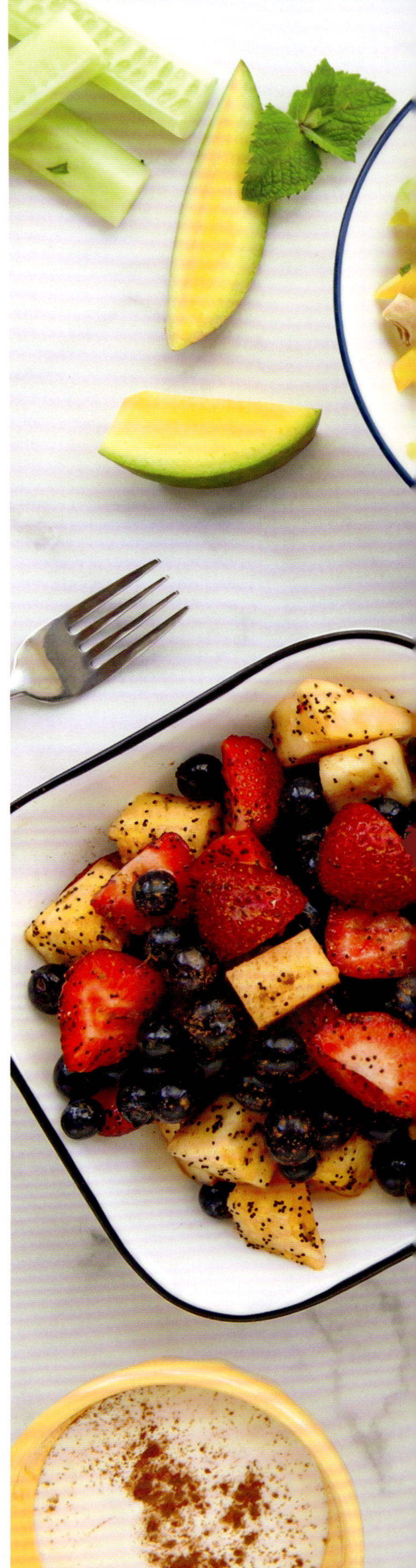

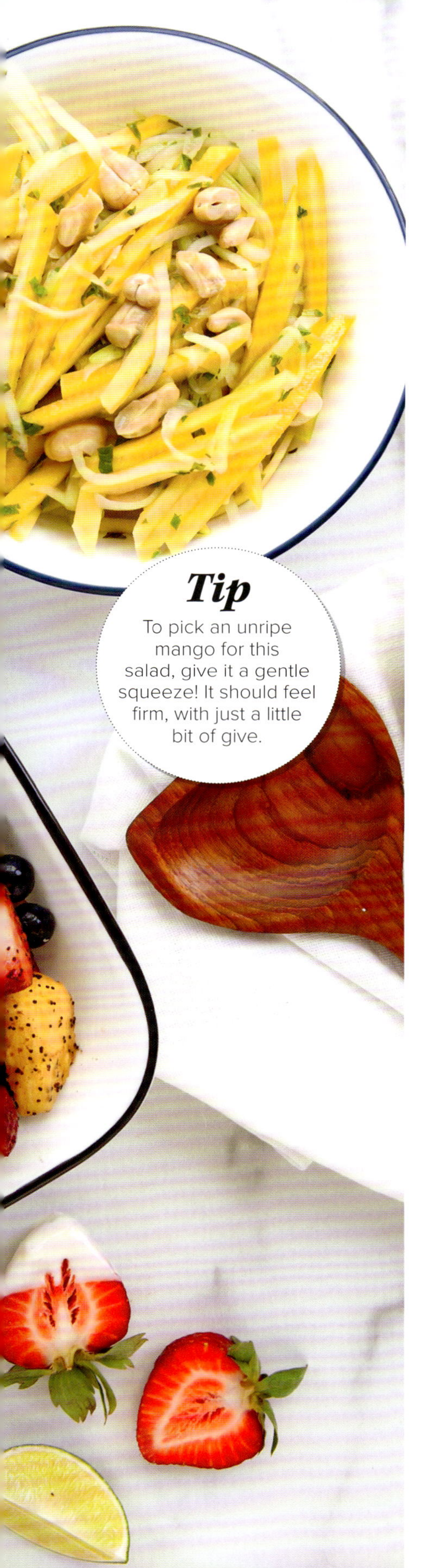

Tip

To pick an unripe mango for this salad, give it a gentle squeeze! It should feel firm, with just a little bit of give.

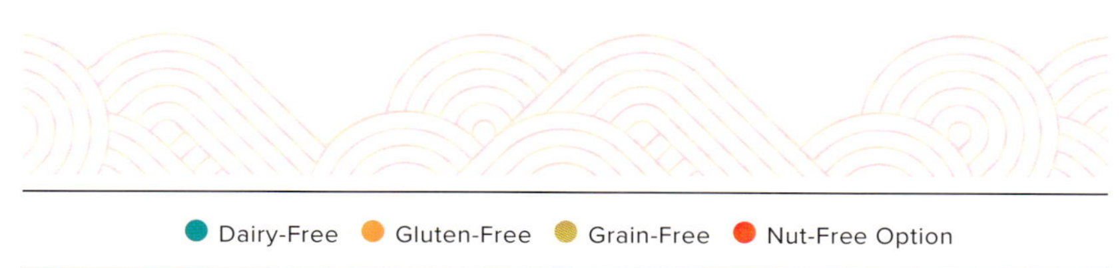

Dairy-Free • Gluten-Free • Grain-Free • Nut-Free Option

Mango Mint Salad

This combo of tart mango, cooling cucumber, and fresh herbs is full of flavour and completely satisfying. Don't be surprised if you eat the whole bowl!

15 MINUTES PREPPING • 0 MINUTES COOKING • MAKES 2 SERVINGS

WHAT YOU NEED:

- 2 mangoes, unripe or partially ripe, sliced into thin strips
- 1 large English cucumber, peeled and sliced into thin strips
- 2 tbsp (30 mL) finely chopped fresh mint
- 2 tbsp (30 mL) finely chopped fresh basil
- 1 ½ tbsp (22 mL) rice vinegar
- 1 tbsp (15 mL) lime juice
- 1 tbsp (15 mL) honey
- ½ tsp and a pinch (2 mL), sea salt
- ½ cup (125 mL) cashews (optional)

HOW TO MAKE IT:

1. In a large bowl, mix together the mint, basil, lime juice, rice vinegar, honey, and sea salt.
2. Add the mango and cucumber, and toss to evenly coat the mixture with the dressing for the salad.
3. Top with cashews (if using) and enjoy immediately.

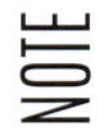

NOTE

To cut an unripe mango for this salad, peel it first. Stand the mango up tall, and slice thin chunks off each side of the mango. Then slice each chunk into thin strips.

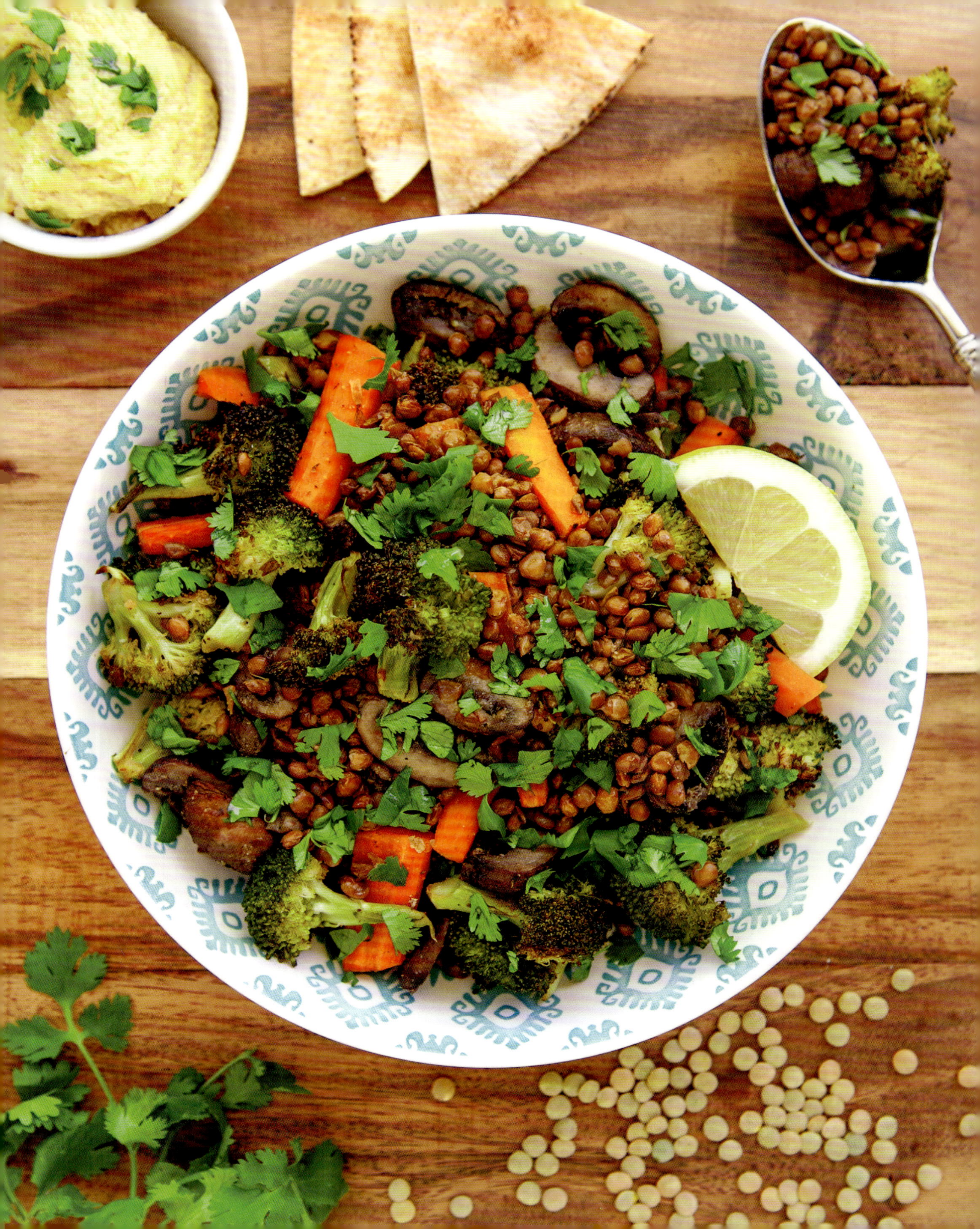

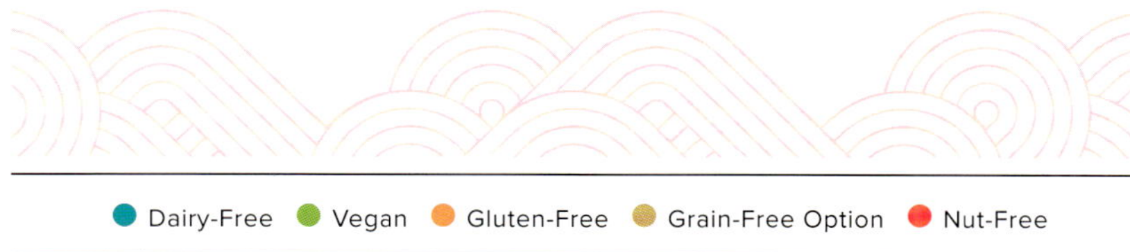

Dairy-Free • Vegan • Gluten-Free • Grain-Free Option • Nut-Free

Sheet Pan Roasted Lentil Bowl

A sheet pan meal featuring one of my favourite prenatal superfoods — lentils. I love this on its own, with a side of hummus and pita wedges, on top of greens or quinoa, or as a side to the Simple Salted Lemon Salmon (page 215).

15 MINUTES PREPPING • 25 MINUTES COOKING • SERVES 2 AS A MEAL, 4 AS A SIDE

WHAT YOU NEED:

- 1 (19 oz/540 mL) can of green or brown lentils, drained and rinsed
- 1 head broccoli, chopped
- 1 (8 oz/225 g) package of cremini mushrooms, chopped
- 3 large carrots, chopped
- 3 tbsp (45 mL) avocado oil
- 1 tsp (5 mL) garlic powder
- 1 tsp (5 mL) cumin
- ½ tsp (2 mL) sea salt
- ¼ tsp (1 mL) pepper
- ¼ cup (60 mL) fresh parsley or cilantro, finely chopped
- Juice of ½ to 1 lemon

HOW TO MAKE IT:

1. Preheat oven to 425°F (220°C) and line a 18 x 13-inch sheet pan with parchment paper.
2. In a large bowl, toss the lentils, broccoli, mushrooms, and carrots in the avocado oil, garlic powder, cumin, salt, and pepper. Transfer to baking sheet and move to oven.
3. Roast for 15 minutes, then give everything a gentle stir. Roast for 10 more minutes, then remove from oven.
4. When ready to eat, top bowl with herbs and lemon juice.

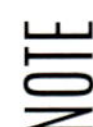

Leftovers are great for breakfast! In a medium skillet, heat 1 tbsp olive oil, then add two scoops of leftover lentils and veggies to one side of the pan, and crack an egg into the other. Cover and cook, 3 to 5 minutes. Top with hot sauce, pink onions (page 87), or salsa.

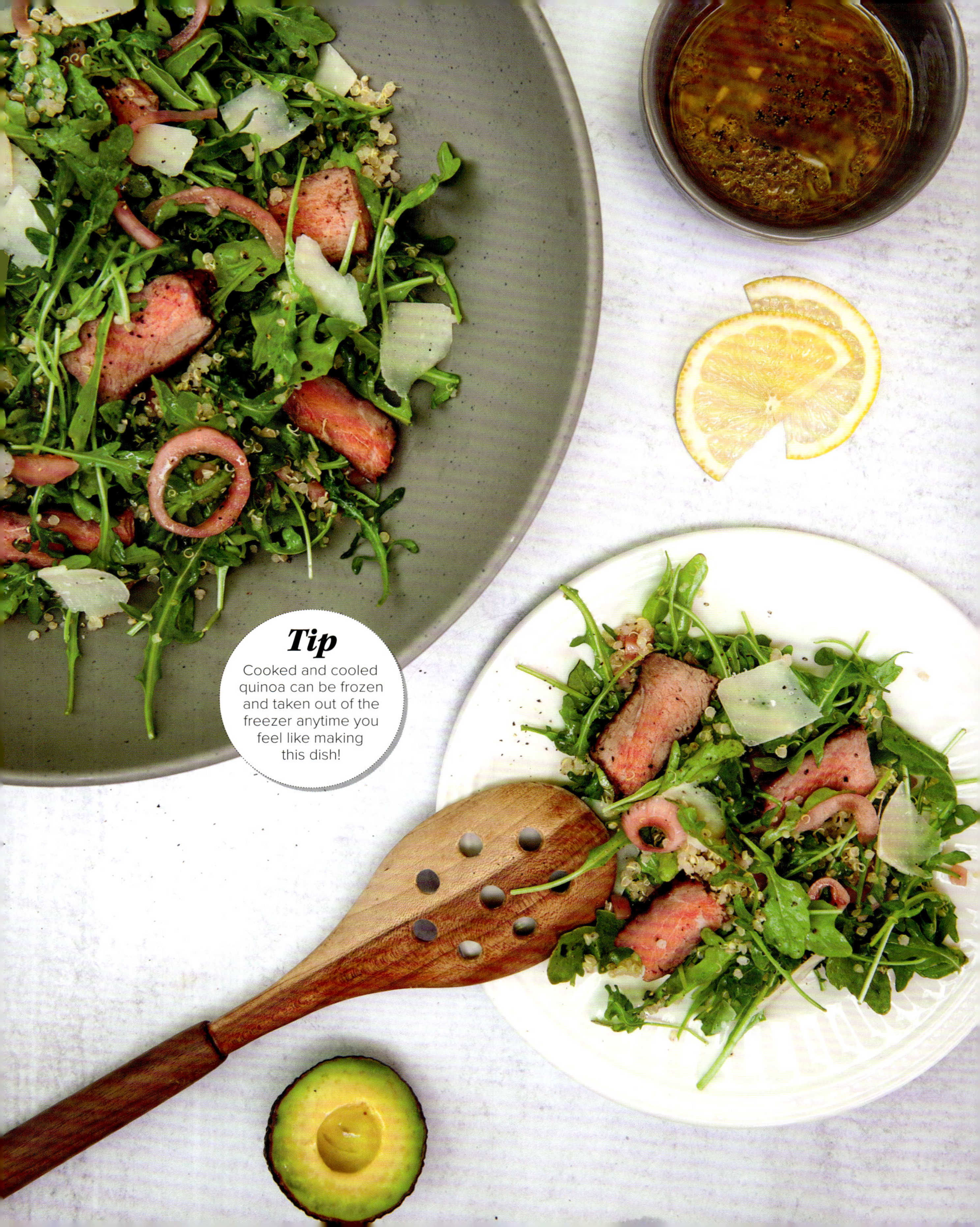
Tip
Cooked and cooled quinoa can be frozen and taken out of the freezer anytime you feel like making this dish!

Gluten-Free • Grain-Free • Nut-Free

Arugula + Quinoa Steak Salad with Lemon Pepper Dressing

This salad brings out the delicious peppery flavour of arugula, balanced with the salty tang of Parmesan cheese, creamy avocado, and flavourful steak. For a delightful vegetarian option, substitute the steak with crispy chickpeas or sautéed mushrooms.

10 MINUTES PREPPING • 25 MINUTES COOKING • SERVES 2 TO 3 AS A MEAL

WHAT YOU NEED:

6 cups (1.5 L) arugula

1¾ cups (435 mL) cooked quinoa

1 (8 oz/225 g) striploin steak

1 avocado, sliced

1 large handful, shaved Parmesan cheese

1 tsp (5 mL) pepper

1 tsp (5 mL) sea salt

For the lemon pepper dressing

⅓ cup (75 mL) lemon juice

¼ cup (60 mL) olive oil

1 shallot, finely sliced (about ¼ cup/60 mL), or use red onion or pink onions (page 87)

¼ tsp (1 mL) pepper

¼ tsp (1 mL) sea salt

HOW TO MAKE IT:

1. Combine the dressing ingredients in a small bowl or glass jar, letting the shallot soften in the salad dressing and pickle a little bit while you make the rest of the salad.
2. Turn grill to high heat, and season steak generously with salt and pepper on both sides.
3. Transfer seasoned steak to the grill, and cook about 15 minutes or until done to your preference.
4. Transfer cooked steak to cutting board and let sit for 10 minutes. Then cut steak into thin slices against the grain.
5. In a large bowl, toss the arugula and quinoa together with all of the dressing, and top with sliced avocado, steak, and Parmesan.

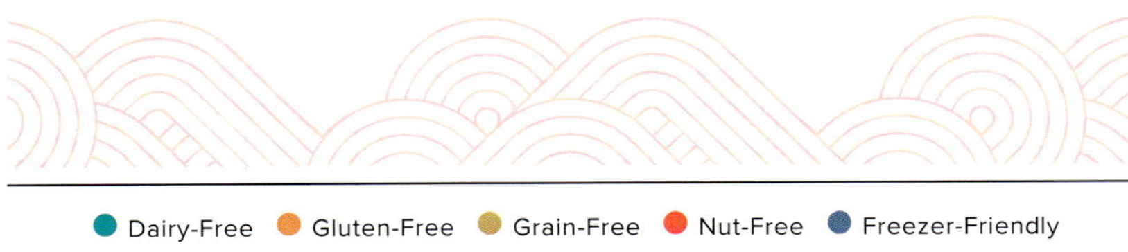

Dairy-Free • Gluten-Free • Grain-Free • Nut-Free • Freezer-Friendly

Greek Chicken Skewers

Greek food is very close to my heart, from growing up with a best friend who is Greek and spending time in Greece watching sunsets and eating gyros. This recipe is my take on souvlaki — flavourful, moist, and perfect with Greek Garlic Kale Salad (page 151) or wrapped up in warm pita with fresh tomatoes and tzatziki.

20 MINUTES PREPPING • 25 MINUTES COOKING • MAKES 8 SKEWERS

WHAT YOU NEED:

- 2 lb (900 g) boneless chicken breast, cut into bite-sized cubes
- ⅓ cup (75 mL) olive oil
- 6 cloves garlic, minced
- 2 tbsp (30 mL) balsamic vinegar
- 2 tbsp (30 mL) lemon juice
- 2 tsp (10 mL) dried oregano
- 1 tsp (5 mL) each of sea salt, onion powder, cumin, and coconut sugar
- Pinch of pepper
- 8 to 10 skewers

HOW TO MAKE IT:

1. In a small bowl, combine oil, garlic, vinegar, lemon juice, and spices.
2. Put cubed chicken into a large bowl or bag, and coat with the marinade (reserving a little to brush on chicken once cooked, if desired). Store in the refrigerator until mealtime (this can be prepared the night before).
3. When almost ready to cook, thread chicken cubes onto each skewer.
4. Transfer chicken skewers to a grill preheated to about 375°F (190°C), and cook for 20 to 25 minutes, flipping occasionally, until chicken is cooked through.

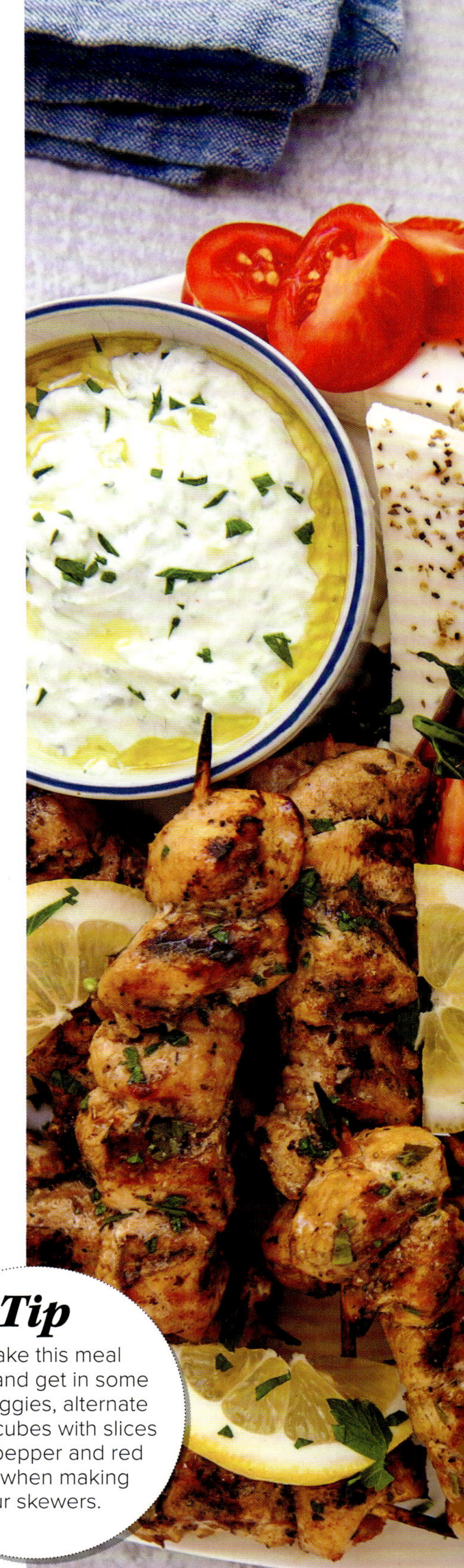

Tip

To make this meal stretch and get in some extra veggies, alternate chicken cubes with slices of bell pepper and red onion when making your skewers.

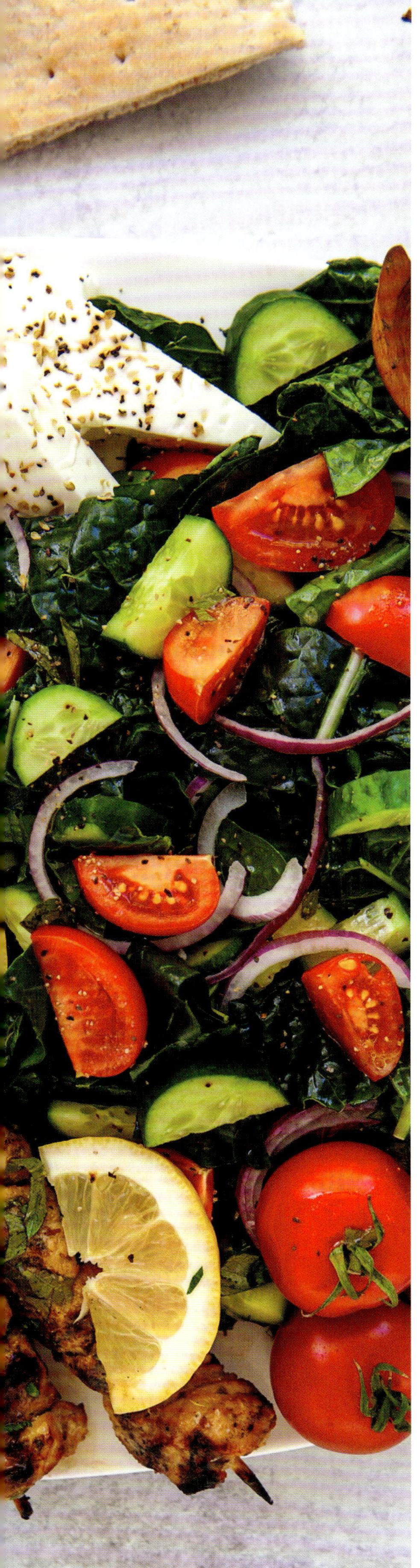

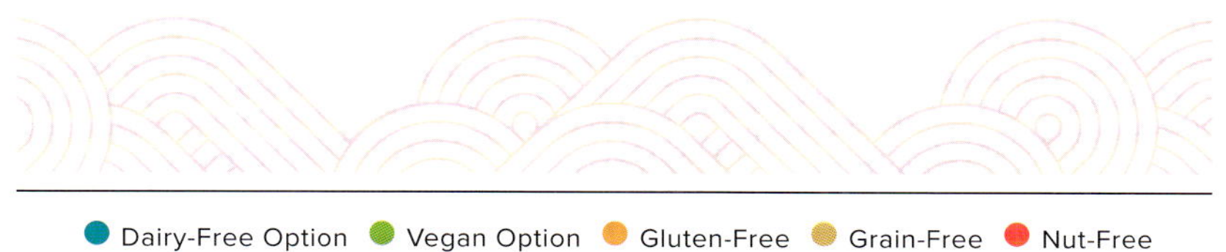

Dairy-Free Option • Vegan Option • Gluten-Free • Grain-Free • Nut-Free

Greek Garlic Kale Salad

Enjoy this garlicky, full-flavour Greek salad with a kale twist. If you have no kale, try it with crunchy romaine lettuce. The Greek salad dressing is one of my favourite dressings of all time, and if you prefer less garlic zing, use 1 garlic clove instead of 2.

15 MINUTES PREPPING • SERVES 2 AS A MEAL OR 4 AS A SIDE

WHAT YOU NEED:

1 bunch kale (I use black/dino kale), destemmed, and chopped

1 tbsp (15 mL) lemon juice

1 tbsp (15 mL) olive oil

Pinch of sea salt

2 cups (500 mL) tomato wedges or cherry tomatoes, halved

2 cups (500 mL) sliced cucumbers

½ cup (125 mL) red onion, finely sliced

(optional) wedge of sheep's milk feta cheese, pasteurized (see Note below)

For the dressing

¼ cup (60 mL) olive oil

2 tbsp (30 mL) white wine vinegar (or use balsamic)

2 garlic cloves, minced

½ tbsp (7 mL) fresh parsley, roughly chopped

½ tsp (2 mL) white miso (or use Dijon mustard)

¼ tsp (1 mL) sea salt

Pinch of pepper

HOW TO MAKE IT:

1. In a small bowl or glass jar, mix together ingredients for the dressing.
2. Add kale to a large bowl and drizzle on the lemon juice, olive oil, and pinch of sea salt. Then give your kale a 3-minute massage (this helps make the kale easier to digest and less bitter).
3. Add veggies, feta (if using), and dressing to salad.

NOTE

Soft cheeses such as feta and goat cheese are moisture-rich and more likely to harbour the listeria bacteria, which can cause a rare but serious infection in pregnant women. Pasteurization reduces this risk. If you choose to eat soft cheeses, look for "pasteurized" on the label.

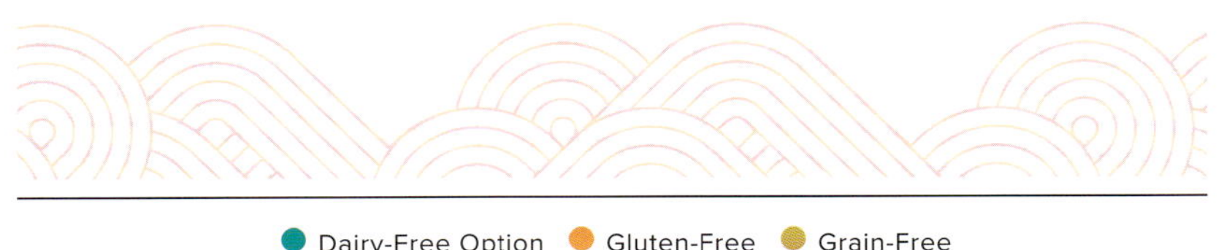

Dairy-Free Option · Gluten-Free · Grain-Free

Skillet Blackened Chicken Thighs with Cashew Chive Dipping Sauce

Kick it up a notch! Make your own blackened seasoning mix to pack in flavour when cooking meat or fish. This recipe is mild, but if you like it hot, add 1/2 to 1 tsp cayenne powder to your mix.

5 MINUTES PREPPING • 25 MINUTES COOKING • SERVES 4

WHAT YOU NEED:

2 tbsp (30 mL) blackened spice mix, or more as needed (see recipe below)

8 bone-in chicken thighs (see Note for boneless thighs)

1 ½ tbsp (22 mL) avocado oil or butter/ghee

For the blackened spice mix

(makes three 2 tbsp (30 mL) servings; keeps well in sealed container for several months)

1 tbsp (15 mL) paprika

1 tbsp (15 mL) coconut sugar

1 tbsp (15 mL) dried thyme

2 tsp (10 mL) onion powder

2 tsp (10 mL) garlic powder

2 tsp (10 mL) sea salt

1 ½ tsp (7.5 mL) black pepper

1 tsp (5 mL) cinnamon

HOW TO MAKE IT:

1. Preheat oven to 425°F (220°C). In a large bowl, gently toss chicken thighs in blackened spice mix.
2. Heat avocado oil or butter/ghee in a large oven-safe skillet over medium-high heat. When oil is hot, add chicken thighs bone-side down and cook, 5 minutes, until chicken is nicely browned. Then flip and cook skin-side down, about 8 minutes.
3. Transfer skillet to oven for about 12 more minutes, or until chicken is fully cooked.

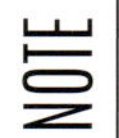
NOTE

For boneless chicken thighs, follow steps 1 and 2 but do not preheat oven. These thighs will not require the oven and will be done in a shorter time.

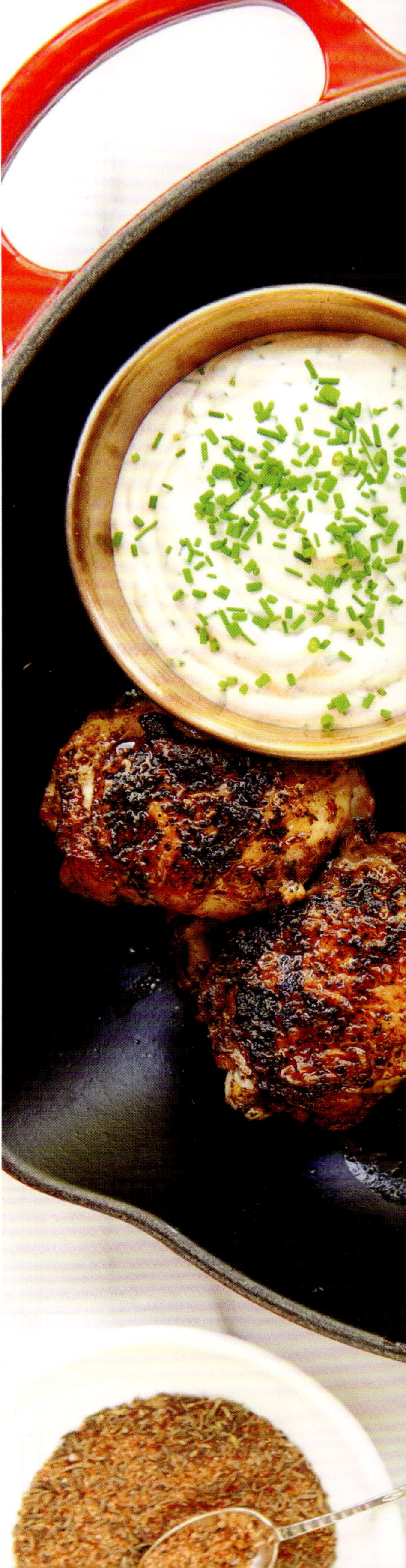

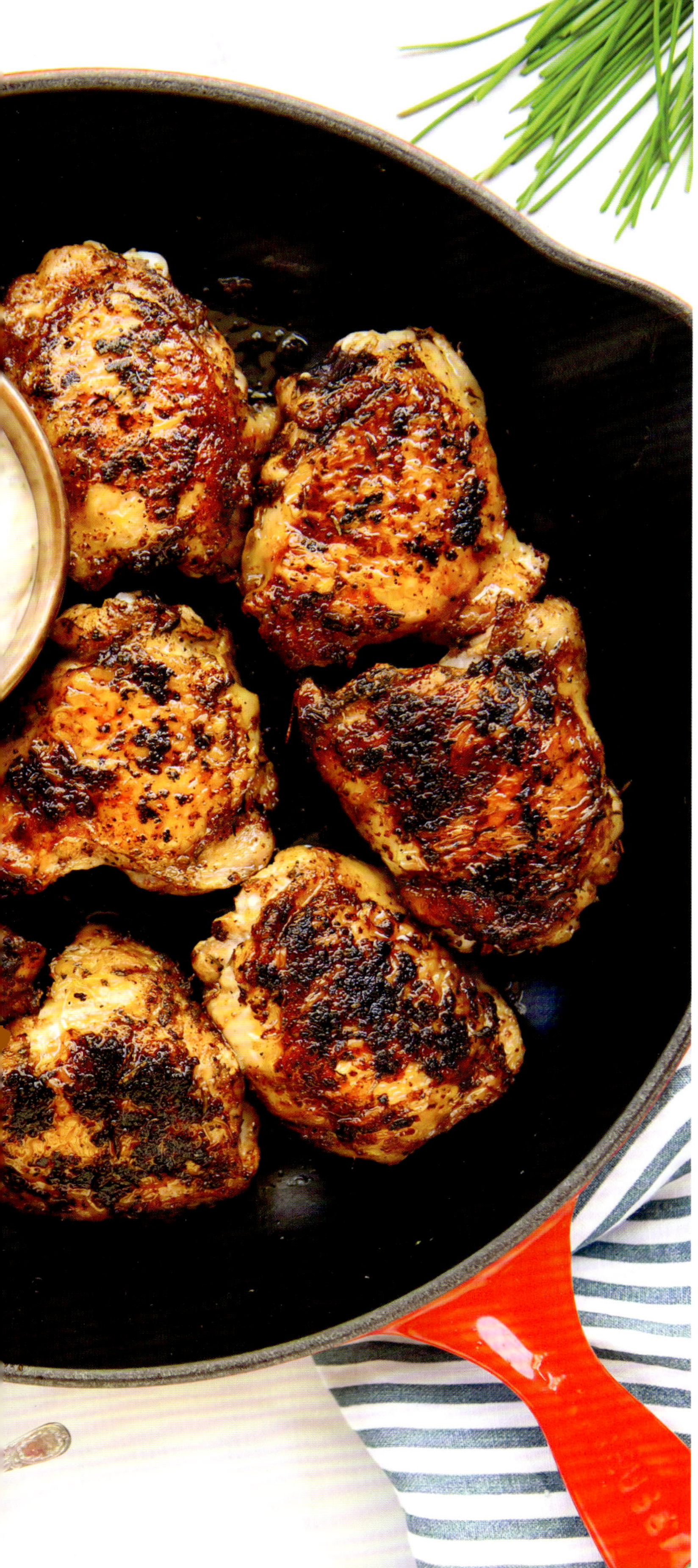

CASHEW CHIVE DIPPING SAUCE

10 MINUTES PREPPING • 5 MINUTES COOKING • MAKES 1 ½ CUPS

WHAT YOU NEED:

1 cup (250 mL) cashews, soaked overnight or in boiling water for 1 to 2 hours, rinsed

½ cup (125 mL) water

1 tbsp (15 mL) lemon juice

2 garlic cloves

½ tsp (2 mL) sea salt

¼ cup (60 mL) thinly sliced chives

HOW TO MAKE IT:

1. Combine the cashews, lemon juice, garlic, and sea salt in a high-speed blender and blend until smooth. Add more salt or lemon juice to your taste. Finally, stir in the chives.

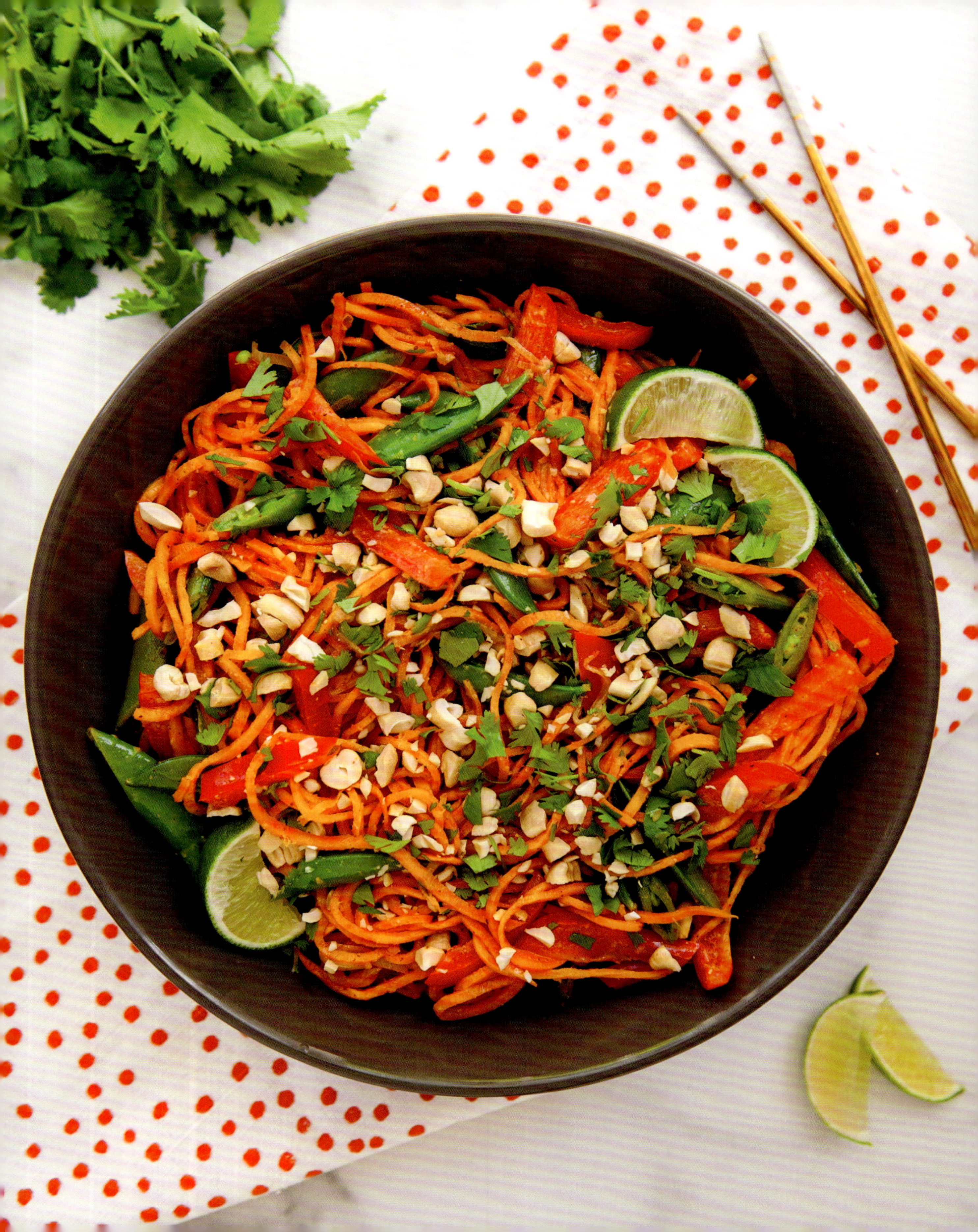

Dairy-Free · Vegan · Gluten-Free · Grain-Free Option

Sweet Potato Pad Thai

This grain-free and veggie-packed version of Pad Thai will keep your blood sugar stable and won't make you uncomfortably full. If you have not tried sweet potato noodles, you're in for a treat. Roasting them in the oven brings out their sweet, slightly caramelized flavour, while keeping an *al dente* texture.

10 MINUTES PREPPING • 10 MINUTES COOKING • SERVES 2 TO 4

WHAT YOU NEED:

8 cups (2 L) sweet potatoes, spiralized

3 tbsp (45 mL) melted coconut oil, divided

2 shallots, thinly sliced

2 cups (500 mL) snap peas, cut in half

2 cups (500 mL) red bell pepper, thinly sliced and cut in half

½ cup (125 mL) cashews, chopped

¼ cup (60 mL) cilantro, chopped

Lime juice, to taste

For the Pad Thai sauce

3 tbsp (45 mL) almond butter

3 tbsp (45 mL) lime juice

2 tbsp (30 mL) tamari (or soy sauce for non-GF)

1 tbsp (15 mL) maple syrup

1 tsp (5 mL) sesame oil

1 tsp (5 mL) minced ginger

2 cloves garlic, minced

¼ tsp (1 mL) sea salt

2 tbsp (30 mL) warm water, to thin

HOW TO MAKE IT:

1. Preheat oven to 425°F (220°C) and line a baking sheet with parchment paper. Then whisk together Pad Thai sauce ingredients in a medium bowl.
2. Add sweet potato spirals to baking sheet and toss with 2 tbsp (30 mL) coconut oil. Transfer to oven and cook, 10 to 12 minutes, until slightly softened and caramelized.
3. While sweet potatoes cook, heat a large skillet over medium heat. Put in remaining 1 tbsp (15 mL) coconut oil, then add chopped shallots and cook for 2 minutes. Throw in the snap peas and bell pepper, and cook for 3 more minutes. Remove from heat and transfer to large bowl.
4. Finally, add cooked sweet potato noodles and Pad Thai sauce to bowl and toss to combine. Finish with cilantro, cashews, and extra lime juice to taste.

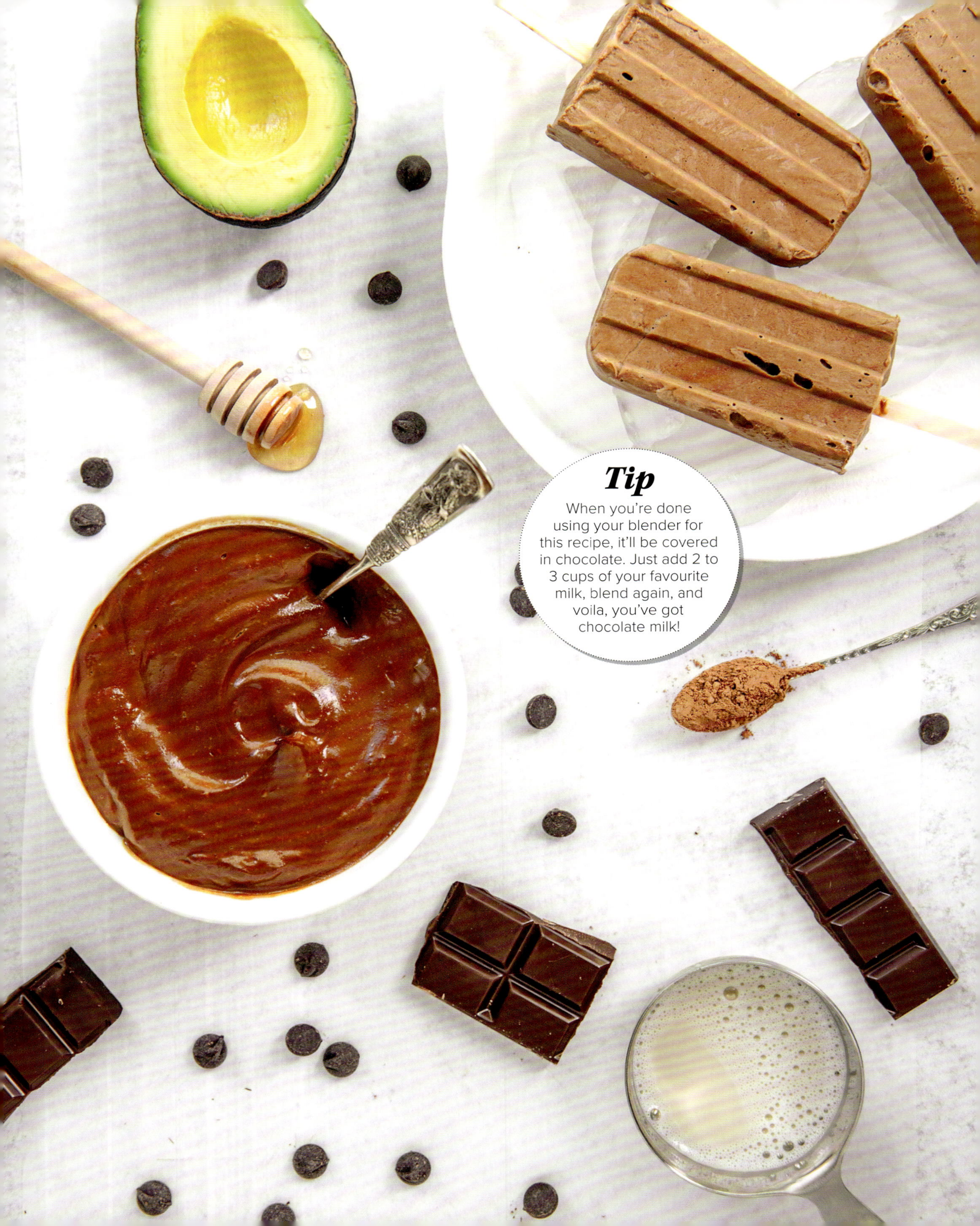
Tip
When you're done using your blender for this recipe, it'll be covered in chocolate. Just add 2 to 3 cups of your favourite milk, blend again, and voila, you've got chocolate milk!

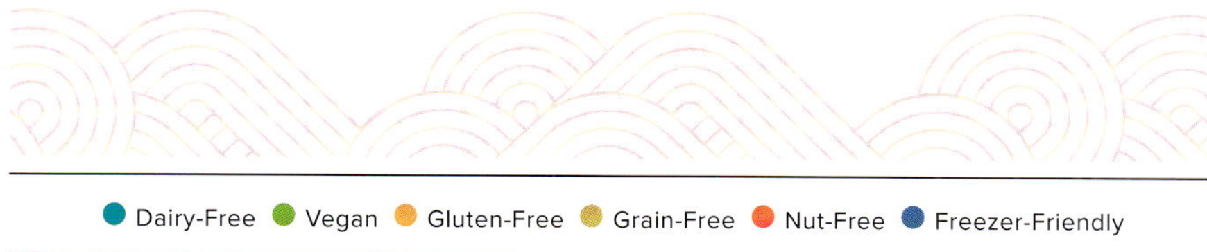

Dairy-Free · Vegan · Gluten-Free · Grain-Free · Nut-Free · Freezer-Friendly

Late-Night Chocolate Avocado Pudding

Here's the perfect snack before bed — it's sweet and comforting, with enough staying power to help you feel good until morning. Can't wait? Eat it straight out of the blender!

5 MINUTES PREPPING • 1 MINUTE BLENDING • MAKES 2 PUDDINGS

WHAT YOU NEED:	HOW TO MAKE IT:
2 small ripe avocados (or 1 large) ¾ cup (175 mL) non-dairy milk ⅓ cup (75 mL) maple syrup ⅓ cup (75 mL) cacao powder 1 tsp (5 mL) vanilla extract Pinch of sea salt 1 to 2 tbsp (15 to 30 mL) hemp hearts (optional)	**1.** Add all ingredients to a high-powered blender and blend on high, about 1 minute, or until smooth and creamy.

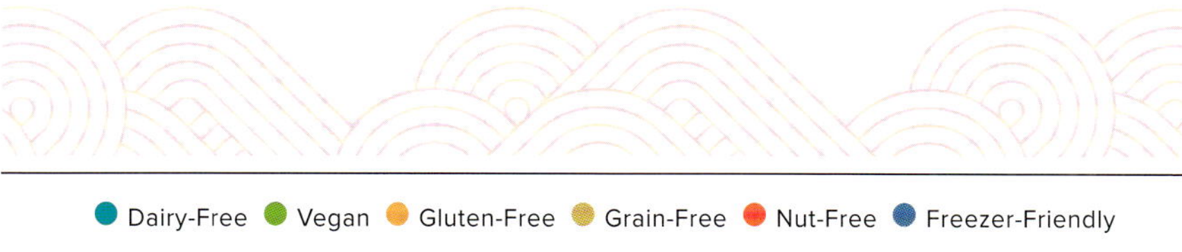

Dairy-Free · Vegan · Gluten-Free · Grain-Free · Nut-Free · Freezer-Friendly

Chocolate Avocado Bliss Bars

When you're in the mood for a chocolatey frozen treat to cool you down on a hot day, this is it! Simply refer to the recipe for Late-Night Chocolate Avocado Pudding. You'll get more than you bargain for — this snack is packed with good fats and protein!

5 MINUTES PREPPING • 3 MINUTES BLENDING AND FILLING • MAKES 5 TO 6 BLISS BARS

HOW TO MAKE IT:

1. Blend up the ingredients for Late-Night Chocolate Avocado Pudding. Then spoon the pudding into ice pop moulds.
2. Transfer to freezer until frozen, about 2 to 4 hours.

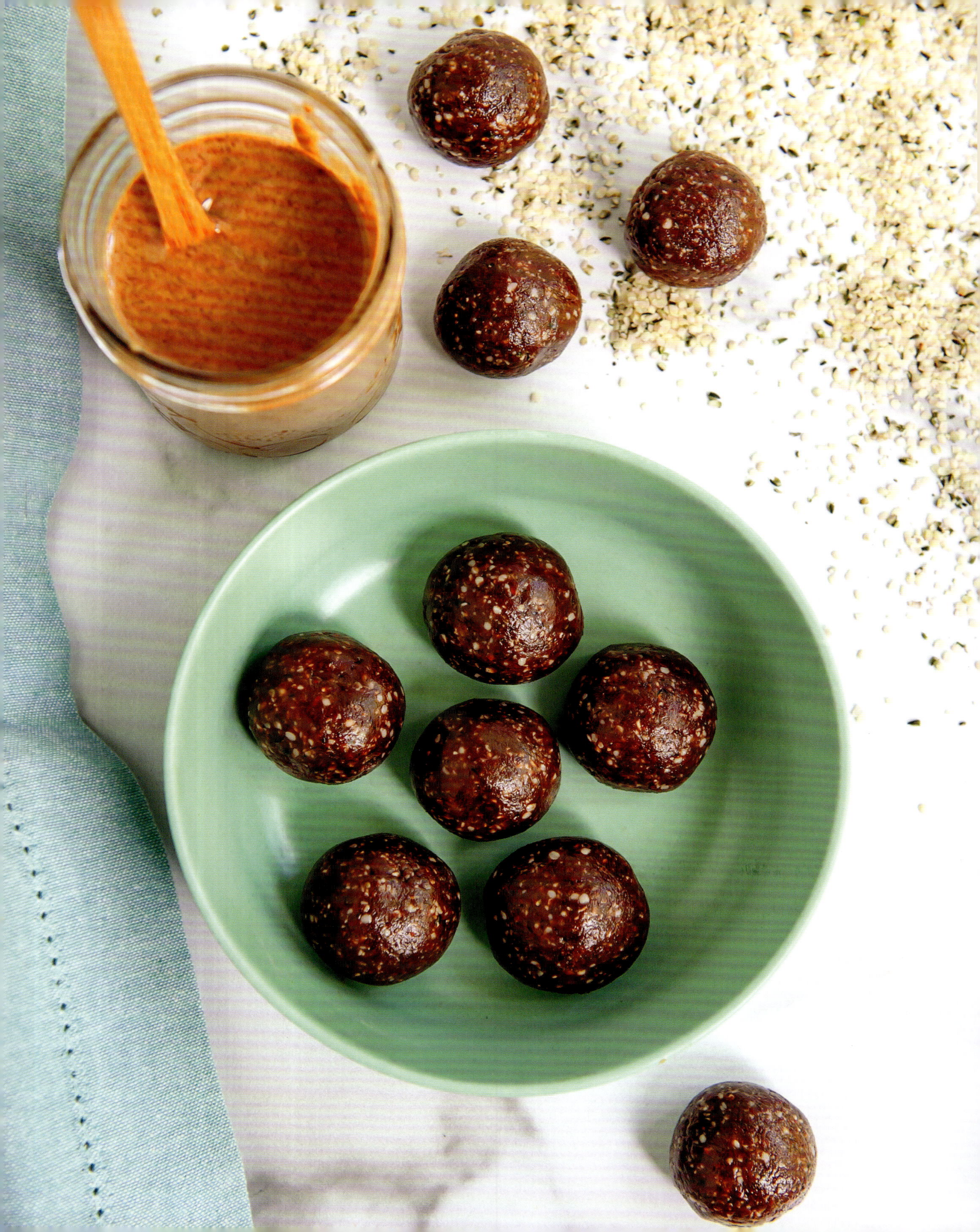

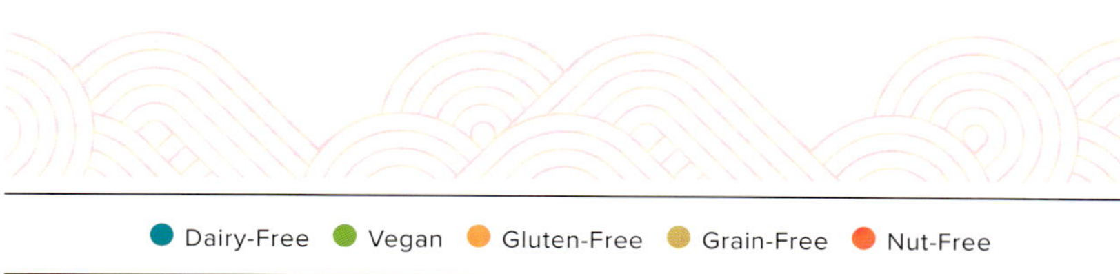

Dairy-Free • Vegan • Gluten-Free • Grain-Free • Nut-Free

Seed Strong Chocolate Energy Balls

These nut-free chocolate energy balls are irresistible, and they provide immune system support, blood sugar control, and antioxidant fuel as well. They're an easy, convenient snack for morning, noon, or night.

5 MINUTES PREPPING • 10 MINUTES ROLLING • MAKES 22 ENERGY BALLS

WHAT YOU NEED:

- 6 medjool dates (about ⅔ cup/150 mL), pitted
- 2 tbsp (30 mL) goji berries (optional)
- ½ cup (125 mL) sunflower seed butter
- ½ cup (125 mL) hemp hearts
- ¼ cup (60 mL) sesame seeds
- ¼ cup (60 mL) maple syrup
- ¼ cup (60 mL) cacao powder
- ½ tsp (2 mL) vanilla extract
- ¼ tsp (1 mL) cinnamon

HOW TO MAKE IT:

1. In a food processor, process the dates and goji berries (if using) until a paste forms.
2. Add remaining ingredients and process until combined. You'll know it's ready when the mixture sticks into a big ball.
3. Roll mixture and form 22 balls.
4. Transfer to refrigerator for one week, enjoying several each day for a pick-me-up!

Link-up

Goji berries are a good add-in to the **Everyday Bone Broth**, page 181.

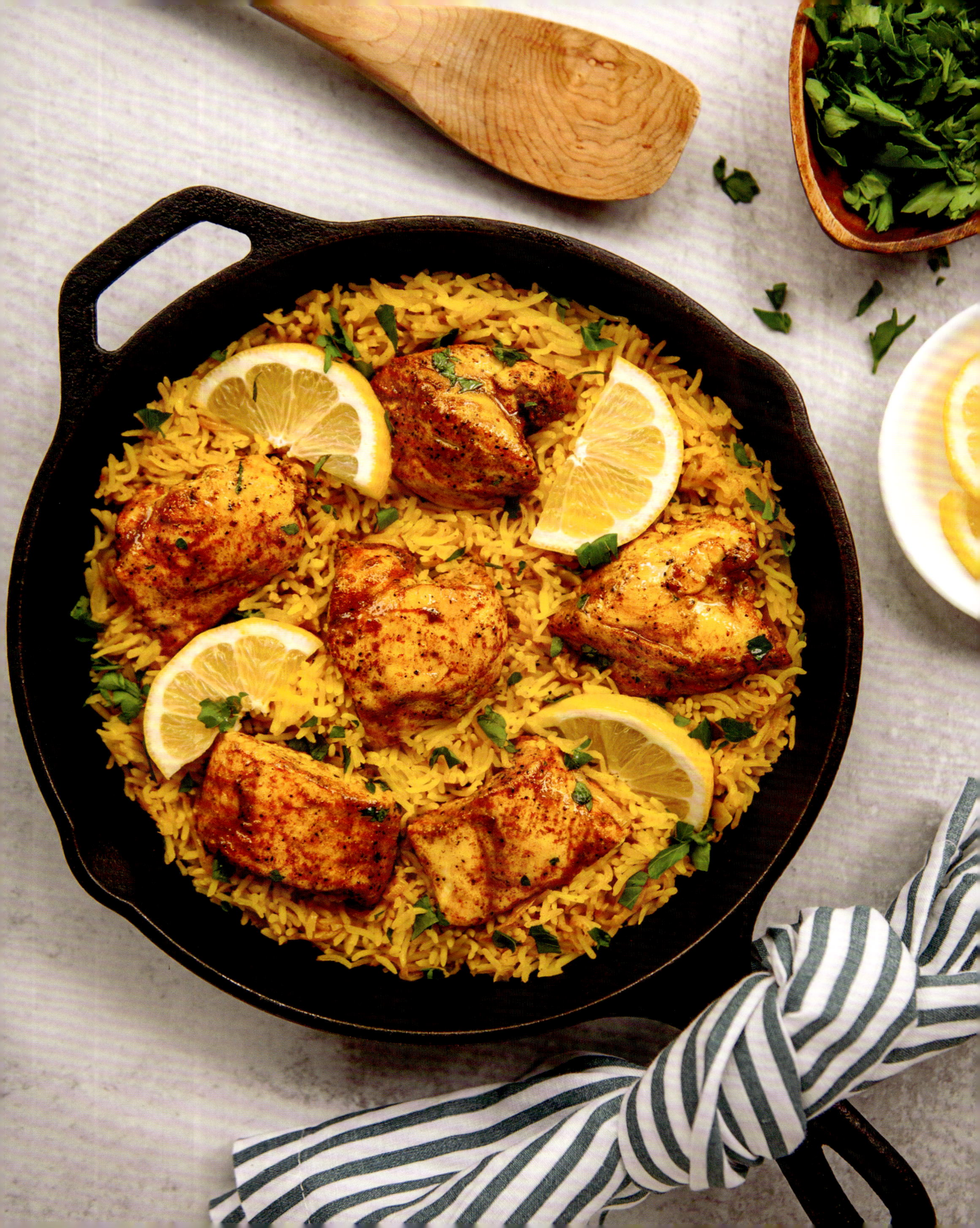

Dairy-Free Option · Gluten-Free · Nut-Free

One-Pan Chicken + Golden Rice

Lemony and bright golden rice with turmeric-spiced chicken thighs is a one-pan meal full of warmth and comfort. Plus, it's flavourful and nutritious.

10 MINUTES PREPPING • 35 MINUTES COOKING • MAKES 3 SERVINGS

WHAT YOU NEED:

2 tbsp (30 mL) butter/ghee or coconut oil, divided

6 chicken thighs (or use 3 large chicken breasts cut in half)

1 small onion, finely diced

2 cloves garlic, minced

2 tsp (10 mL) turmeric

1 ½ tsp (7.5 mL) cumin

¾ tsp (4 mL) sea salt

½ tsp (2 mL) ground ginger

½ tsp (2 mL) pepper

3¼ cups (810 mL) no-salt-added chicken broth

1 ½ cups (375 mL) basmati rice

¼ cup (60 mL) lemon juice (from 1 lemon)

Fresh cilantro, for serving

HOW TO MAKE IT:

1. Stir spices together in a small bowl.
2. In a large bowl, gently toss chicken with ½ of the spice mix, reserving the rest.
3. In a large pan, heat 1 tbsp (15 mL) of the butter/ghee over medium-high heat. When hot, brown chicken, about 3 minutes per side, then turn heat down to medium and transfer chicken to a plate.
4. Add the remaining 1 tbsp (15 mL) butter/ghee to the pan, and sauté the onion and garlic for 3 minutes until onion is translucent and softened. Add remaining spices and cook, 1 minute.
5. Pour in the broth, rice, and lemon juice and bring it to a simmer. Return chicken to pan, turn heat to low, and cover.
6. Let dish simmer for 15 to 18 minutes until rice is cooked and liquid has been absorbed. Remove pan from heat, sprinkle on cilantro, and enjoy!

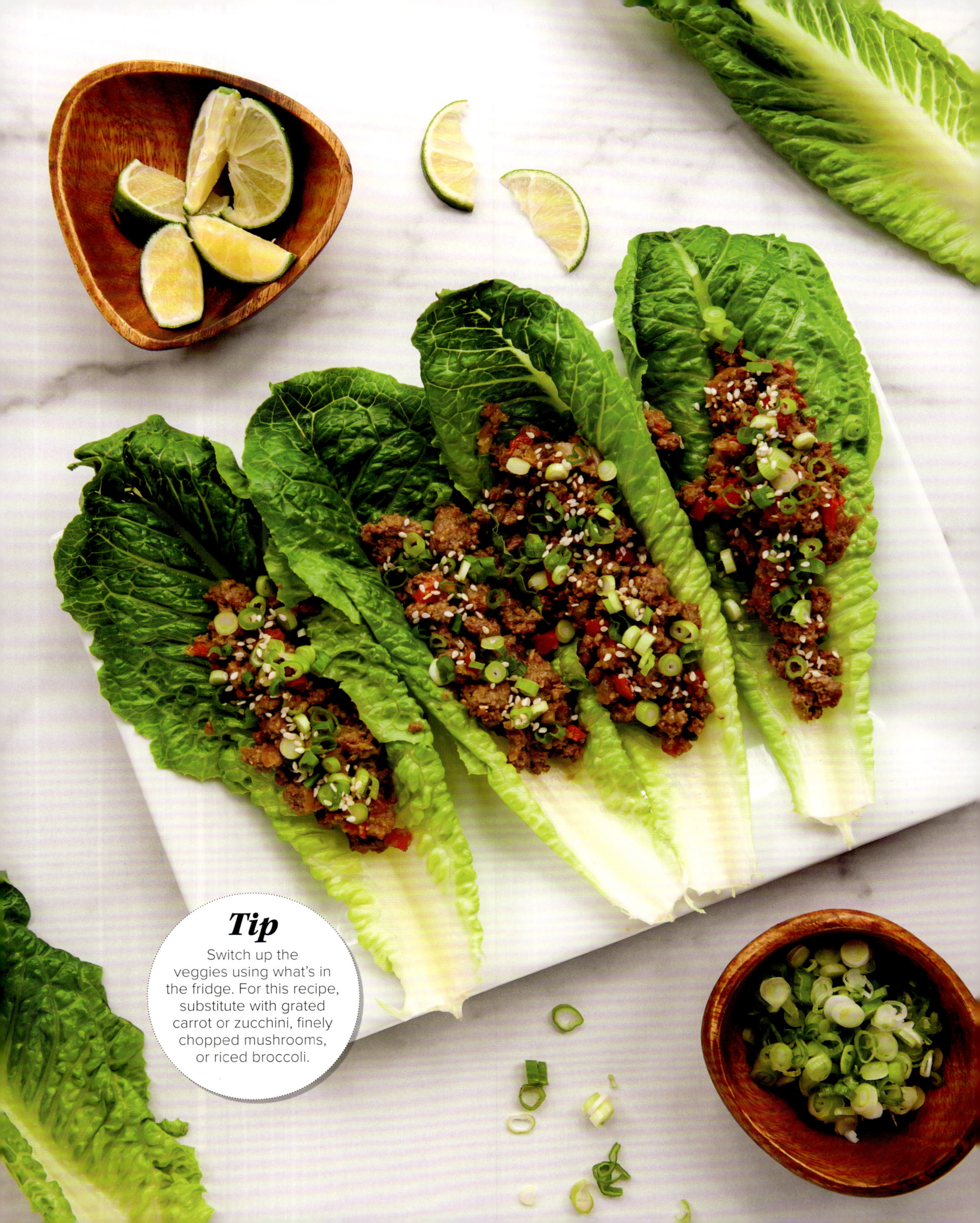

Tip

Switch up the veggies using what's in the fridge. For this recipe, substitute with grated carrot or zucchini, finely chopped mushrooms, or riced broccoli.

Dairy-Free • Gluten-Free • Grain-Free • Nut-Free

Romaine Calm Lettuce Wraps

In the final weeks of pregnancy, you'll look forward to easy meals that pack in the nutrients and keep you feeling good. These lettuce wraps can easily last for several days. Just keep the lettuce separate until ready to eat.

15 MINUTES PREPPING • 15 MINUTES COOKING • MAKES 2 TO 4 SERVINGS

WHAT YOU NEED:

For the wraps

1 head romaine lettuce (or use Boston/butter lettuce), leaves removed and washed

1 lb (450 g) pastured ground beef (or use ground chicken)

1 tbsp (15 mL) avocado oil

2 cloves garlic, minced

1 small onion, finely chopped

2 tsp (10 mL) fresh ginger, minced

½ cup (125 mL) cauliflower rice

½ cup (125 mL) red bell pepper, finely chopped

4 to 6 green onions, finely sliced, divided

For the sauce

¼ cup (60 mL) tamari (or use soy sauce for non-GF)

1 tbsp (15 mL) rice vinegar

1 tbsp (15 mL) maple syrup

1 tsp (5 mL) sesame oil

For topping (optional)

Sesame seeds, lime juice, or hot sauce

HOW TO MAKE IT:

1. Mix together sauce ingredients in a small bowl.
2. Heat avocado oil in a large pan over medium-high heat. When hot, add the beef and brown, breaking up with a wooden spoon, about 5 to 7 minutes.
3. Add garlic, ginger, onion, cauliflower rice, and bell pepper to the pan and cook, about 3 minutes, until vegetables start to soften.
4. Pour sauce into pan and cook until heated through, about 2 minutes, then remove from heat.
5. When ready to eat, use a spoon to add a large scoop of filling into the middle of each romaine leaf, then sprinkle with green onions and optional toppings. Roll or fold over either end of the lettuce and take a big bite!

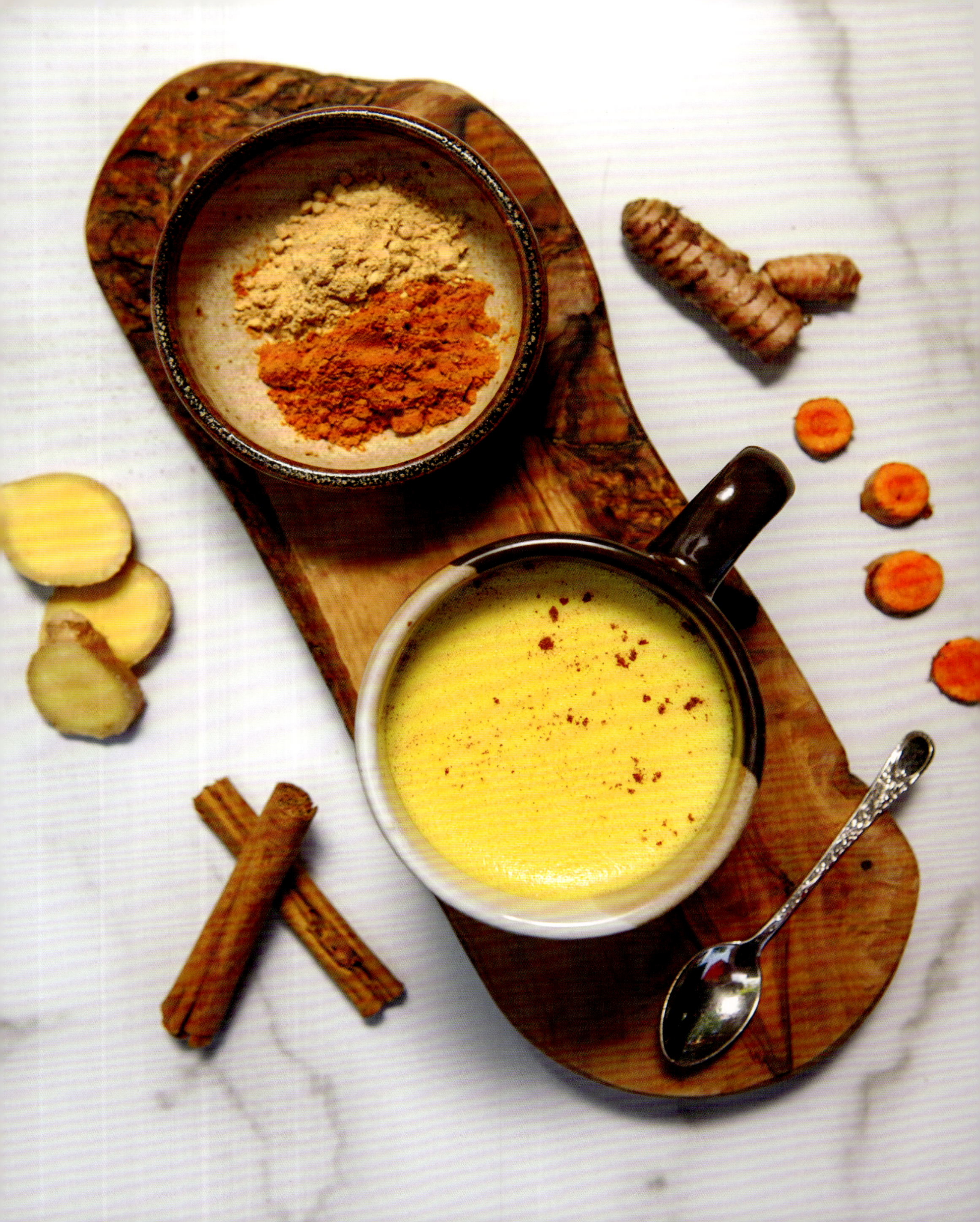

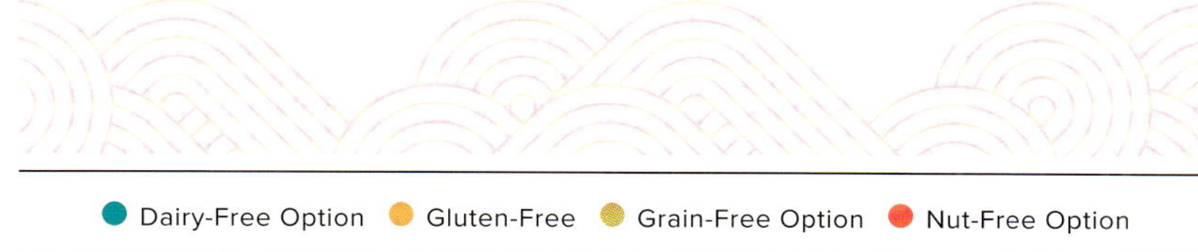

● Dairy-Free Option ● Gluten-Free ● Grain-Free Option ● Nut-Free Option

Golden Milk Latte

Soothing, warming, and nutrient-rich, this latte is the perfect addition to your evening routine, especially if falling asleep is getting harder or getting hungry occurs more frequently late at night. To get the most out of the beneficial health properties of turmeric, don't skip the coconut oil or pepper — they help your body absorb as much curcumin as possible (curcumin is the main medicinal component of turmeric).

5 MINUTES PREPPING • 5 MINUTES COOKING • MAKES 1 LARGE LATTE

WHAT YOU NEED:	HOW TO MAKE IT:
2 cups (500 mL) milk of choice (I like coconut milk best) ½ to 1 tbsp (7 to 15 mL) coconut oil ½ tbsp (7 mL) honey 1 tsp (5 mL) ground turmeric ¼ tsp (1 mL) ground ginger ¼ tsp (1 mL) cinnamon Pinch of pepper	1. Add all ingredients to a small saucepan and whisk to combine while bringing the latte to a slow simmer. Continue to whisk, about 2 to 3 more minutes, until silky and hot. 2. Remove from heat and enjoy.

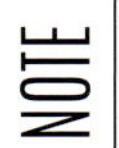

NOTE: If you're using a low-fat milk, you'll likely want to use the full tbsp of coconut oil for a satisfying and creamy latte.

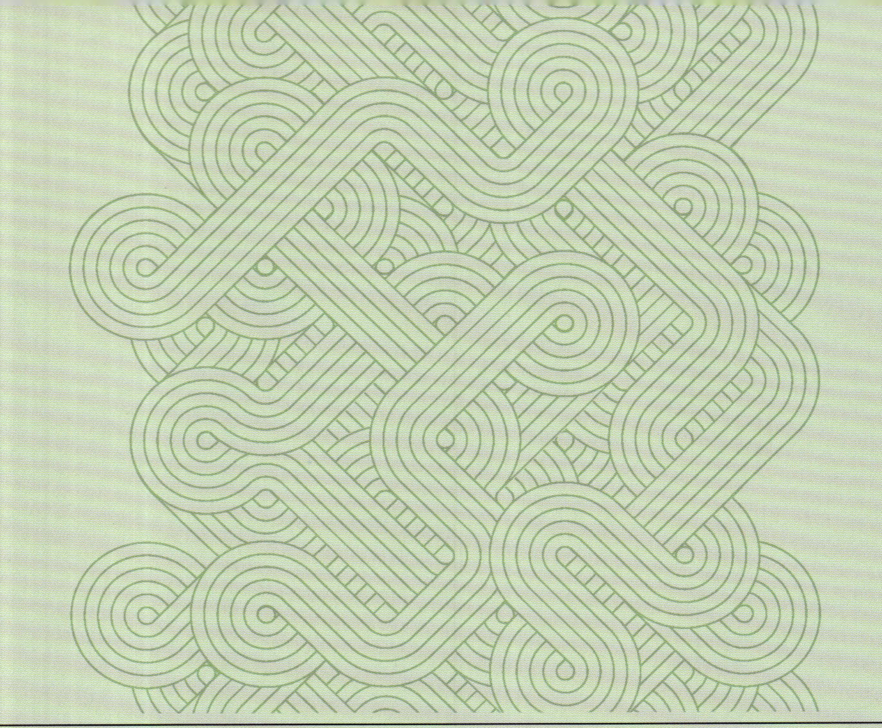

TRIMESTER 4: POSTPARTUM

(BABY'S HERE)

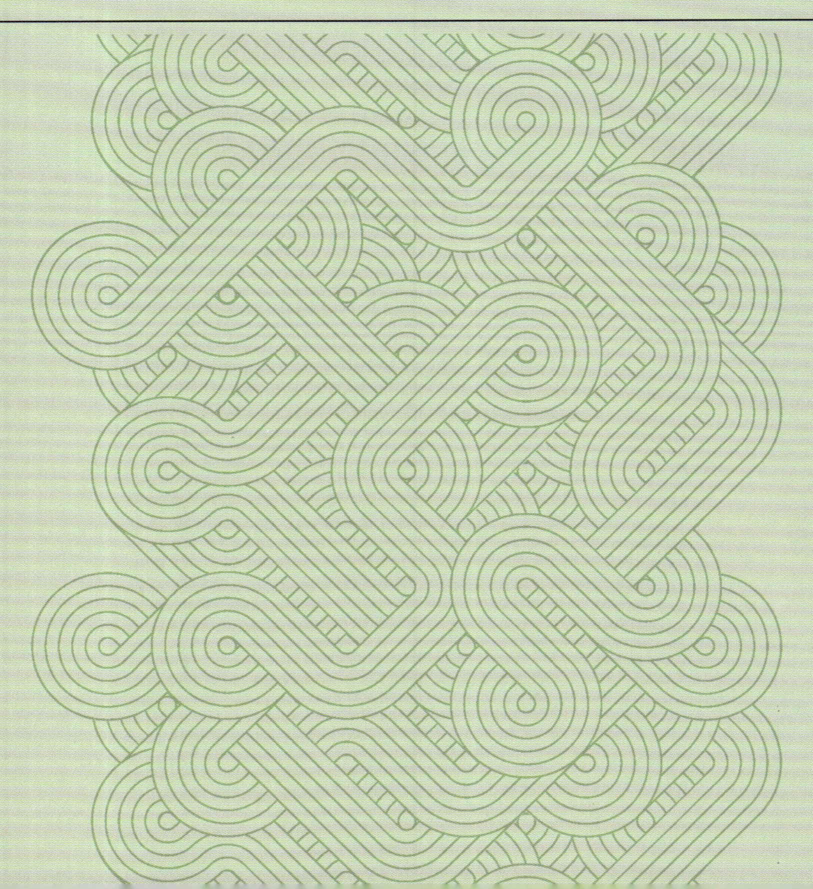

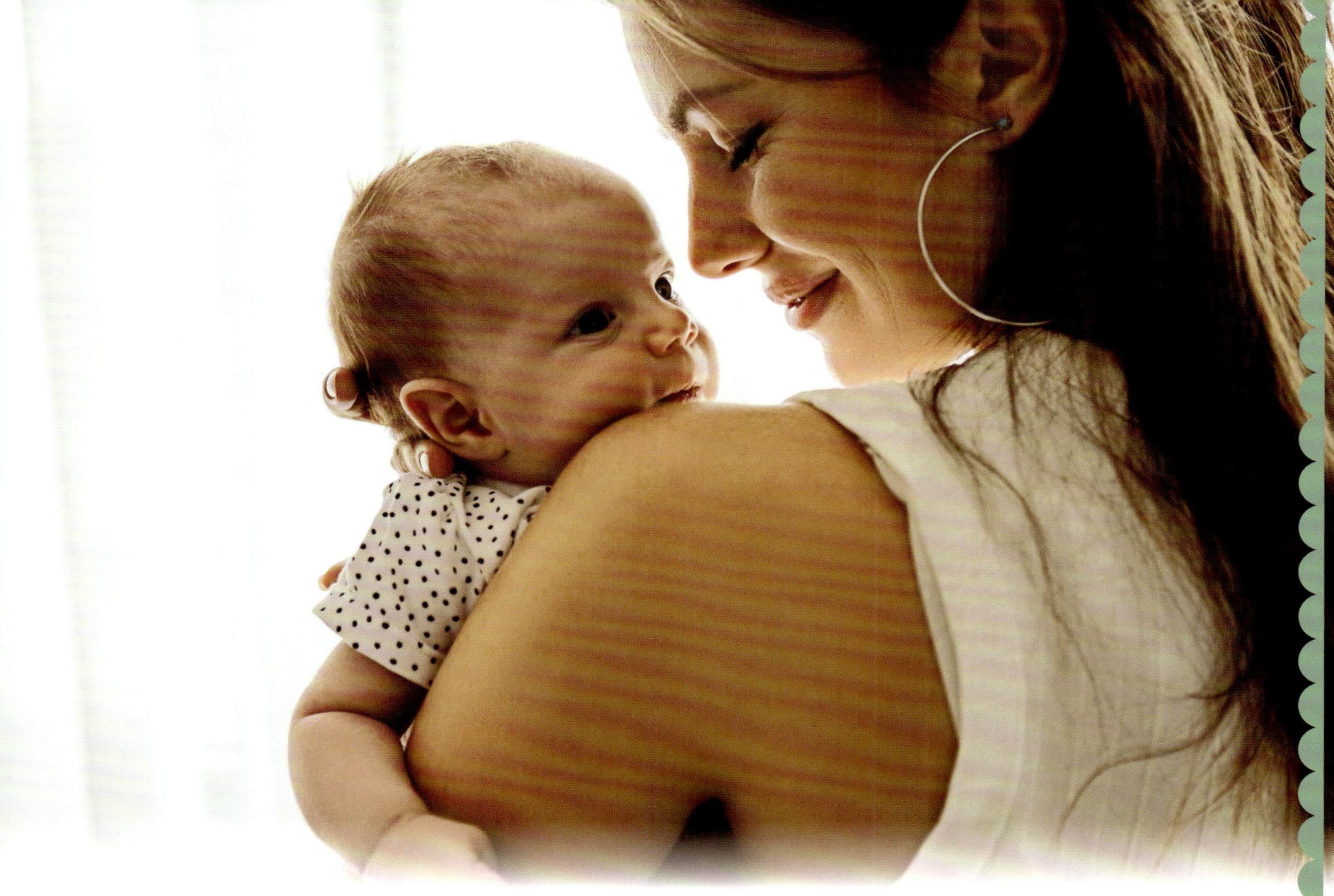

YOU MATTER *too*

YOU DID IT, MAMA!

You got through nine months of physical transformation and emotional turmoil, and you brought a baby into this world.

Now that baby is here (or babies as the case may be), attention is showered on your little one. Of course, baby deserves it. The birth of a baby is one of life's most important events, but so is being a new mom. You merit the same love, comfort, and care being showered on your baby. After going through a major life-changing experience, your body is now shifting to postpartum mode — producing breast milk, shrinking the uterus back to size, adjusting to changes in hormones, and managing new demands on your energy.

As a postpartum doula, I know that you need to heal from the physical strains of childbirth, have sufficient sleep, and eat well. In this postnatal period, you deserve more attention and support than ever before. So, rest and nest, take care of yourself, eat nourishing food, regain your health, and enjoy mothering.

Postpartum Self-Care

New motherhood can be overwhelming. and how you feel matters. That's why postpartum self-care is just as important as mothering. Your health and well-being are a priority — the better you feel, the more you'll be able to adjust and thrive in your new role. Postpartum self-care involves taking time to recover — with nourishing meals, rest, support, and fresh air — and giving yourself permission to nest, which could mean:

- Not returning to your usual routine right away
- Easing up on laundry, cleaning, and cooking
- Ignoring other people's expectations of you
- Staying in bed, napping and resting, and taking frequent breaks during the day
- Dealing with uncomfortable emotions your way (it's okay to be sad, disappointed, frustrated, or to miss your old life — this doesn't mean you love your baby any less, it just makes you human)

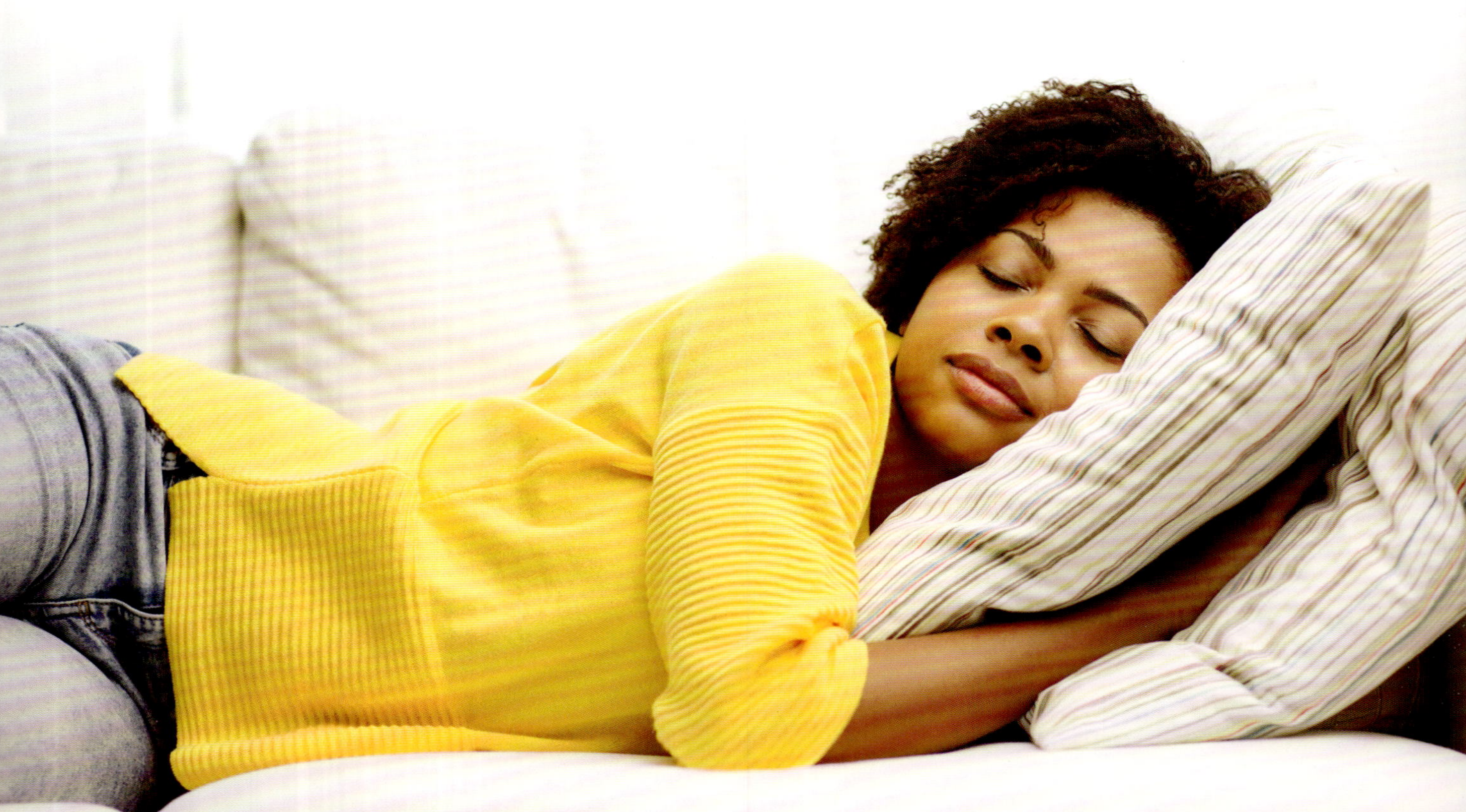

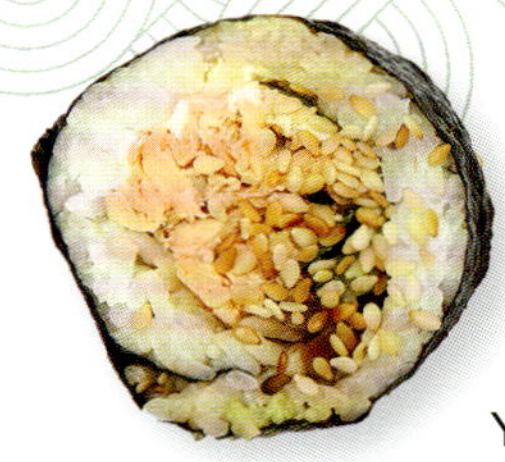

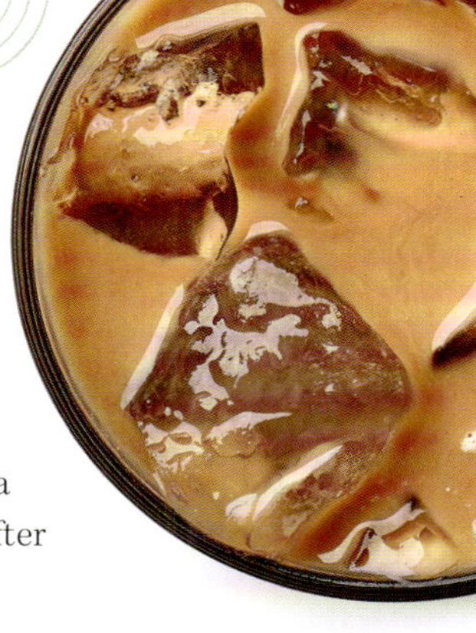

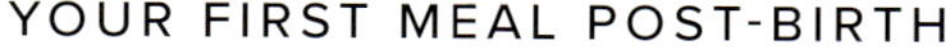

YOUR FIRST MEAL POST-BIRTH

For your first meal after giving birth — eat whatever you like! If there's something that you've been craving or a first meal that you've been dreaming about — have that. Ask a partner or loved one to make it or go pick it up. Toast and tea will work too — just remember to have a larger meal soon after because you'll need the energy.

Here's a tip for you: Have that much-craved meal with a large drink and a side of fibre. Add some veggies, greens, or berries. Why? Because you really, really, really don't want to get constipated. Have some fibre on the first day postpartum, get your system rolling again, and you'll be thankful you did.

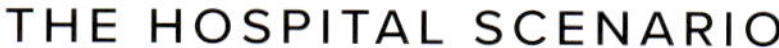

THE HOSPITAL SCENARIO

Not all new moms get to go home soon after baby is born. It might be, for a variety of reasons, that baby and/or mom need a longer stay in the hospital post-birth. If this is the case, it would be ideal if the hospital offers healthy, delicious meals to support a new mom's recovery. However, it is more likely that hospital food may not be as nutritious as you'd like.

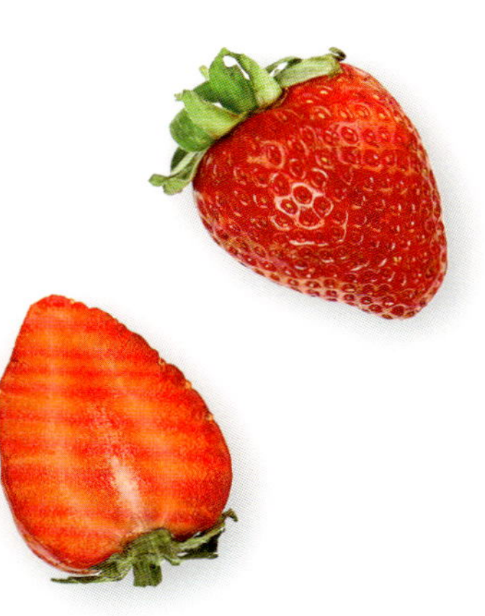

Here are some ideas for keeping you (and your family) nourished and well-fed when you need to extend your stay in the hospital:

- Supplement hospital food with bone broth, brought from home in an insulated container (a useful tip is making broth in advance and storing it in individual glass jars in the freezer). Broth is the first food I'd recommend making prior to baby's birth.
- Have friends or family members bring you meals or snacks from outside the hospital, whether home-cooked or purchased from a store or restaurant. Fresh fruit is always good for you.
- If you have other kids, consider asking your parents, family members, or friends to drop off dinners or lunch-box staples for your family at home. This will be a big relief for you.

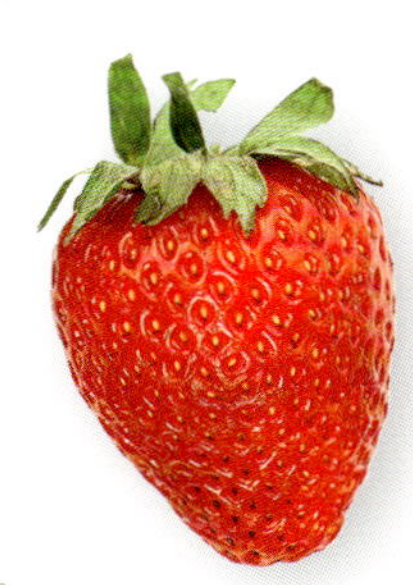

Postpartum Nourishment

There's not much left in the tank! The nutrient depletion that happens during pregnancy is one of the reasons that feeding a new mom nourishing and nutrient-rich meals is so important in all cultures.

Food plays many important roles post-birth:

- It replenishes the energy and nutrient stores that were depleted during your pregnancy.
- It supplies the building blocks for healing and tissue repair that take place after birth.
- It can provide emotional comfort.
- It gives your body the energy and nutrients it needs for the production of breast milk.
- It is a time-honoured way to show love and kindness to someone who has just delivered a baby.

Postpartum nourishment is not about "getting your body back" (a body you never lost, by the way) or supporting breastfeeding (all moms deserve good nourishing food whether they are breastfeeding, pumping, or formula feeding).

As a new mom, you need to be eating and drinking enough to support the healthy functioning of your body and mind. Nothing will drain you faster than attempting to function in a sleep-deprived state with no energy in the tank.

Grabbing something easy and eating what you can with one hand while baby naps on your chest is real-life postpartum. It can also be easy to forget to eat, especially when you don't feel up to cooking or even walking to the refrigerator. If you find yourself forgetting to eat, not having time to eat, or always in search of a meal or snack, now is the time to get help.

Accept help, even if it is baby 2, 3, 4, or 10. You *can* do all of the things you used to do, but now is the time to channel your energy to resting, recovering, and mothering your infant. A friend or family member can help you stay healthy and nourished by prepping and cooking you some meals or by holding baby while you eat a full meal and have a moment to yourself. If you don't have support people around, it may be worthwhile to consider the support of a postpartum doula, an in-home cook, or a meal delivery service. Any of these options is a short-term investment with big payout to your health and well-being.

Nutrient status of a new mom

How does a low nutrient supply make you feel? Probably extra tired, foggy-brained, and a little overwhelmed and frustrated. The good news is that eating a wide variety of nutrient-dense food will top up your tank and increase your energy level, speed up your healing, support breastfeeding, and possibly protect you against perinatal mood disorders such as postpartum depression.

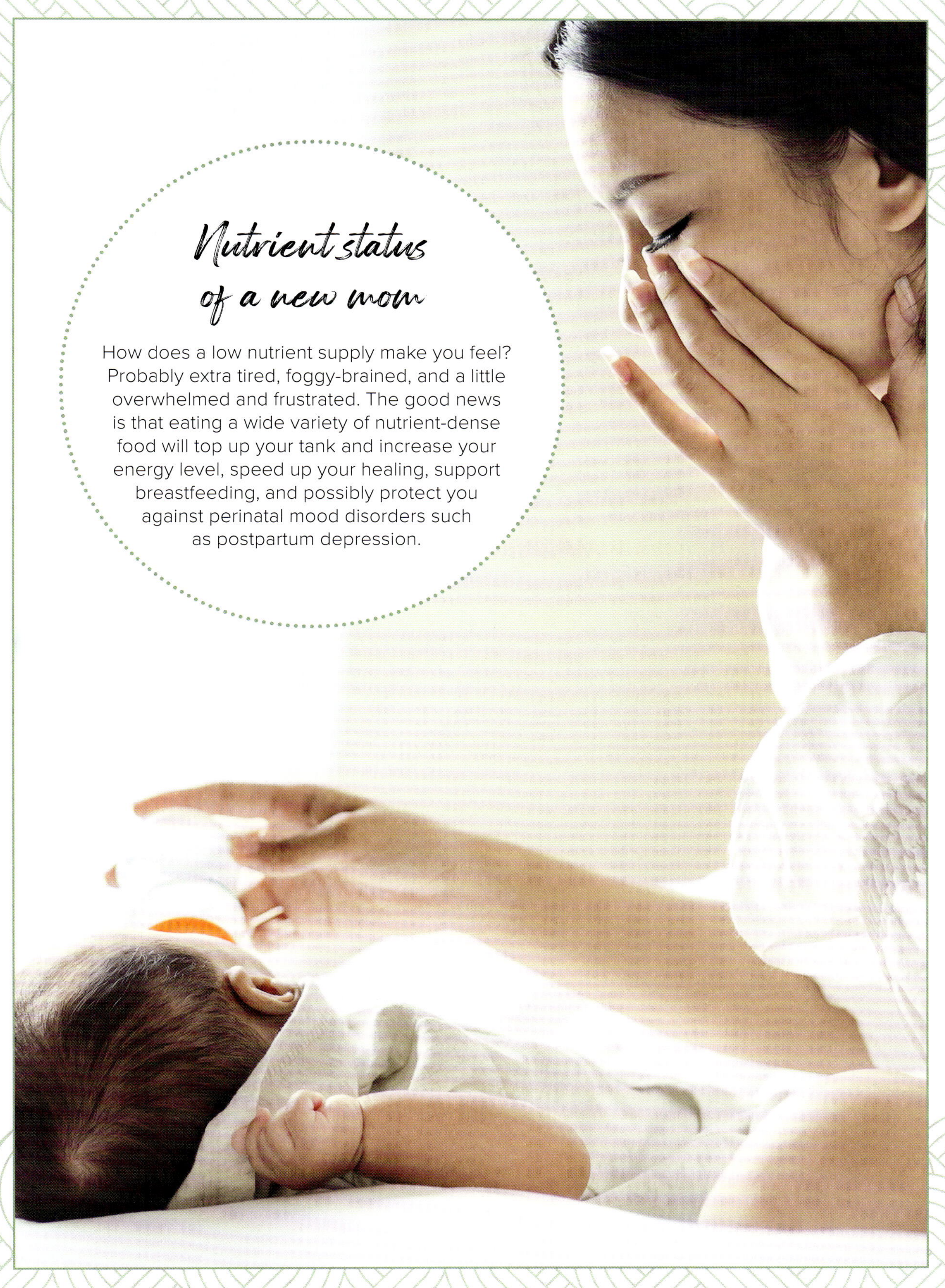

Healing Traditions

There is general consensus that it's important to nourish a mother back to health after she has given birth. Worldwide, there are many cultural traditions for how to nourish the new mom after childbirth. Countries and cultures vary on what healing foods and drinks are, but many of them agree on this: *Warm, liquid-based meals (soups, stews, and broths) are ideal for new mothers.*

Soups, stews, porridges, broths, congee, and other liquid-heavy meals are comforting and provide much-needed hydration and electrolyte replenishment for both recovery and milk production. Warm soupy meals also include cooked, soft veggies and meat. These foods are easy on your digestive system. They allow your body to absorb the nutrients effortlessly and to focus its energy on healing and recovery.

BROTH IT

Broth-based meals are also powerhouses of nutrition and contain exactly the types of nutrients your body needs to heal. When a broth is made by slowly simmering bones, the minerals, gelatin, collagen, and amino acids from the connective tissues infuse into the broth. When your body tissues are stressed or impaired from giving birth, these are the exact ingredients they need to repair and rebuild.

After childbirth, you may have a weakened pelvic floor or a sluggish digestive system, which can make constipation even more uncomfortable. Warm, soupy meals help your digestive system to bounce back, and the servings of broth, veggies, and legumes provide the hydration and fibre you need.

These meals are not only nourishing but also easy to make. Soups, stews, and broths can all be made ahead of time, kept in the freezer, and defrosted as needed. These meals are also ideal for friends and family to make and drop off, fresh. They can be stored for a week in the refrigerator, and you can have your support person heat some up when you're hungry. Keeping an insulated container full of hot broth at your bedside is a wonderful idea. The broth will help to keep you hydrated and satiated, and it's packed with nutrients that you need.

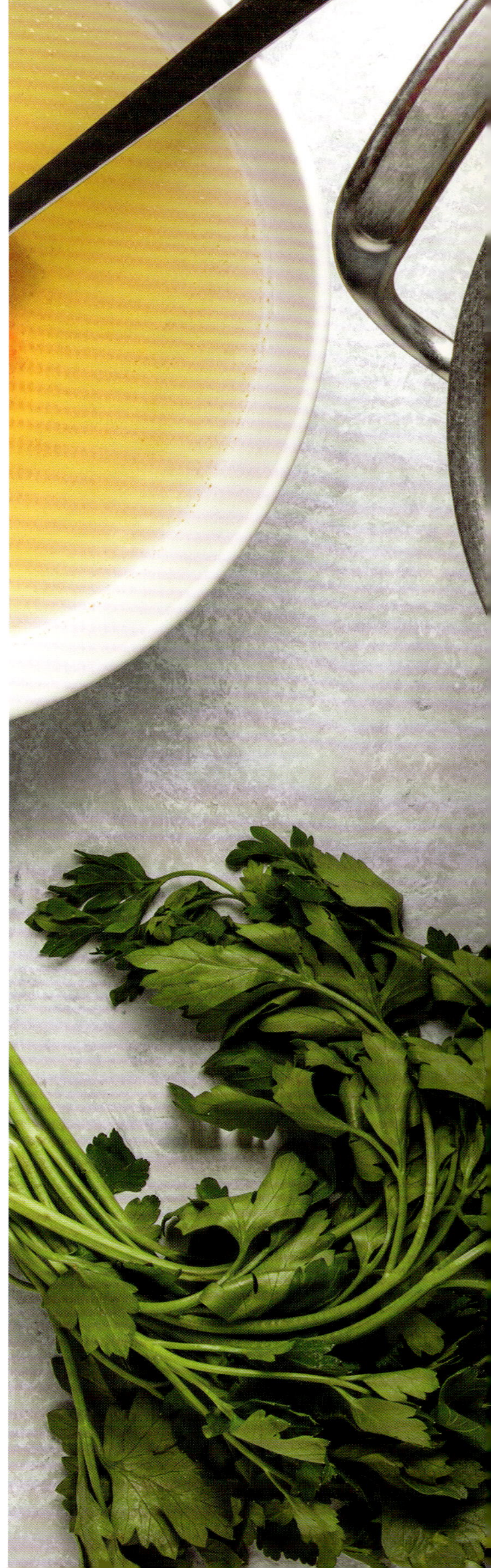

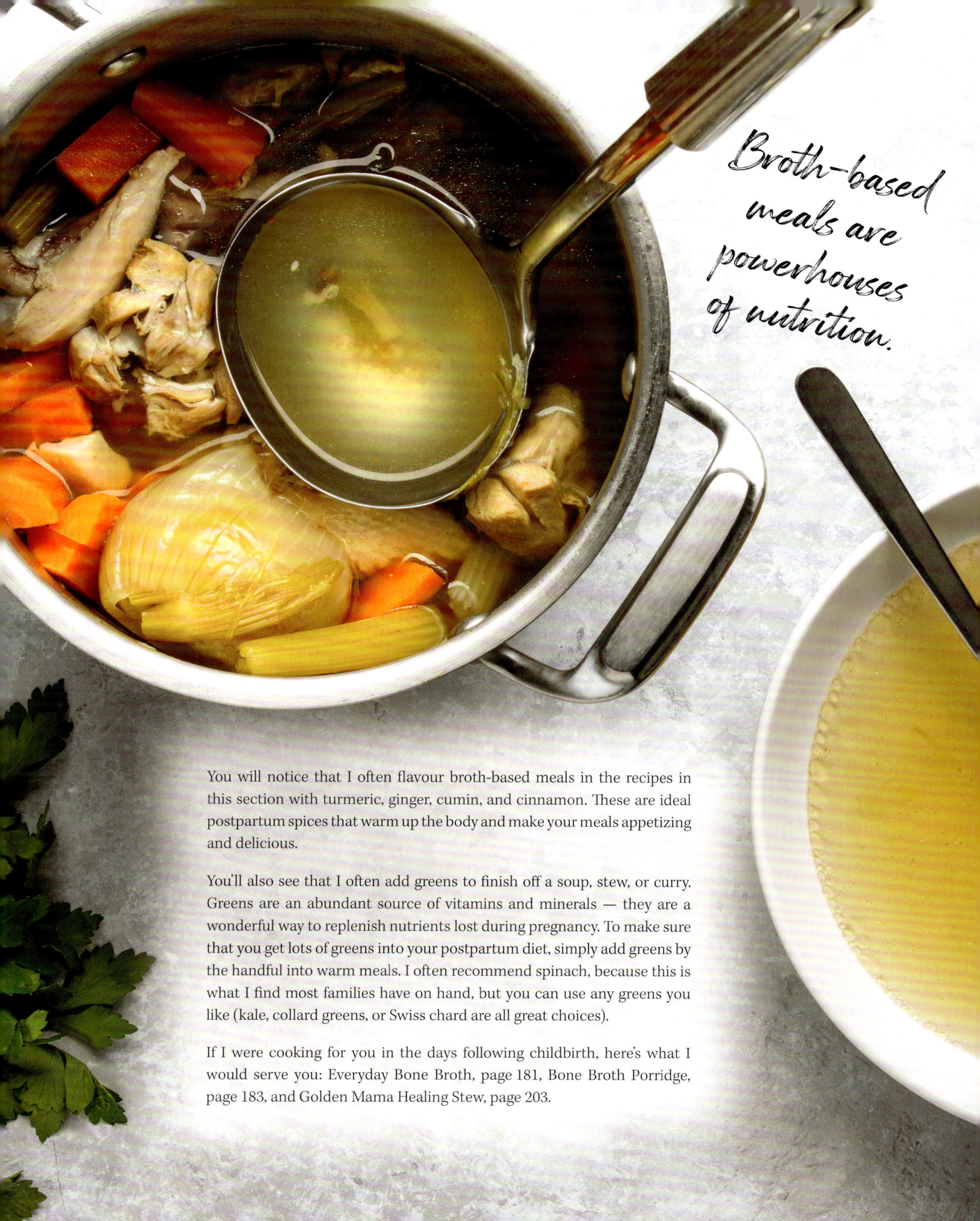

You will notice that I often flavour broth-based meals in the recipes in this section with turmeric, ginger, cumin, and cinnamon. These are ideal postpartum spices that warm up the body and make your meals appetizing and delicious.

You'll also see that I often add greens to finish off a soup, stew, or curry. Greens are an abundant source of vitamins and minerals — they are a wonderful way to replenish nutrients lost during pregnancy. To make sure that you get lots of greens into your postpartum diet, simply add greens by the handful into warm meals. I often recommend spinach, because this is what I find most families have on hand, but you can use any greens you like (kale, collard greens, or Swiss chard are all great choices).

If I were cooking for you in the days following childbirth, here's what I would serve you: Everyday Bone Broth, page 181, Bone Broth Porridge, page 183, and Golden Mama Healing Stew, page 203.

Foods That Support Postpartum Healing

Post-birth healing is hugely supported by the foods you eat, especially those rich in protein, fat, and iron. As you know by now, bone broth (and meals made with it) is my top postpartum pick because it's rich in collagen-forming amino acids that support tissue healing (as are meals made from bone-in meats such as pulled pork or chicken thighs). Animal products are also high on the list of postpartum healing foods because they are rich in protein and iron. Childbirth involves blood loss, even if it is natural and goes smoothly. Iron replenishes the blood in your body by supporting your body to make red blood cells.

PUMP UP IRON AND PROTEIN

Red meat, poultry, legumes, spinach, and seeds are all excellent sources of iron, which will not only support healing but also increase your postpartum energy levels by helping to replenish your iron stores (iron deficiency is common by the time the third trimester rolls around). Pair iron-rich foods with those high in vitamin C (bell peppers, citrus, sweet potatoes, broccoli, and strawberries). Vitamin C, in addition to being crucial for wound healing, helps your body absorb iron.

Protein is your body's building block for tissue repair.

Protein is your body's building block for tissue repair. Remember that lesson in gym class about how a protein-rich meal after exercise helps muscles to rebuild and get stronger? The same idea applies after childbirth. Protein is key, so carry on incorporating your favourite protein-rich staples into your meals, whether those are animal sources or vegetarian.

And don't forget the fat — fat supports healing by helping your body absorb nutrients and store crucial energy that you need.

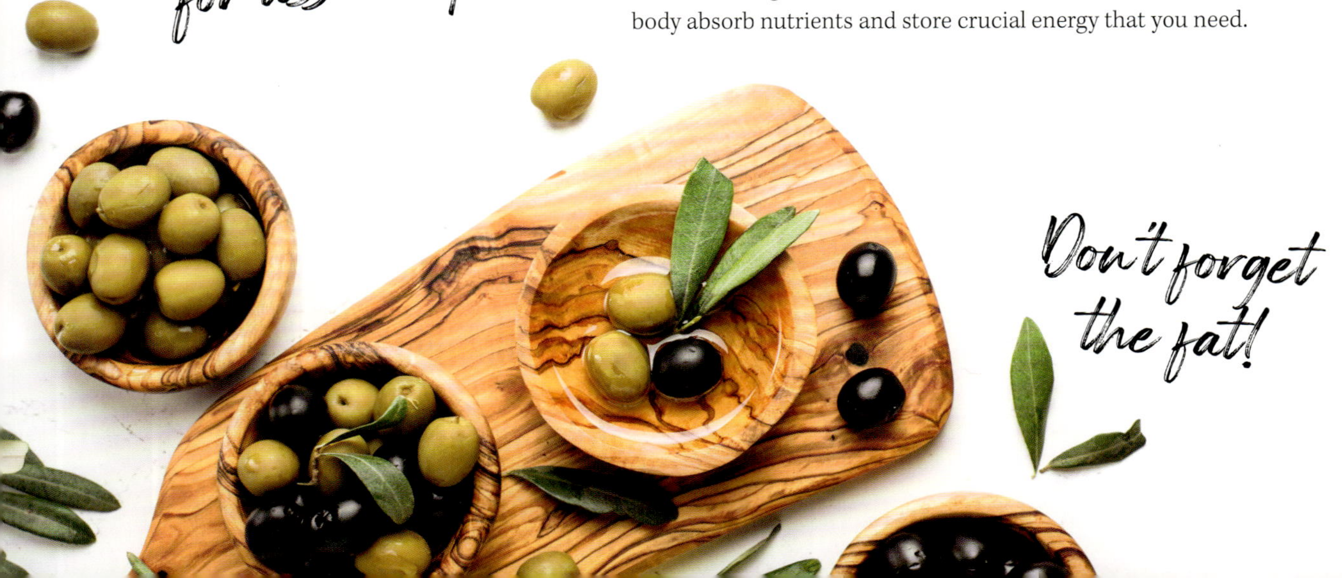

Don't forget the fat!

KEEP DRINKING

Staying hydrated is crucial for healing too. The feeling of thirst is actually your body alerting you to get more liquid into your system, which is especially important after childbirth.

Drinking enough water can help you feel less fatigued, cloudy-brained, irritable, and confused. It can help you regulate your mood, control your body temperature, and keep your gastrointestinal system functioning efficiently. Have your favourite water bottle with you all the time. Also keep in mind that there are other options — bone broth, teas, smoothies, ice infusions, and smoothie pops can help you stay hydrated. So can lots of fruit and vegetables.

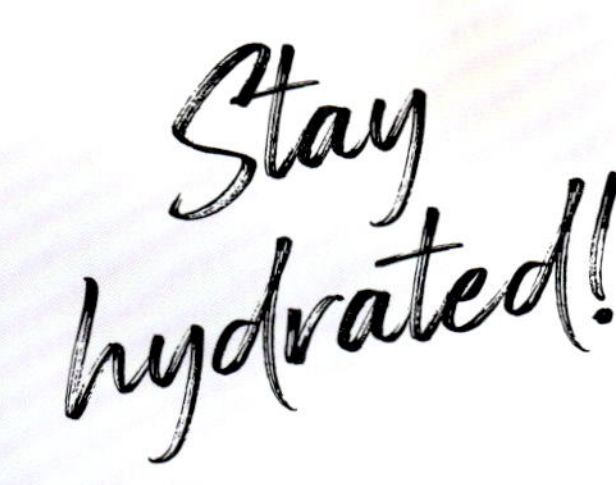

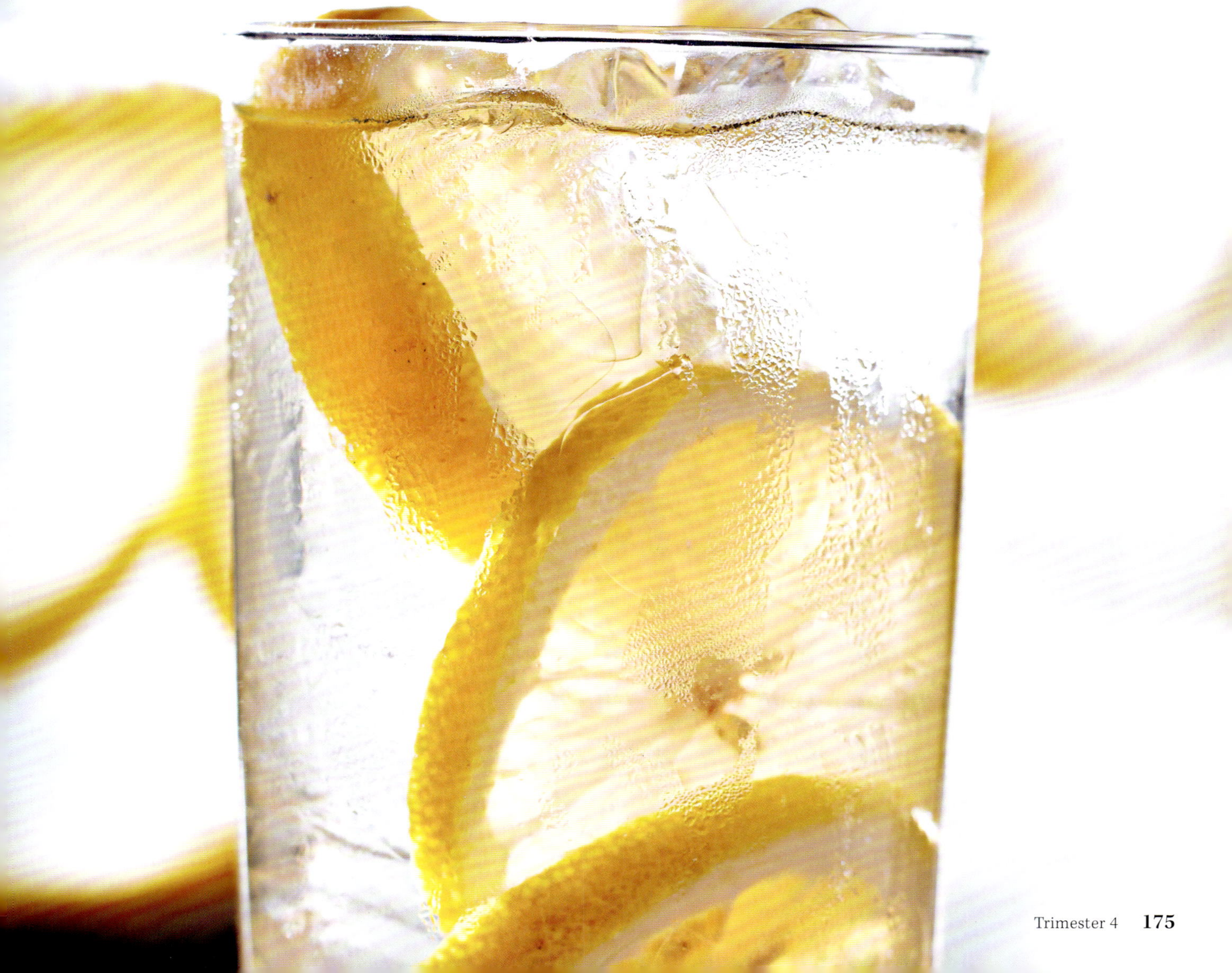

Foods That Support Breastfeeding

Here's a look at how food and nutrition can support breastfeeding — producing milk, optimizing its nutrition, and learning how foods and herbs can help with milk supply. But take note of this: *The most important thing for a postpartum breastfeeding diet isn't a supplement, a herb, or oats. It's straight-up calories (and water).*

MILK SUPPLY

Eating enough food, no matter what that food is, and drinking enough water are the most important things you can do to support your milk supply. Yes, you do need more calories while breastfeeding than you do during pregnancy. Now's not the time to eat less (so try to ignore messages about postpartum weight loss and diets). It is in fact a time to eat more — which is why I've included so many simple meals and nutrient-dense snacks to make in the early days postpartum.

And this is key: Eat intuitively and follow your hunger cues. Trust your body! If you find yourself always hungry, eat more food and increase your fat intake. You can do this simply by adding a splash of olive oil, a sliced avocado, a scoop of coconut oil or ghee, or nuts and seeds to your meals.

GALACTAGOGUES

You have likely heard of galactagogues — a group of drugs, herbs, and foods thought to induce or boost milk supply. Galactagogues are thought to work by stimulating the hormones involved in lactation. They have become increasingly popular among women when first-line remedies such as pumping or feeding more frequently (and getting in enough food and water) haven't increased milk supply sufficiently.

Pharmaceutical galactagogues require a prescription. It's best to discuss these with a healthcare professional.

Herbal galactagogues are herbs in supplement form, taken in amounts much higher than what's used in culinary applications (such as tea or baked goods). Popular herbal supplements include blessed thistle, fenugreek, fennel, alfalfa, marshmallow root, and goat's rue. If you'd like to try out herbal galactagogues in supplement form, talk to a qualified healthcare professional.

Culinary galactagogues are the herbs and foods used in smaller amounts to make teas, meals, and snacks. Popular culinary galactagogues include teas with herbs such as fenugreek and fennel, and meals and snacks made with oats, flax, almonds, ginger, garlic, cilantro, cumin, and hops. Check out the Little Lactation Cookies on page 201, and brew yourself some warming Ginger Tea with Fennel + Goji Berries on page 193.

NUTRIENT-RICH BREAST MILK

The food you eat not only helps you meet energy requirements for breast milk production but may actually contribute toward making breast milk more nutrient-rich. The amount of some vitamins and minerals in breast milk appears to be related to mom's dietary intake. What a good reason to prioritize eating healthy, nourishing food!

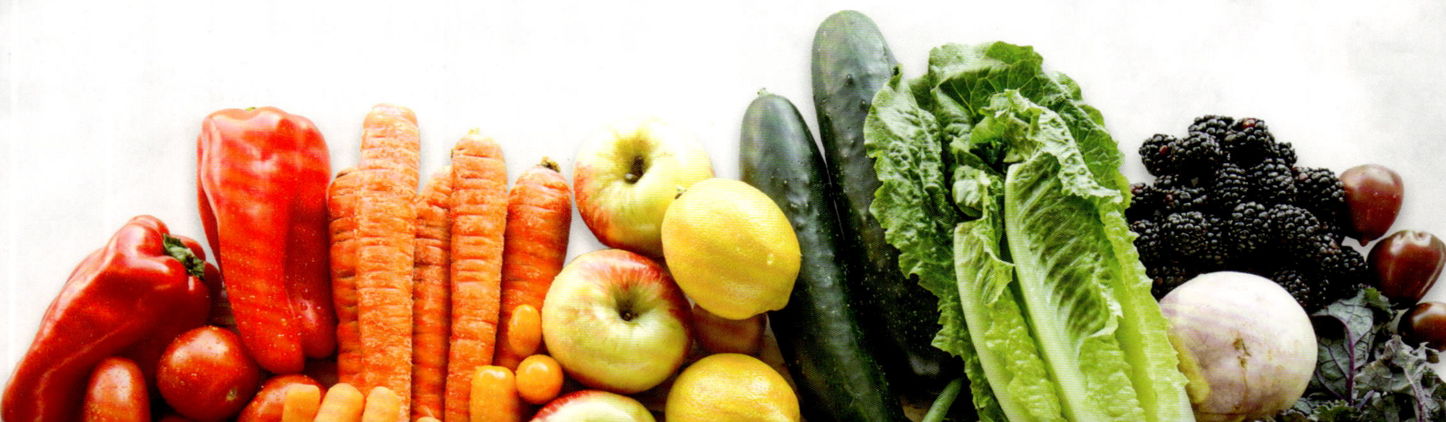

Salmon is an excellent source of DHA.

Want to give your milk a boost? Start with DHA (the important omega-3 fatty acid) and vitamin B12. Research shows that breastfeeding mothers who regularly eat foods high in DHA have higher levels of DHA in their breast milk, increasing what's available to support baby's brain development. The absolute best food source of DHA is fatty fish such as salmon.

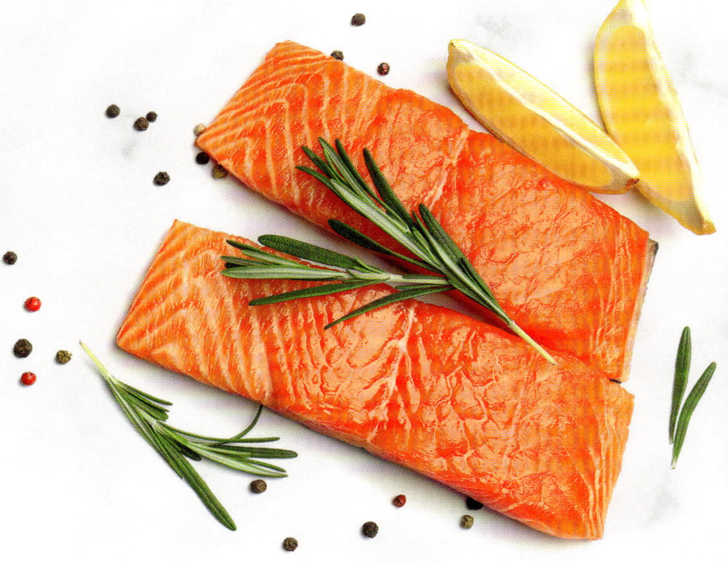

Vitamin B12 is another nutrient crucial for infant neurological development. Natural food sources of vitamin B12 are almost exclusively found in animal products including meat, dairy, and eggs, which is another reason why animal proteins are high on my list of excellent postpartum foods. The amount of B12 you consume may directly affect the amount of B12 in your breast milk. If you're a vegetarian or vegan, talk to a healthcare professional if you're considering a supplement.

Foods for Good Mood

Certain nutrients are essential for our nervous system and mood regulation. Nutrient deficiencies in the body brought on through pregnancy and breastfeeding may make some postpartum moms more likely to experience perinatal mood disorders, which can come up at any time in the first year after baby's birth.

Research is ongoing, but the reports we do have suggest that certain nutrients, namely fatty acids (DHA, omega-3 fatty acids, and a low omega-6 to omega-3 ratio), vitamin D, zinc, and possibly other minerals such as selenium and calcium can protect against postpartum depression. Studies have found that mothers with higher levels of these nutrients are less likely to experience perinatal mood disorders.

If that sounds overwhelming, know that eating a variety of colourful, wholesome foods is likely sufficient to get in those essential fats, vitamins, and minerals. In fact, several studies have looked at the impact of an overall "healthy" diet compared to one that is more processed and have found a healthy diet to be protective against postpartum depression. Adding a fish oil or a vitamin D supplement to your diet may be something of interest, but do consult a healthcare professional for personal advice.

Of course, experiencing perinatal mood disorders does not mean you are not eating healthfully enough. We have yet to fully understand how nutrients interact with the hormonal changes, lifestyle changes, and complex biochemical processes going on in the body of a postpartum mom. For now — it's food for thought. There's never a bad reason for nourishing yourself with wholesome, real food.

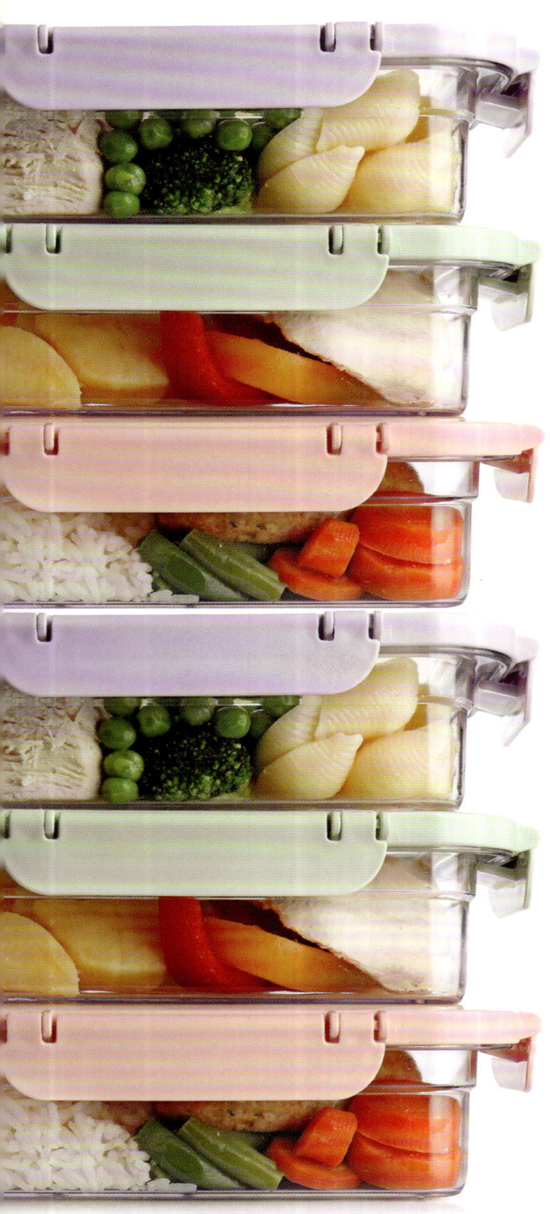

Postpartum Meal Guidelines

Beyond the beneficial impact that nutrition can have on postpartum life, the reality is that food preparation — shopping for groceries, figuring out what to eat, prepping ingredients, and cooking meals — can cause stress in a household with a newborn. Below are my four top meal guidelines to help make the postpartum period a more positive and less challenging experience.

- **A little prep goes a long way.**

  Have a baby-prep cooking weekend before baby's arrival, as described on page 126, so that freezer meals can make up a large portion of your meal plan for the first little while or can be a support as needed, depending on the help you have.

- **Cook once, eat more.**

  Meals should be batch-friendly and freezer-friendly. The energy and effort put into making a meal should pay off two- or three-fold so that cooking needs to be done only every few days. Consider doubling any recipe you make (or someone else makes for you) so that half of it can be put away in the freezer.

- **Food gets priority on your postpartum wish list.**

  If you're getting comfortable asking for help and letting loved ones know how they can be of support, ask for food. It could be groceries, prepped meals, or even better than that — a meal train organized by a friend, involving friends who rotate and bring you meals from week to week.

- **Stock up on snacks.**

  In the early postpartum days in order to eat, you need food you can just grab. I'm a big fan of having homemade snacks always available. Oat bars, muffins, energy balls, chia puddings, or granola in the house make nutritious snacking easy. Check out the recipes for these snacks in this book.

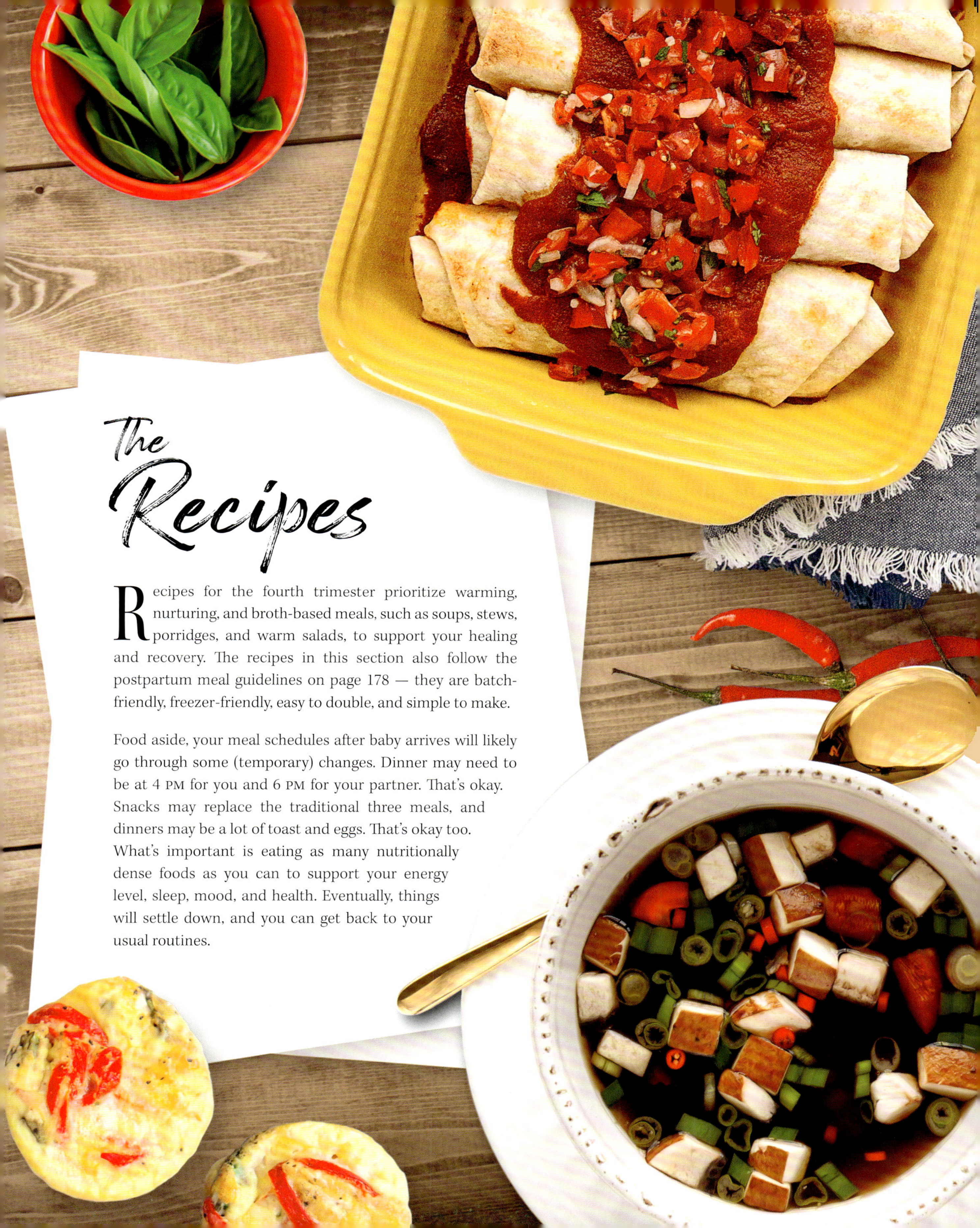

The Recipes

Recipes for the fourth trimester prioritize warming, nurturing, and broth-based meals, such as soups, stews, porridges, and warm salads, to support your healing and recovery. The recipes in this section also follow the postpartum meal guidelines on page 178 — they are batch-friendly, freezer-friendly, easy to double, and simple to make.

Food aside, your meal schedules after baby arrives will likely go through some (temporary) changes. Dinner may need to be at 4 PM for you and 6 PM for your partner. That's okay. Snacks may replace the traditional three meals, and dinners may be a lot of toast and eggs. That's okay too. What's important is eating as many nutritionally dense foods as you can to support your energy level, sleep, mood, and health. Eventually, things will settle down, and you can get back to your usual routines.

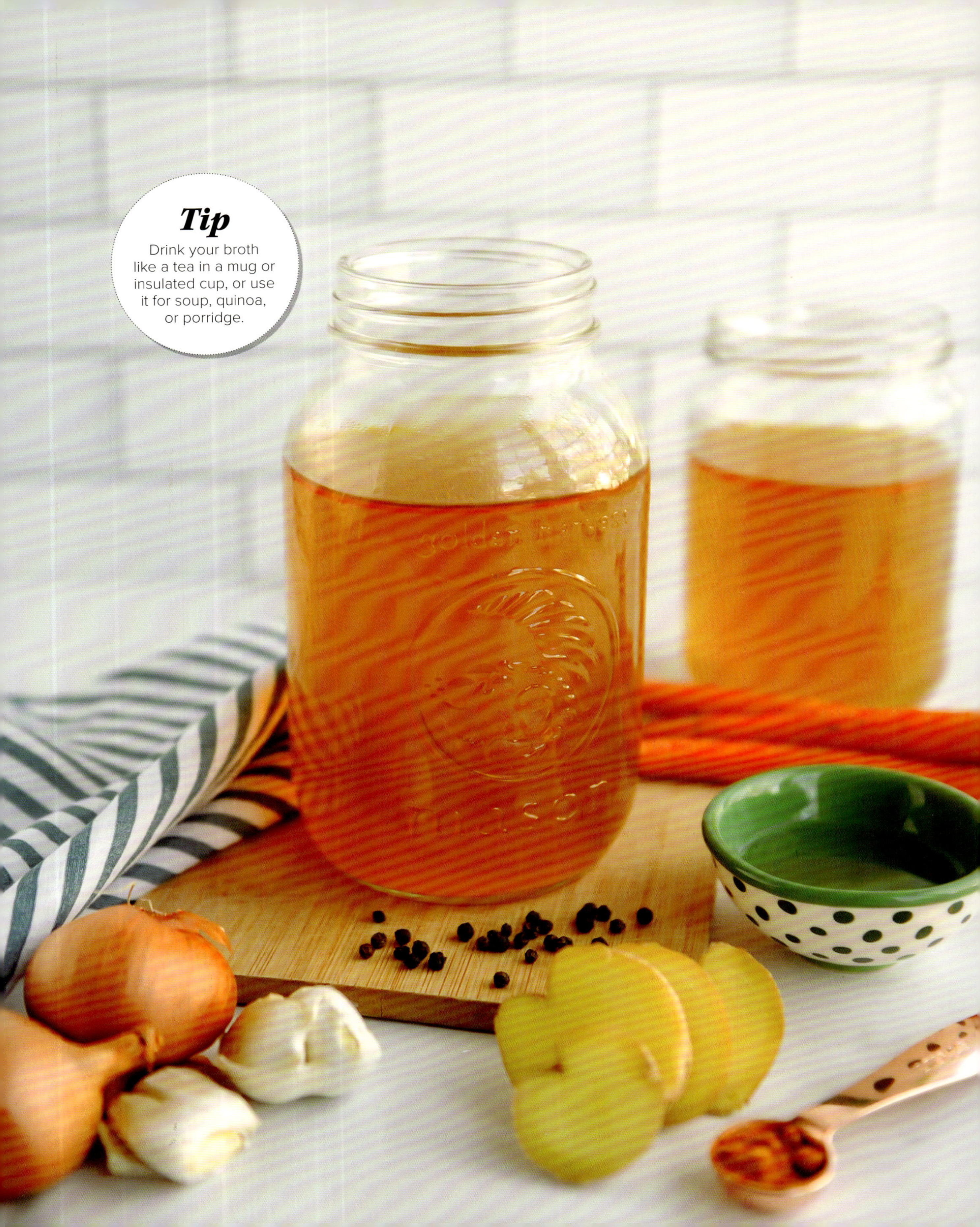

Tip

Drink your broth like a tea in a mug or insulated cup, or use it for soup, quinoa, or porridge.

Dairy-Free · Gluten-Free · Grain-Free · Nut-Free · Freezer-Friendly

Everyday Bone Broth

Bone broth is a postpartum healing tonic — one that I wish would be served to new mothers after delivery as hospital policy. When bones are simmered over a long time with a bit of acid, easily absorbable minerals and amino acids such as the collagen-forming gelatin infuse into the broth. All those minerals mean bone broth is like an electrolyte replacement beverage — without the food colouring.

I often roast a chicken once a week and save the bones for this broth. Although this recipe calls for chicken bones, you can substitute with beef, pork, turkey, or fish bones. A favourite is beef marrow bones, which can be roasted before being added to the pot or slow cooker.

5 MINUTES PREPPING • 24 HOURS COOKING • MAKES 3 TO 5 LARGE JARS

WHAT YOU NEED:

1 to 3 organic chicken carcasses

1 onion, skin removed and roughly chopped

6 garlic cloves, peeled

1-inch (2.5-cm) piece ginger, peeled and sliced

1 tbsp (15 mL) apple cider vinegar

Pinch of peppercorns

Water

Optional

Peeled and roughly chopped carrots, mushrooms, leftover herbs, and a tsp (5 mL) of turmeric or a small handful of goji berries for colour and an anti-inflammatory boost

HOW TO MAKE IT:

1. In a large pot or slow cooker, add the bones and cover with water. Add the onion, garlic, ginger, apple cider vinegar, peppercorns, and any other optional ingredients you have on hand.
2. Turn slow cooker to low or burner to medium and bring to a simmer. Skim off any foam that floats to the surface. Let broth simmer gently for about 24 hours on low heat.
3. When you're done simmering your broth, remove all bones/veggies and strain. Here's how I do it: First, put a large bowl (or your compost bag/bin) on the counter. Using tongs, remove as much of the bones/veggies as you can and place in the bowl/bag. Then, set up several large glass jars on the counter. One at a time, place a funnel in a glass jar, then place a fine-mesh sieve on top. Using a soup ladle, transfer the broth into the jar (any remaining pieces will stay on your sieve and can be discarded into your bowl/bag), stopping when you're 1 inch (2.5 cm) from the top.
4. Let broth cool on the counter, then move to refrigerator. When cold, transfer any broth you aren't planning on using right away to the freezer.

Link-up

Bone broth is excellent for these other recipes in this book: **Bone Broth Porridge**, **Golden Mama Healing Stew**, and **Rosemary Chicken Noodle Soup**.

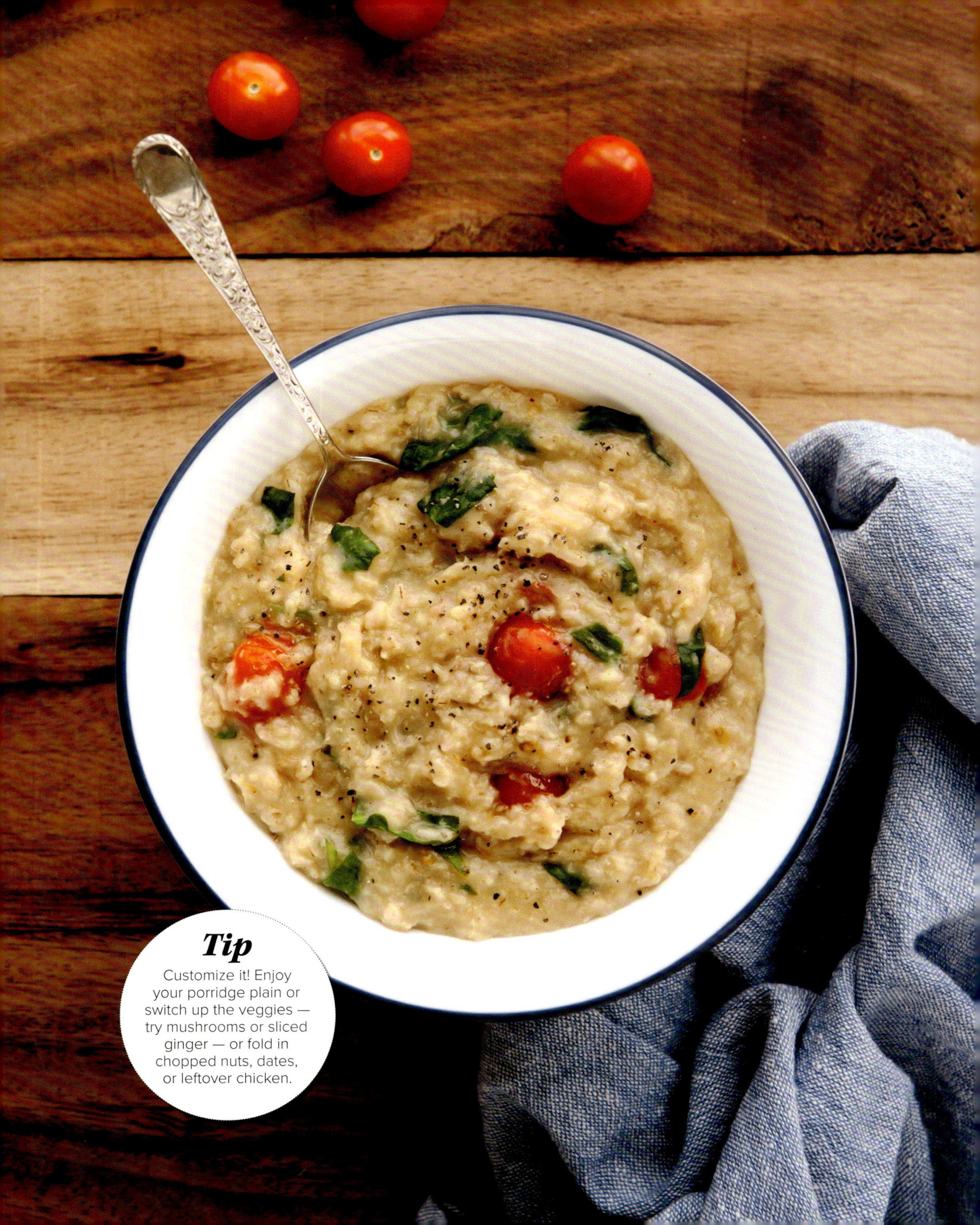

Tip

Customize it! Enjoy your porridge plain or switch up the veggies — try mushrooms or sliced ginger — or fold in chopped nuts, dates, or leftover chicken.

● Gluten-Free ● Nut-Free

Bone Broth Porridge with Cherry Tomatoes + Greens

Porridge made with bone broth is warming and comforting, and it provides replenishment to support recovery and milk production. Enjoy this simple porridge, anyway you like it, in the days following baby's birth. It's gentle on your digestive system and helps your body to focus its energy on healing.

5 MINUTES PREPPING • 10 MINUTES COOKING • MAKES 2 SERVINGS

WHAT YOU NEED:

- 1 tbsp (15 mL) ghee/grass-fed butter
- 1 shallot, thinly sliced
- ½ cup (125 mL) cherry tomatoes, halved
- ½ cup (125 mL) baby spinach, roughly chopped or torn
- 2 cups (500 mL) bone broth (Everyday Bone Broth, page 181, or store-bought)
- 1 cup (250 mL) rolled oats
- ¼ tsp (1 mL) cumin
- ¼ tsp (1 mL) sea salt
- Pinch of pepper

HOW TO MAKE IT:

1. Warm ghee or butter over medium heat in a small pot.
2. Add shallot and cherry tomatoes and sauté, 2 to 3 minutes.
3. Add broth, oats, salt, cumin, and pepper, and bring porridge to a simmer. Cook, about 5 minutes, until oats are creamy. Stir in spinach and cook until just wilted, about 30 seconds.

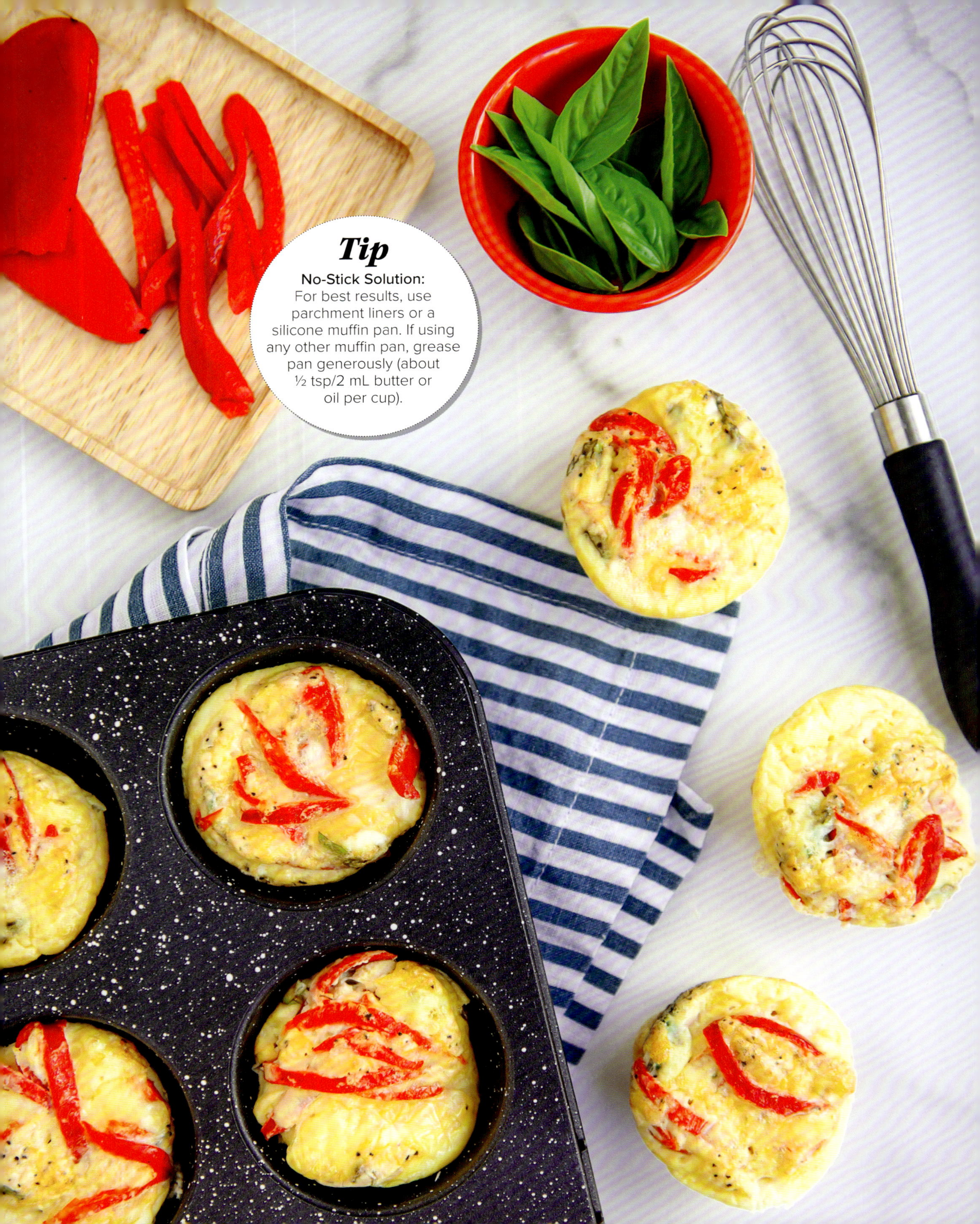

Tip

No-Stick Solution: For best results, use parchment liners or a silicone muffin pan. If using any other muffin pan, grease pan generously (about ½ tsp/2 mL butter or oil per cup).

● Dairy-Free ● Gluten-Free ● Grain-Free ● Nut-Free

Red Pepper Basil Egg Cups

This is one of many easy recipes for new moms. In every egg cup recipe I've ever seen, there's an additional step that requires an extra pan (to clean) and extra time (to precook the veggies or meat). I've eliminated that step completely by using ingredients that require zero precooking. This is breakfast for several days — appetizing and nourishing.

5 MINUTES PREPPING • 20 MINUTES COOKING • MAKES 12 EGG CUPS

WHAT YOU NEED:

10 large eggs

½ tsp (2 mL) sea salt

¼ tsp (1 mL) garlic powder

¼ tsp (1 mL) pepper

2 roasted red peppers, from a jar (about ¾ cup/175 mL), thinly sliced

1 heaping tbsp (20 mL) fresh basil, finely chopped

HOW TO MAKE IT:

1. Line or grease a muffin pan if necessary (after consulting the No-Stick Solution), and heat oven to 350°F (180°C).
2. In a large bowl, whisk the eggs, sea salt, garlic powder, and pepper together.
3. Portion egg mixture into prepared muffin pan until each cup is about half-full, then distribute the roasted red peppers and basil into each cup.
4. Transfer to oven and bake, about 20 minutes, or until the top looks just set (it may still have a tiny bit of liquid on top).
5. Cool, remove egg cups from muffin pan, and store in the refrigerator, 3 to 4 days.

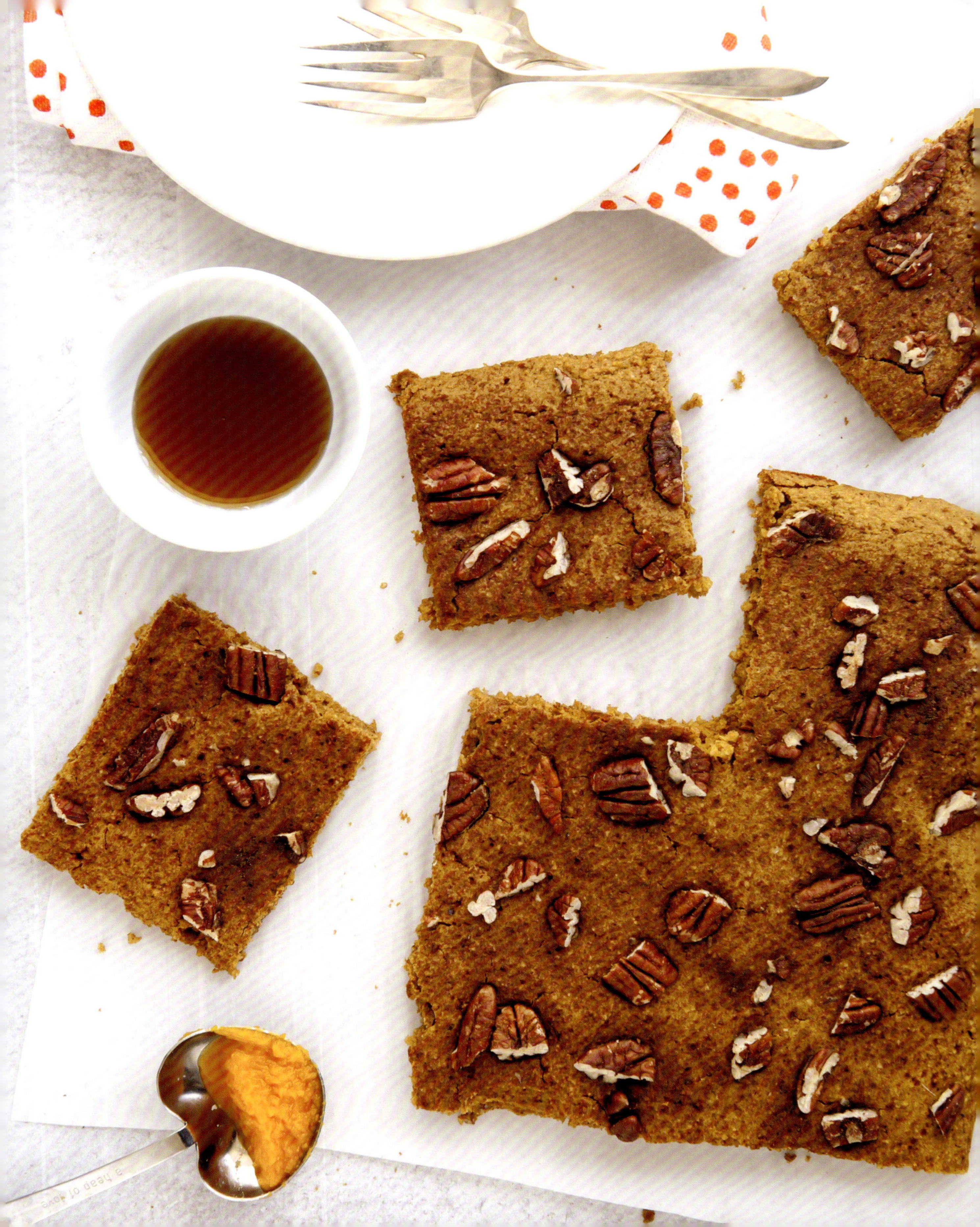

Dairy-Free · Gluten-Free · Nut-Free Option · Freezer-Friendly

Sheet Pan Pumpkin Pancakes

I love pancakes, but standing over the stove for half an hour to cook them is hard for a new mom. Enter sheet pan pancakes: simply pour the batter onto a lined baking sheet, pop it in the oven, and you're done. Perfect pancakes are ready in half the time. The addition of pumpkin in this sugar-free recipe provides an extra boost of vitamin C, iron, fibre, and beta carotene.

15 MINUTES PREPPING • 10 MINUTES COOKING • MAKES 6 TO 8 SERVINGS

WHAT YOU NEED:

Dry ingredients

3 ¼ cups (810 mL) oat flour (use whole wheat flour for non-GF)

1 ½ tsp (7.5 mL) baking powder

1 ½ tsp (7.5 mL) baking soda

1 ½ tsp (7.5 mL) sea salt

2 tbsp (30 mL) cinnamon

1 tsp (5 mL) nutmeg

1 tsp (5 mL) ground ginger

Optional toppings:

¾ cup (175 mL) chopped pecans

Cinnamon sugar: mix together 1 ½ tsp (7.5 mL) coconut sugar and ½ tsp (2 mL) cinnamon

Wet ingredients

1 ½ tbsp (22 mL) lemon juice

1 ½ tsp (7.5 mL) vanilla

1 ½ cup (375 mL) non-dairy milk

1 cup plus 1 tbsp (265 mL) pumpkin purée

3 eggs

3 tbsp (45 mL) coconut oil, melted

HOW TO MAKE IT:

1. Heat oven to 425°F (220°C) and line a 18 × 13-inch sheet pan with parchment paper.
2. Mix dry ingredients together in large bowl.
3. Mix wet ingredients together in medium bowl, then pour over dry ingredients and stir to combine.
4. Pour pancake mix onto prepared sheet pan and use a spatula to evenly spread it across the pan. Sprinkle on pecans and cinnamon sugar, if using.
5. Bake for about 10 minutes, or until centre is cooked, and enjoy! Leftovers can be separated by sheets of parchment paper in an airtight container or bag and kept in the freezer.

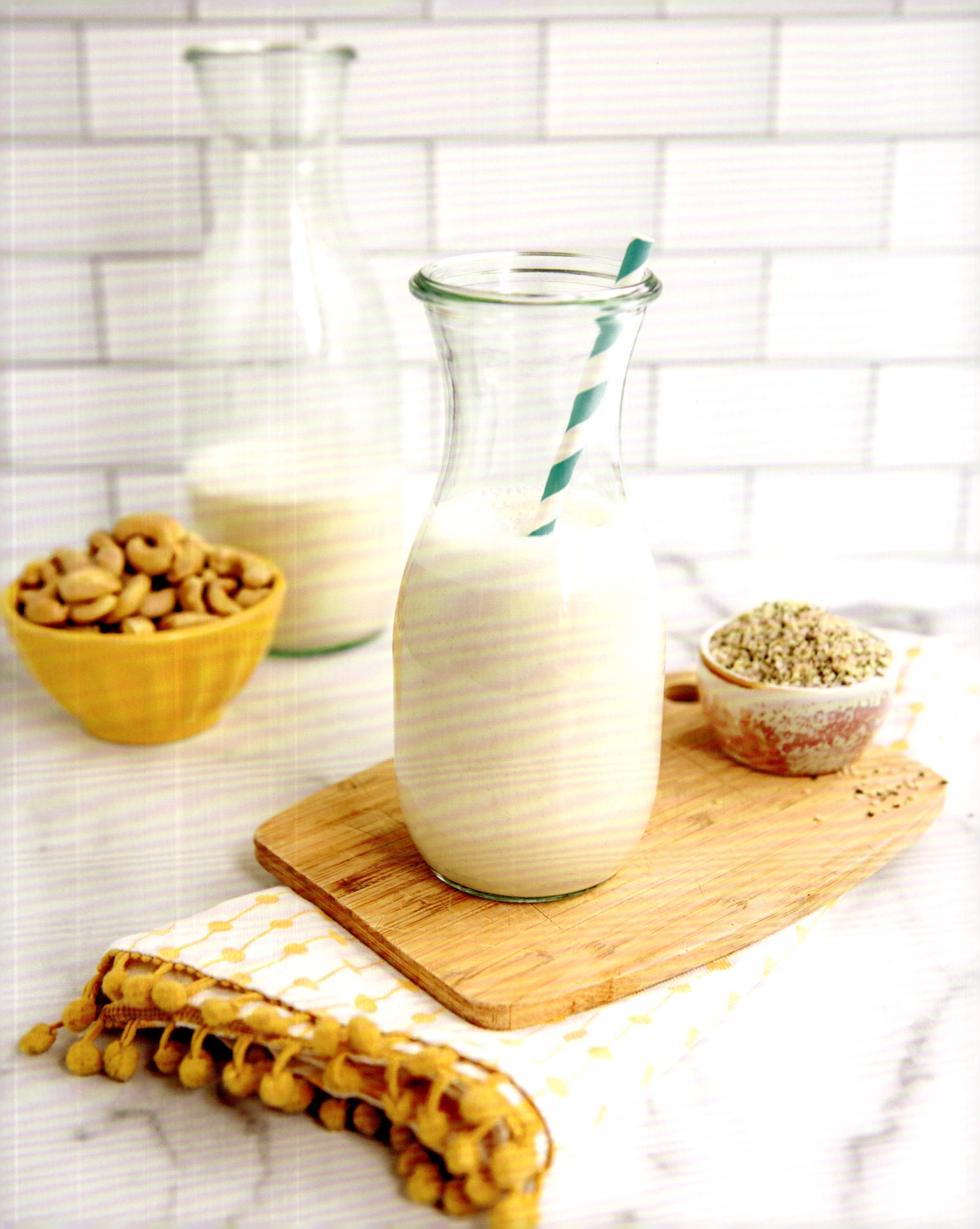

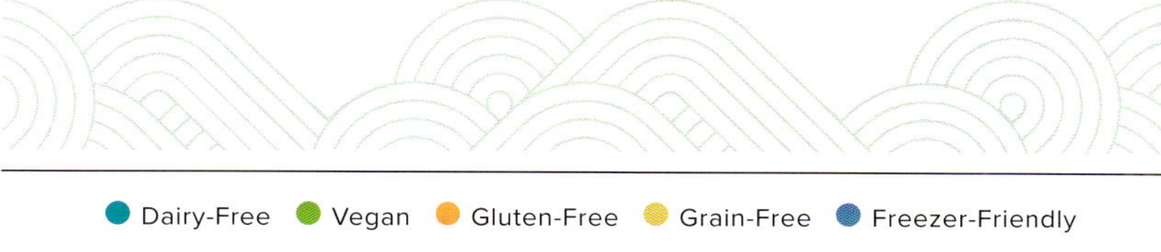

Dairy-Free · Vegan · Gluten-Free · Grain-Free · Freezer-Friendly

Cashew Hemp Milk

If you've never tried your hand at homemade milk, this is the perfect starting place. Cashews and hemp hearts blend up so well you don't even need a nut milk bag. Perfect in a smoothie or straight from the glass for a protein and nutrient-rich drink.

30 MINUTES PREPPING • 1 MINUTE COOKING • MAKES 3 CUPS (750 ML)

WHAT YOU NEED:	HOW TO MAKE IT:
¾ cup (175 mL) cashews, soaked in boiling water for 30 minutes ¼ cup (60 mL) hemp hearts 1 to 2 medjool dates, pits removed 3 cups (750 mL) water Pinch of sea salt	1. Add all ingredients to a high-powered blender and blend on high, about 1 minute, or until smoothly combined. 2. If desired, pour milk through a nut milk bag, cheesecloth, or clean dish towel to remove the small amount of sediment that remains. 3. Enjoy, and keep leftovers in the fridge for 3 days.

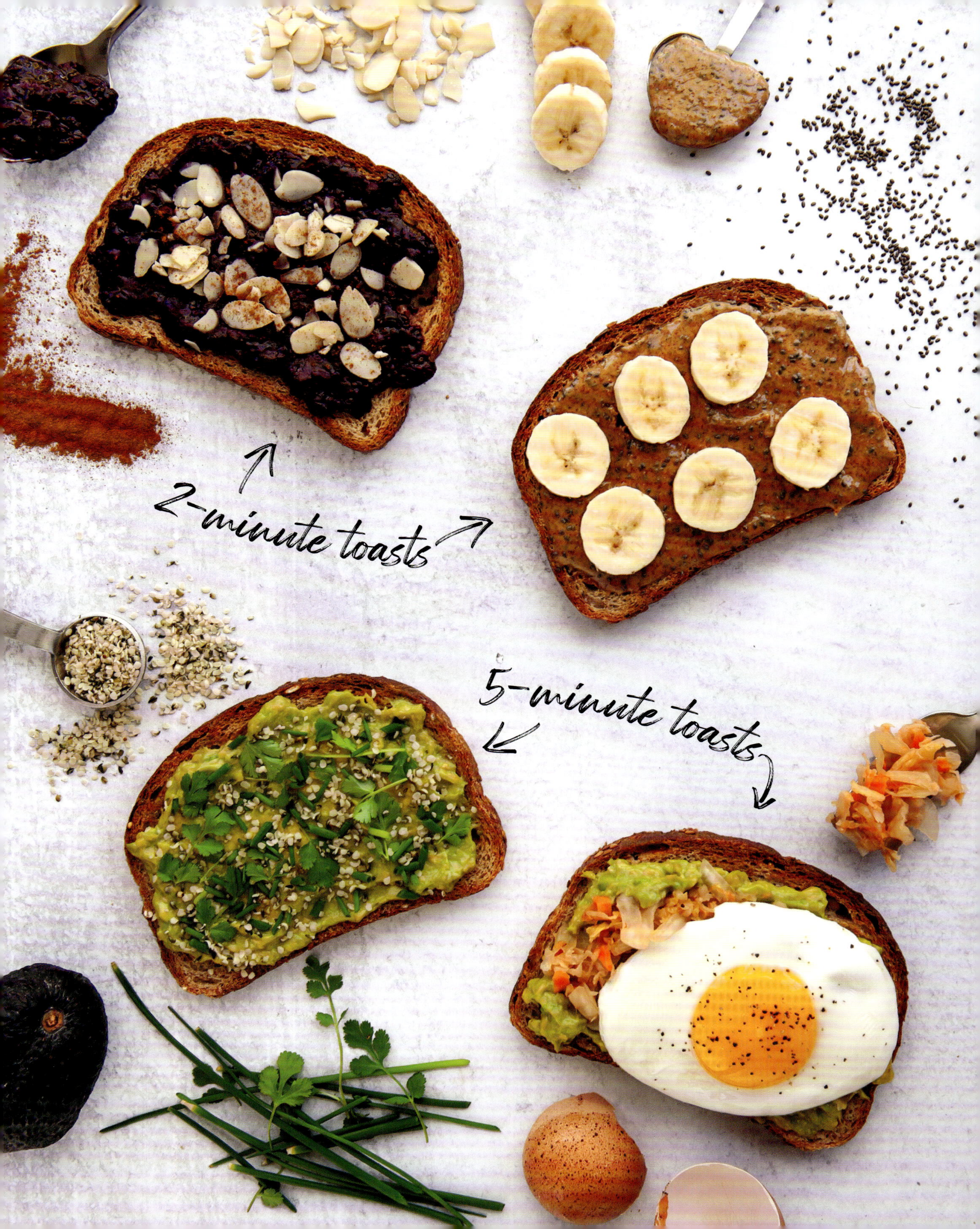

2-minute toasts
5-minute toasts

Gluten-Free Option

Toast with the Most

Let's face it: What's postpartum life without toast being a major food group? I ate my share of toasts round-the-clock. Here are some inspirations for boosting this postpartum staple, and in two or five minutes you'll be rewarded with toast that packs in the nutrients.

2-MINUTE TOASTS

Berry Cinnamon Crunch

WHAT YOU NEED:

1 tbsp (15 mL) ghee or butter

2 tbsp (30 mL) chia jam (see page 42)

2 tbsp (30 mL) sliced almonds

Sprinkle of cinnamon

HOW TO MAKE IT:

Spread ghee/butter and chia jam across your toast and top with almonds and cinnamon.

Chia Butter + Banana Treat

WHAT YOU NEED:

¼ cup (60 mL) almond butter

1 ½ tsp (7.5 mL) chia seeds

½ banana, sliced

HOW TO MAKE IT:

Spread almond butter on toast, then sprinkle on the chia seeds, swirling around with a spoon to mix in the chia seeds (optional). Top with banana slices.

5-MINUTE TOASTS

Herb-a-cado

WHAT YOU NEED:

½ large or 1 small avocado

2 tbsp (30 mL) fresh herbs of choice (cilantro, parsley, basil, chives) or use chopped spinach

1 tbsp (15 mL) hemp hearts

Sprinkle of sea salt

HOW TO MAKE IT:

Mash avocado onto toast, then top with herbs, hemp hearts, and sea salt.

The Works

WHAT YOU NEED:

1 tbsp (15 mL) olive oil

1 egg

½ large or 1 small avocado

2 tbsp (30 mL) kimchee (or substitute sauerkraut)

Sprinkle of sea salt

HOW TO MAKE IT:

Fry egg in pan coated with olive oil, covering to cook for 4 minutes, or until done to your preference. Meanwhile, mash avocado onto toast, sprinkle with sea salt, then top with kimchee. Finish with egg on top.

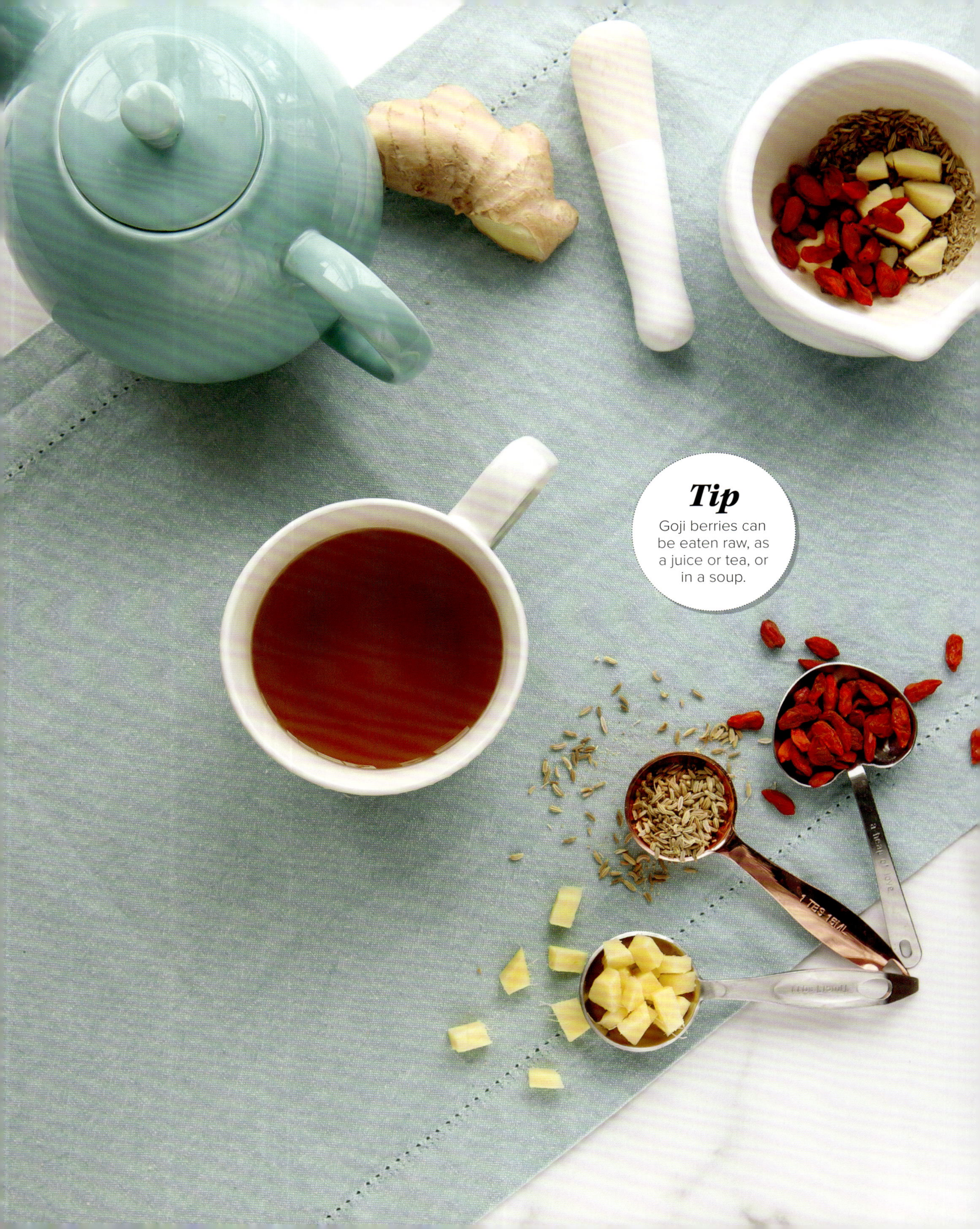
Tip
Goji berries can be eaten raw, as a juice or tea, or in a soup.

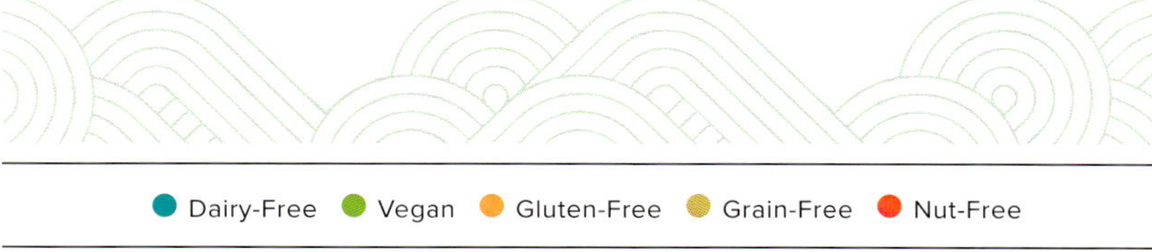

Dairy-Free · Vegan · Gluten-Free · Grain-Free · Nut-Free

Ginger Tea with Fennel + Goji Berries

A caffeine-free herbal tonic that supports the digestive system, provides antioxidants, and boosts immunity. This sweet ginger tea is as soothing as it is health promoting. Drink it in the morning or afternoon after a meal.

5 MINUTES PREPPING • 15 MINUTES COOKING • MAKES 2 SERVINGS

WHAT YOU NEED:	HOW TO MAKE IT:
3 ½ cups (875 mL) water 1 tbsp (15 mL) fennel seeds, lightly crushed with the back of a chef's knife or mortar and pestle for about a minute until fragrant 1 tbsp (15 mL) peeled and sliced ginger 1 tbsp (15 mL) goji berries	1. In a small pot, bring the water to a boil. Add fennel seeds, ginger, and goji berries, and simmer, 10 to 15 minutes. Strain and enjoy, storing leftovers in a small glass jar.

Link-up

Prep extra ginger so that it's ready for the **Miso Mineral Soup** (page 207) or **Heal in a Curry** (page 209).

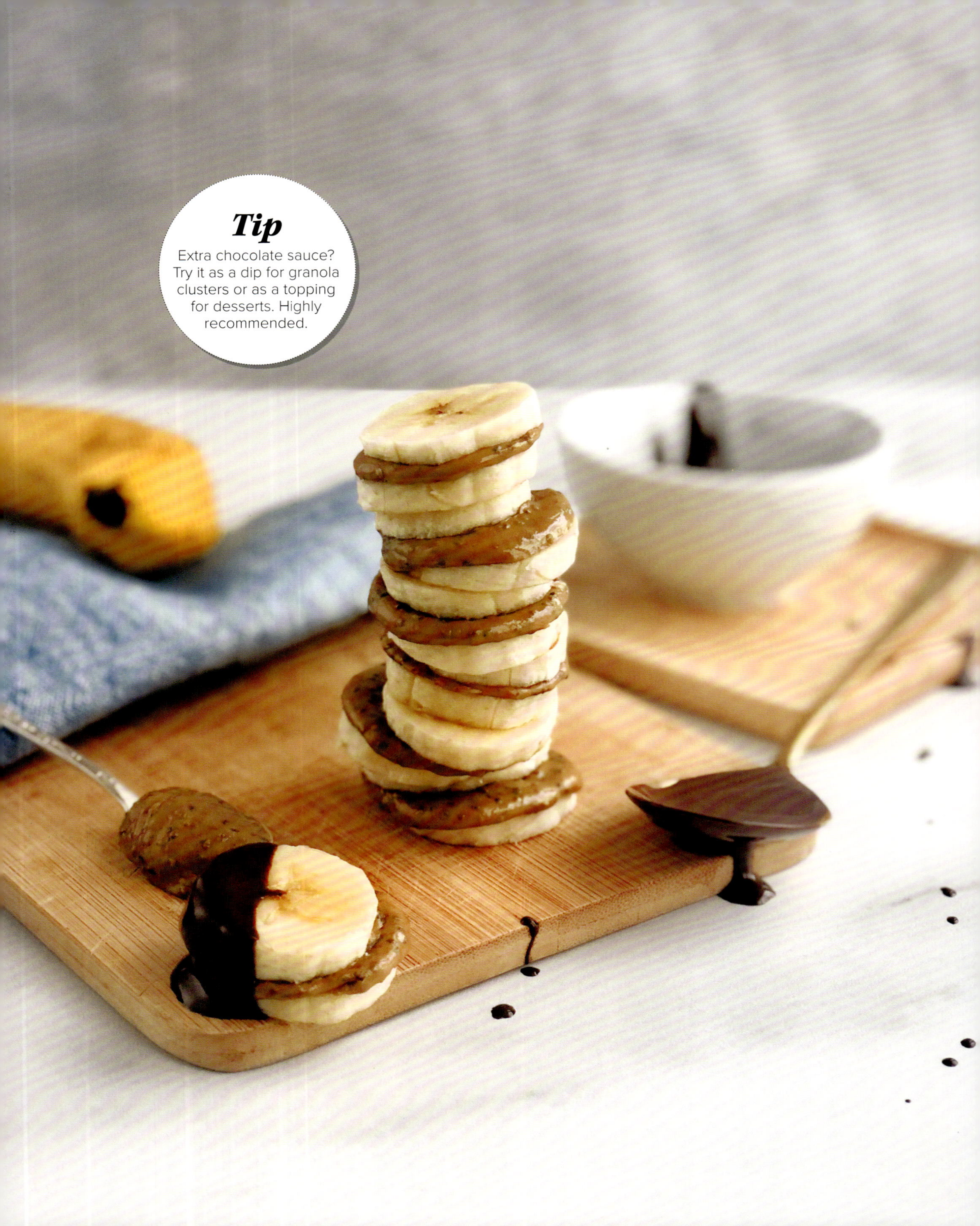
Tip
Extra chocolate sauce? Try it as a dip for granola clusters or as a topping for desserts. Highly recommended.

Dairy-Free Option · Vegan Option · Gluten-Free · Grain-Free
Nut-Free Option · Freezer-Friendly

Chia Butter + Chocolate Banana Bites

A super easy snack with a few upgrades: sandwiching almond butter between banana slices increases the protein and fat in your snack, stirring chia seeds into your almond butter ups the omega-3 fats and fibre, and dipping the whole thing in chocolate makes you feel good, and what's better than that? Bonus — you can stick these in the freezer — chocolate-dipped or plain — grabbing a couple every time you need a sweet snack.

10 MINUTES PREPPING • MAKES 16 BITES

WHAT YOU NEED:

2 bananas

⅓ cup (75 mL) nut or seed butter of choice

1 tbsp (15 mL) chia seeds

Pinch of sea salt (optional)

Chocolate dip (optional)

¼ cup (60 mL) chocolate chips (non-dairy or regular)

1 heaping tsp (6 mL) coconut oil

HOW TO MAKE IT:

1. If freezing, line a baking tray with parchment paper and set aside.
2. Slice bananas into slices, and stir nut butter, chia seeds, and sea salt (if using) together in a small bowl.
3. Make your banana bites: spread about ½ tsp (2 mL) chia butter mixture on one slice of banana, and top it with a second slice. Repeat until all of your banana slices have been buttered and paired up.
4. If freezing, place banana bites on baking tray and move to the freezer for an hour or two until frozen.
5. Make the chocolate dip (if using). Melt the chocolate chips and coconut oil together on low heat. If eating fresh — dip and enjoy!
6. If freezing, remove the banana bites from the freezer and dip or drizzle with the chocolate sauce. Place back in the freezer until set, about an hour. Enjoy straight from the freezer (take out a couple of minutes before you want to eat).

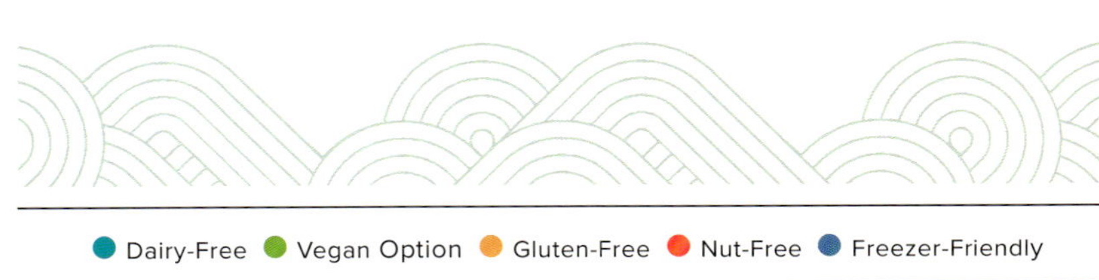

Dairy-Free • Vegan Option • Gluten-Free • Nut-Free • Freezer-Friendly

Apple Pie Oat Bars

Naturally sweetened, soft and chewy homemade oat bars are wonderful to have on hand. I keep mine by the batch in the freezer, transferring a handful of bars to the counter on a weekly basis for an easy snack.

10 MINUTES PREPPING • 25 MINUTES COOKING • MAKES ONE 8 × 8-INCH PAN OF BARS

WHAT YOU NEED:

Dry ingredients

1 cup (250 mL) oat flour (or substitute whole wheat flour for non-GF)

1 cup (250 mL) thick rolled oats

2½ tbsp (37 mL) ground flax

2 tsp (10 mL) cinnamon

½ tsp (2 mL) nutmeg

½ tsp (2 mL) fine sea salt

Wet ingredients

2½ tbsp (37 mL) coconut oil, melted

1 cup (250 mL) apple sauce

3 tbsp (45 mL) maple syrup or honey

½ tsp (2 mL) vanilla extract

HOW TO MAKE IT:

1. Heat oven to 350°F (180°C), and line an 8 × 8-inch pan with parchment paper.
2. In a large bowl, mix together dry ingredients.
3. In a medium bowl, combine wet ingredients.
4. Pour wet mix into dry bowl and stir to combine until smooth. Using a spatula, slide mixture into prepared pan. To even out the top of the oat bars, smooth mixture out with spatula, or place another sheet of parchment paper on top and press lightly.
5. Move pan to oven and bake, about 25 minutes, or until edges are just starting to turn golden.
6. Remove from oven, and score into bars with a serrated knife. Store in airtight container on the counter for a few days, in the fridge for about a week, or a couple of months in the freezer.

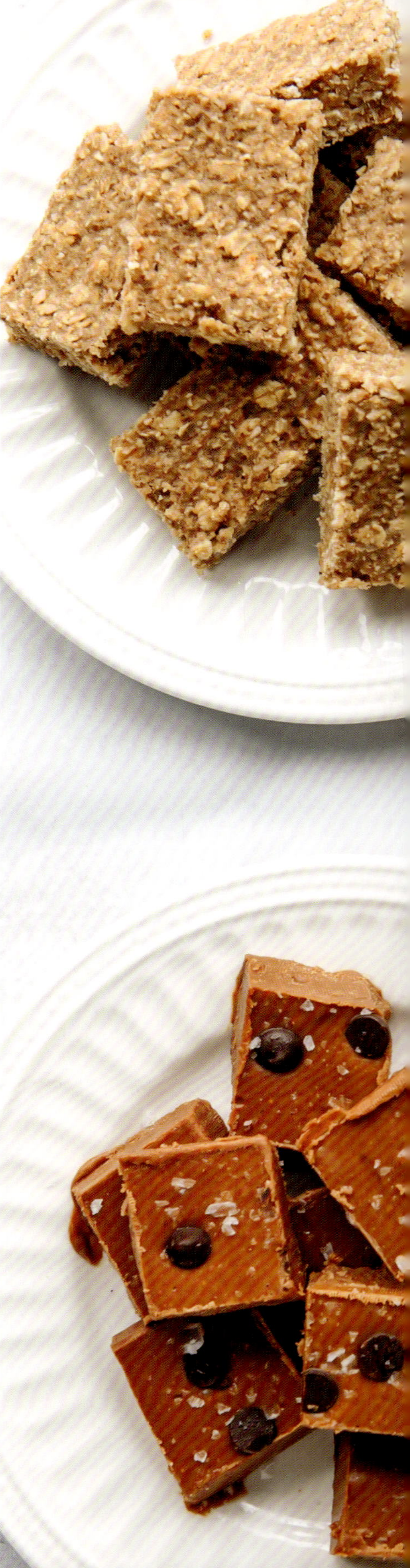

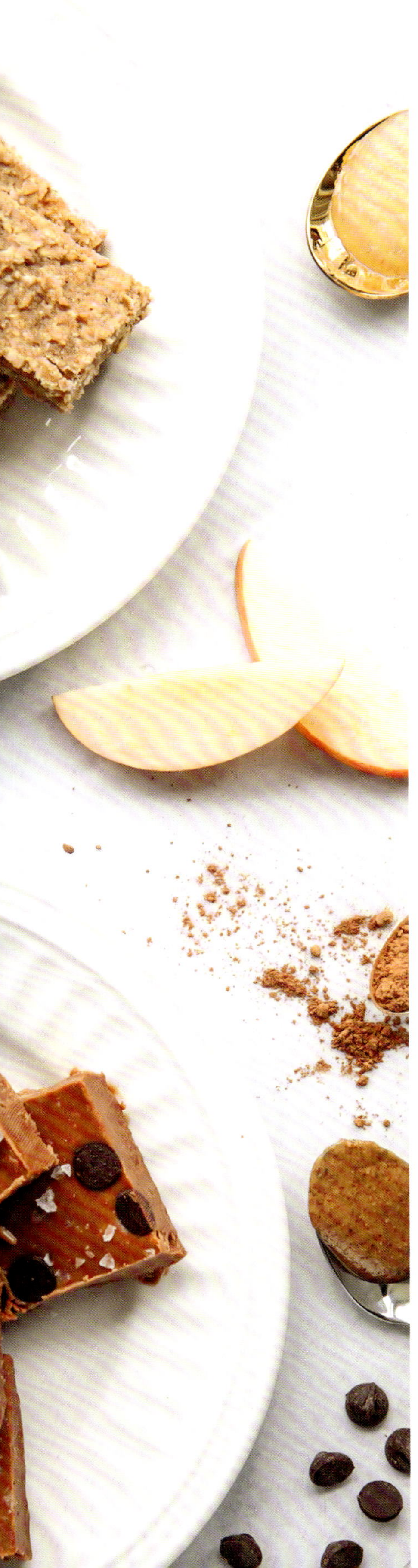

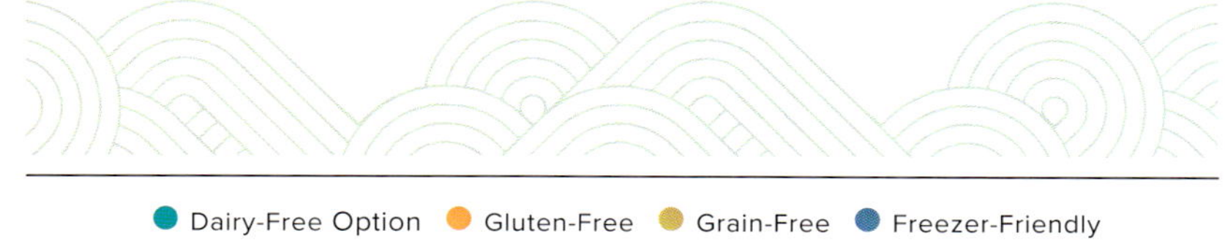

● Dairy-Free Option ● Gluten-Free ● Grain-Free ● Freezer-Friendly

Mama's Freezer Fudge

Sometimes you just need a sweet snack that you can grab, ready-to-go, from the freezer. Besides satisfying your sweet tooth, these have lasting power thanks to the peanut butter, tahini, and coconut oil. If you don't have tahini, you can just use extra peanut butter, but I've added it here to give this snack a selenium and calcium boost.

15 MINUTES PREPPING • MAKES ONE 8 × 5-INCH PAN

WHAT YOU NEED:	HOW TO MAKE IT:
1 cup (250 mL) organic peanut butter or almond butter 3 tbsp (45 mL) tahini ⅓ cup (75 mL) coconut oil, melted ¼ cup (60 mL) honey or maple syrup 3 tbsp (45 mL) cacao powder 1 tbsp (15 mL) dairy-free or regular chocolate chips (optional) Pinch of coarse sea salt (optional)	**1.** Line an 8 × 5-inch loaf pan with parchment paper. **2.** In a large bowl or food processor, mix together the peanut butter, tahini, coconut oil, honey or maple syrup, and cacao powder until smooth and combined. **3.** Pour mixture into prepared pan and use a spatula to make sure you get all of the fudge mix out of the bowl and to evenly smooth out the fudge in the pan. **4.** Sprinkle on chocolate chips and sea salt, if using. **5.** Move pan to freezer until frozen, about 2 hours. **6.** Remove fudge from pan, score into squares, and freeze in a freezer-safe container or bag, about 1 to 2 months.

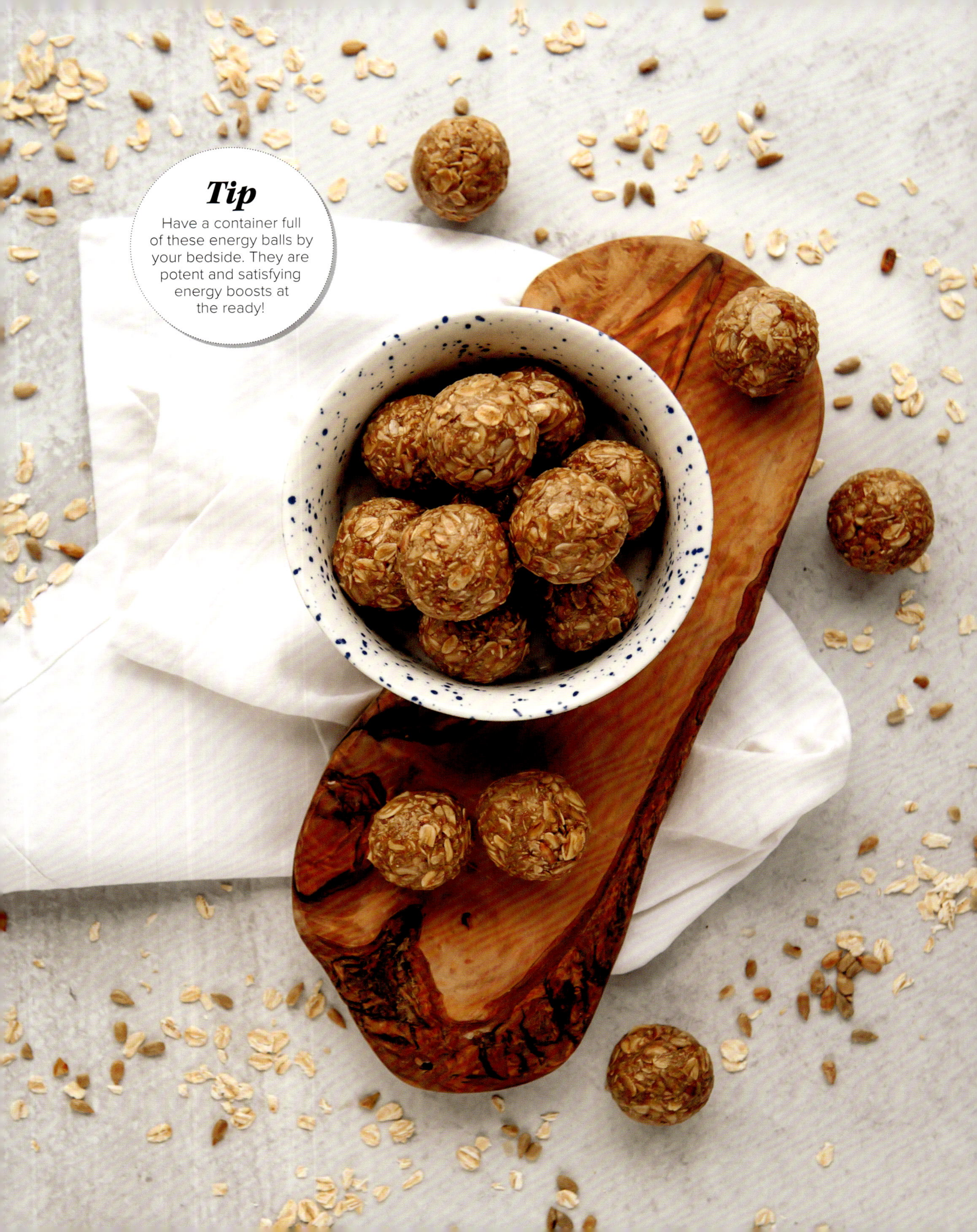
Tip
Have a container full of these energy balls by your bedside. They are potent and satisfying energy boosts at the ready!

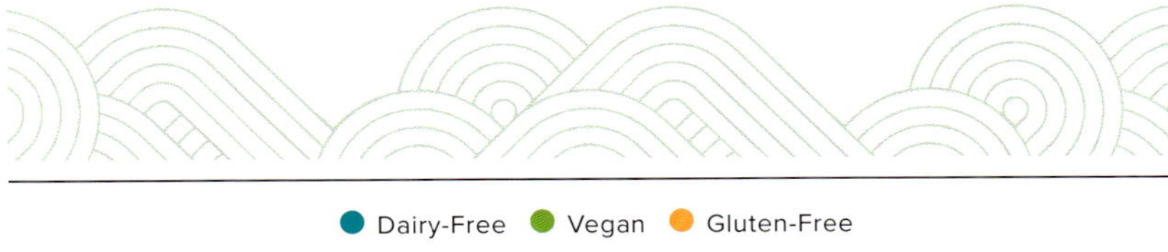

Dairy-Free · Vegan · Gluten-Free

Sunflower Flax Energy Balls

This is an energy-boosting snack for new moms — anytime of day or night. These energy balls contain several foods thought to be milk-boosting galactagogues — oats, flax, and almonds. What's better than a power snack packed with protein, fibre, good carbs, and healthy fats?

15 MINUTES PREPPING • MAKES 28 BITES

WHAT YOU NEED:	HOW TO MAKE IT:
1 ¾ cups (425 mL) rolled oats ¾ cup (175 mL) sunflower seed butter (or nut/seed butter of choice) ½ cup (125 mL) maple syrup ½ cup (125 mL) sunflower seeds ¼ cup (60 mL) chopped walnuts ¼ cup (60 mL) sliced almonds ¼ cup (60 mL) ground flaxseed	1. Add all ingredients to a large bowl and combine. 2. Chill mixture in fridge for about an hour, then roll into balls. Store energy balls in large glass container in the fridge for about a week and enjoy!

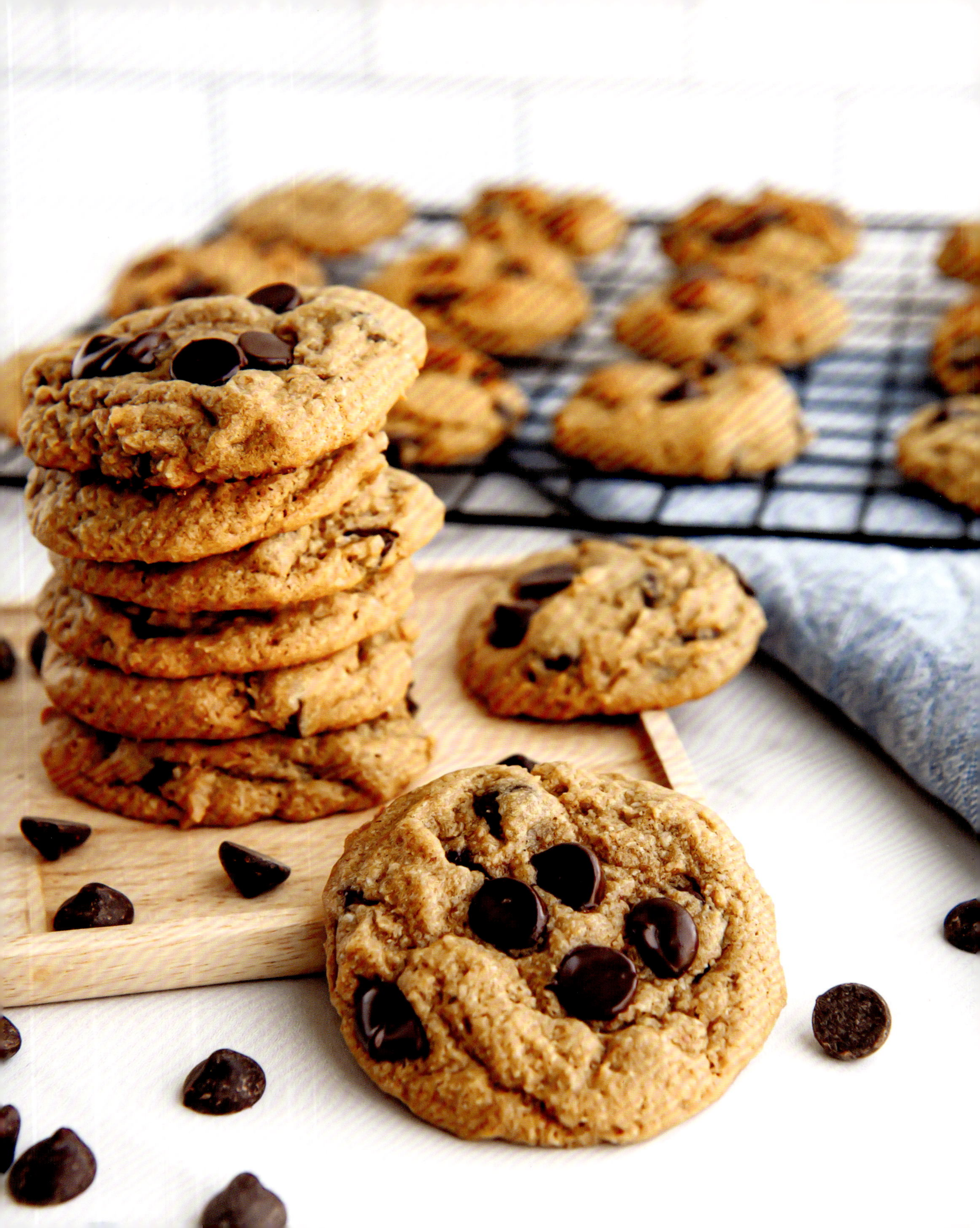

Gluten-Free • Freezer-Friendly

Little Lactation Cookies

The science is out on how much foods and herbs truly help with milk supply, but what is rock solid is that nursing moms absolutely need calories and water. What's also important for breastfeeding is less stress for moms, and we know chocolate chip cookies are a great stress reducer! So, enjoy these delicious cookies (which are free of refined sugar and pack in some protein) and take a moment for you. You deserve it!

15 MINUTES PREPPING + 30 TO 60 MINUTES CHILLING • 10 MINUTES COOKING • MAKES 48 LITTLE / 24 REGULAR COOKIES

WHAT YOU NEED:

- ½ cup (125 mL) butter, soft and room temperature but not liquid
- 1 large egg
- 1 ½ tsp (7.5 mL) vanilla
- ¾ cup (175 mL) coconut sugar
- 1 ¼ cup (310 mL) almond flour
- 1 cup (250 mL) oat flour (or substitute whole wheat flour for non-GF)
- ½ tsp (2 mL) baking powder
- ½ tsp (2 mL) baking soda
- ½ tsp (2 mL) sea salt
- ½ to ¾ cup (125 to 175 mL) chocolate chips (dairy-free or regular)

HOW TO MAKE IT:

1. In a medium bowl, cream together the softened butter, egg, vanilla, and coconut sugar using a hand mixer or spatula.
2. In a large bowl, sift together the flours, baking powder, baking soda, and sea salt, then pour in the wet mixture and stir to combine.
3. Stir in chocolate chips, then preheat oven to 350°F (180°C) and refrigerate your cookie dough for 30 to 60 minutes.
4. Using a tablespoon (for regular-sized cookies) or ½ tablespoon (for little cookies), portion the cookie dough onto 1 to 2 baking stones or baking sheets lined with parchment paper.
5. Transfer cookies to oven and bake, about 9 to 12 minutes. Let cookies cool on pan for 5 minutes, then transfer cookies to cooling rack. Store in an airtight container for a week, or freeze in a freezer-safe container or bag for several months.

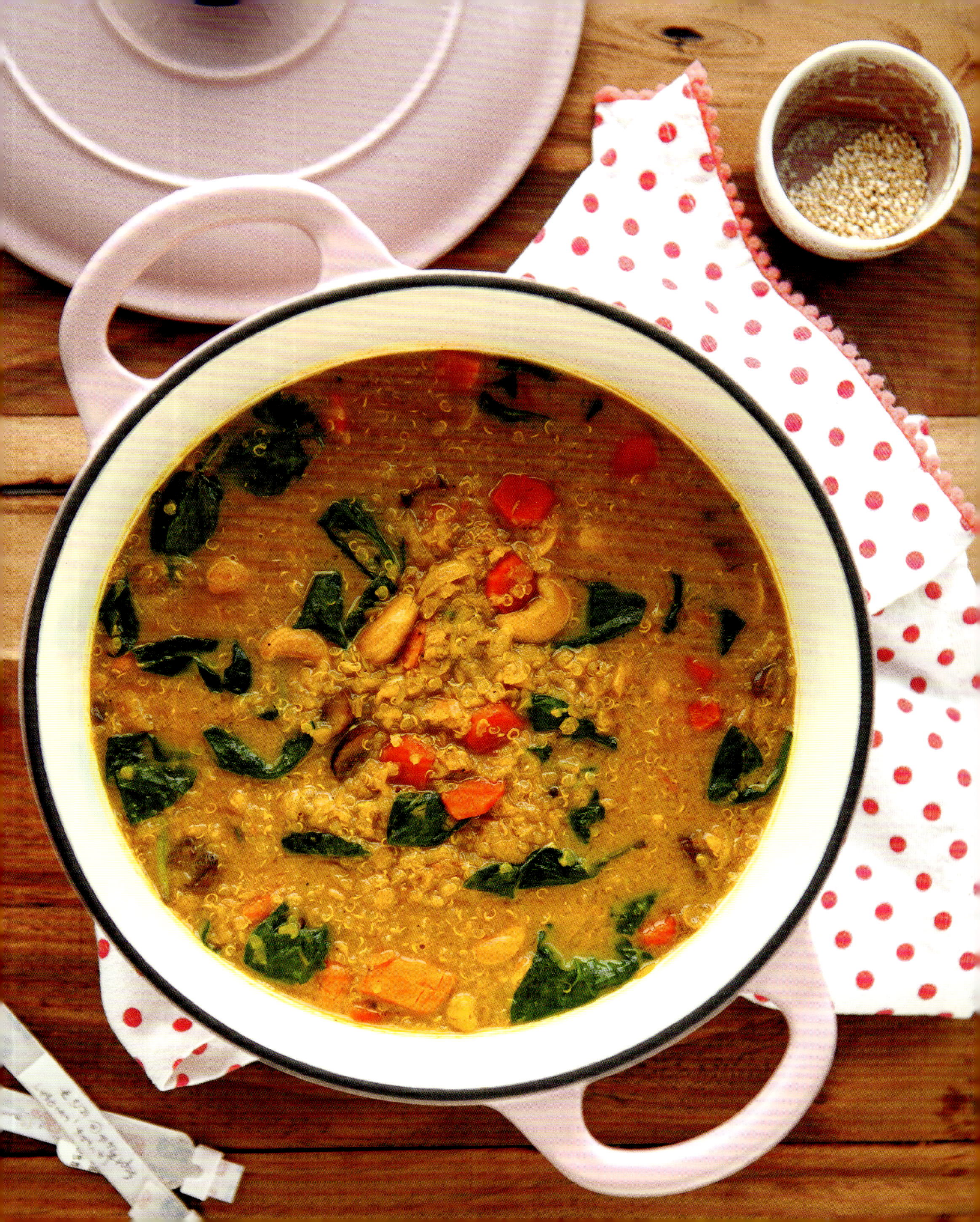

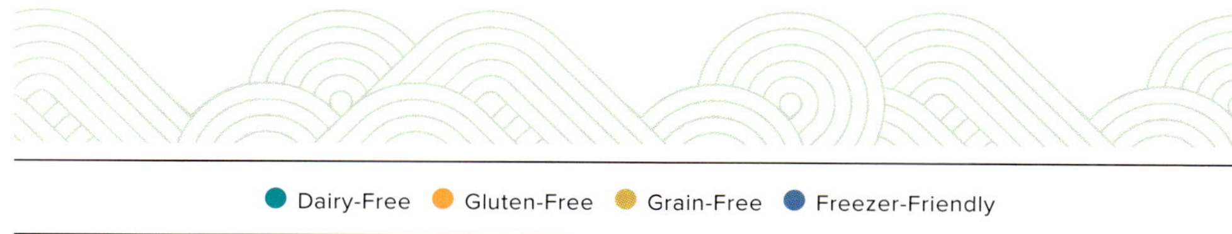

Dairy-Free • Gluten-Free • Grain-Free • Freezer-Friendly

Golden Mama Healing Stew

This is the ultimate post-birth meal: warm, bone broth-based, gentle on your digestive system, and packed with vitamins, proteins, and fats you need for recovery. The ingredient list is long, but this is easy to throw together and makes enough to feed a crowd (or just you, for a week straight).

This stew (which can be turned into a soup with an extra cup or two of broth added) is ideal to make and freeze before baby is born. It's also my favourite to bring to friends in their early postpartum days.

20 MINUTES PREPPING • 45 MINUTES COOKING • MAKES 4 TO 6 SERVINGS

WHAT YOU NEED:

- 1 ½ tbsp (22 mL) olive oil
- 2 cloves garlic, minced
- 1 medium/large onion, diced
- 1-inch (2.5-cm) piece of ginger, minced
- 2 tsp (10 mL) cumin
- 2 tsp (10 mL) turmeric
- ½ tsp (2 mL) cinnamon
- ½ tsp (2 mL) sea salt
- ¼ tsp (1 mL) pepper
- 5 to 6 cups (1.25 to 1.5 L) Everyday Bone Broth, page 181, or store-bought, low-sodium chicken broth
- 2 medium/large carrots, peeled and sliced
- 1 large sweet potato, peeled and cubed
- 1 ½ cups (375 mL) mushrooms, chopped
- ½ cup (125 mL) raw cashews
- ½ cup (125 mL) uncooked red lentils, rinsed
- ½ cup (125 mL) uncooked quinoa, rinsed
- 1 can (13.5 oz/400 mL) full-fat coconut milk
- 1 cup (250 mL) spinach, loosely packed

HOW TO MAKE IT:

1. In a large pot, heat the olive oil over medium heat, add the onion, garlic, and a pinch of salt, and sauté for about 5 minutes, or until the onion has softened.
2. Add the ginger and spices and cook for 1 minute, stirring frequently, then add the broth, carrots, sweet potato, mushrooms, and cashews, and bring to a boil. Simmer, uncovered, for 15 minutes.
3. Drop in the quinoa and lentils, reduce heat to low, and cook, covered, until lentils and quinoa are soft and cooked, about 15 to 20 minutes.
4. Finish up with the coconut milk and spinach and cook for 5 more minutes, then turn off the heat and enjoy. Leftovers can be kept in large glass jars or containers for a week in the refrigerator or several months in the freezer.

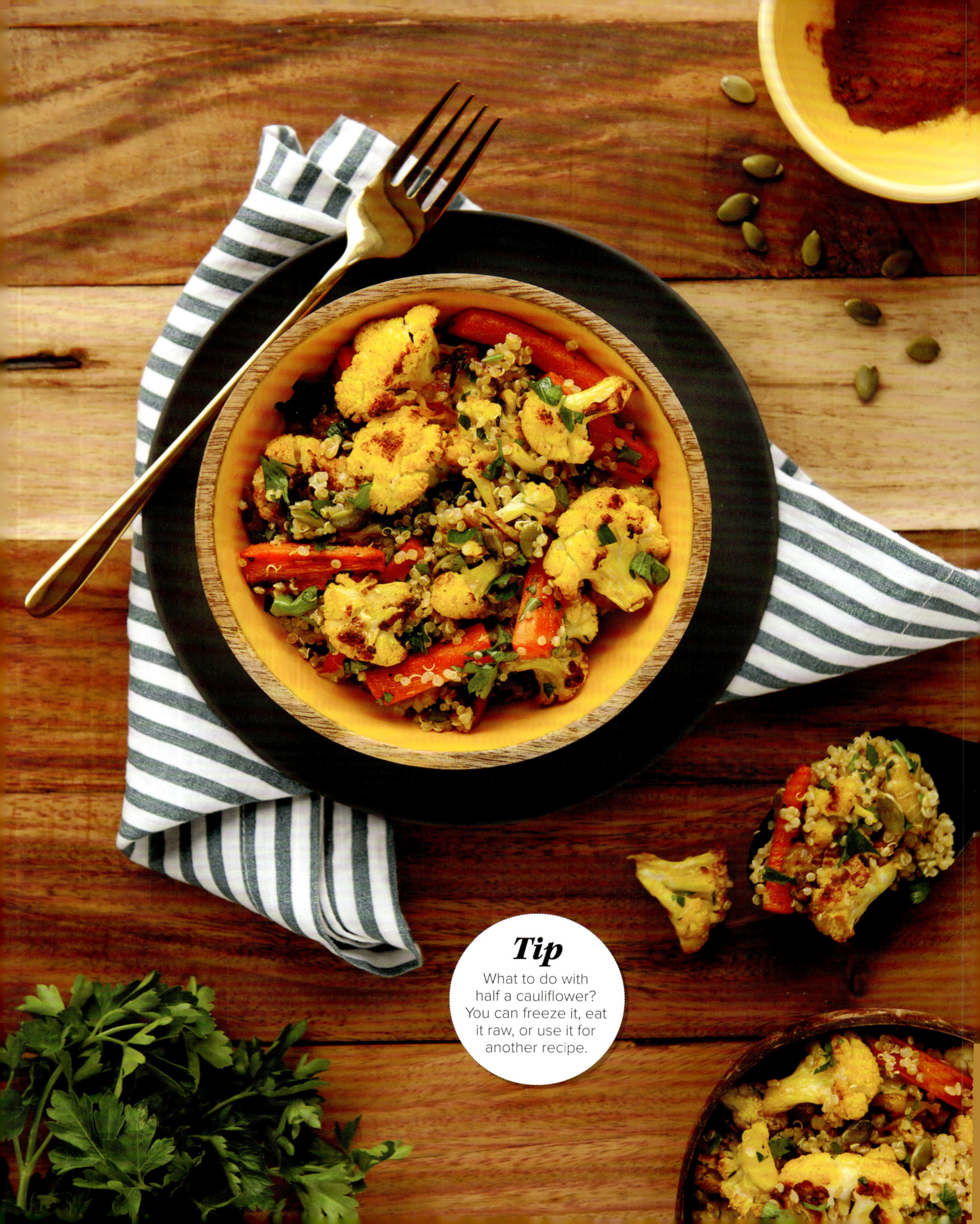

Tip

What to do with half a cauliflower? You can freeze it, eat it raw, or use it for another recipe.

Dairy-Free · Vegan Option · Gluten-Free · Grain-Free · Nut-Free

Warm Golden Cauliflower + Carrot Salad with Cinnamon Maple Dressing

If there ever was a salad equivalent to a warming, good-for-the-soul soup, this is it. Golden roasted veggies in a sweet cinnamon maple dressing, with a hint of freshness and crunch from the parsley and pepitas, make this salad a crowd pleaser or a just-for-you meal that keeps well for several days. This cinnamon maple dressing is SO good you'll want to make extra and drizzle it on everything (try it on roasted fall veggies such as squash and sweet potatoes).

20 MINUTES PREPPING • 30 MINUTES COOKING • MAKES 3 TO 4 SERVINGS

WHAT YOU NEED:

For the salad

½ large head of cauliflower, chopped into bite-sized pieces

3 carrots, halved lengthwise and sliced into small finger-sized strips

2 shallots, thinly sliced

2 tbsp (30 mL) avocado oil, plus another ½ tbsp (7 mL) if needed

1 tsp (5 mL) turmeric powder

½ tsp (2 mL) fine sea salt

½ tsp (2 mL) cumin

¼ tsp (1 mL) pepper

⅔ cup (150 mL) quinoa, uncooked

1 ¼ cups (310 mL) broth or water

3 tbsp (45 mL) parsley, chopped

3 tbsp (45 mL) pepita seeds (pumpkin seeds)

For the cinnamon maple dressing

⅓ cup plus 1 tbsp (90 mL) olive oil

3 tbsp (45 mL) apple cider vinegar

1 tbsp (15 mL) maple syrup

½ tsp (2 mL) cinnamon

¼ tsp (1 mL) fine sea salt

HOW TO MAKE IT:

1. Heat oven to 425°F (220°C) and line a baking sheet with parchment paper.
2. Transfer chopped cauliflower, carrots, and shallots to a large bowl. Top with avocado oil, sea salt, pepper, turmeric, and cumin, and toss with wooden spoon until veggies are evenly coated with oil and spices. Add another ½ tbsp (7 mL) avocado oil if veggies look a bit dry.
3. Pour veggies onto prepared pan and transfer to oven. While veggies are roasting, combine quinoa and broth or water in a medium saucepan and bring to a boil. Cover with lid, turn burner to your lowest setting, and cook, 17 minutes, or until quinoa is fluffy and has absorbed all the water.
4. While quinoa and veggies cook, prepare cinnamon maple dressing by combining ingredients in a small jar or bowl.
5. Veggies are done when they look nice and caramelized, with tops flecked with a golden-brown crust, about 25 to 30 minutes.
6. Mix roasted veggies, quinoa, and dressing together, and top with chopped parsley and pepita seeds.

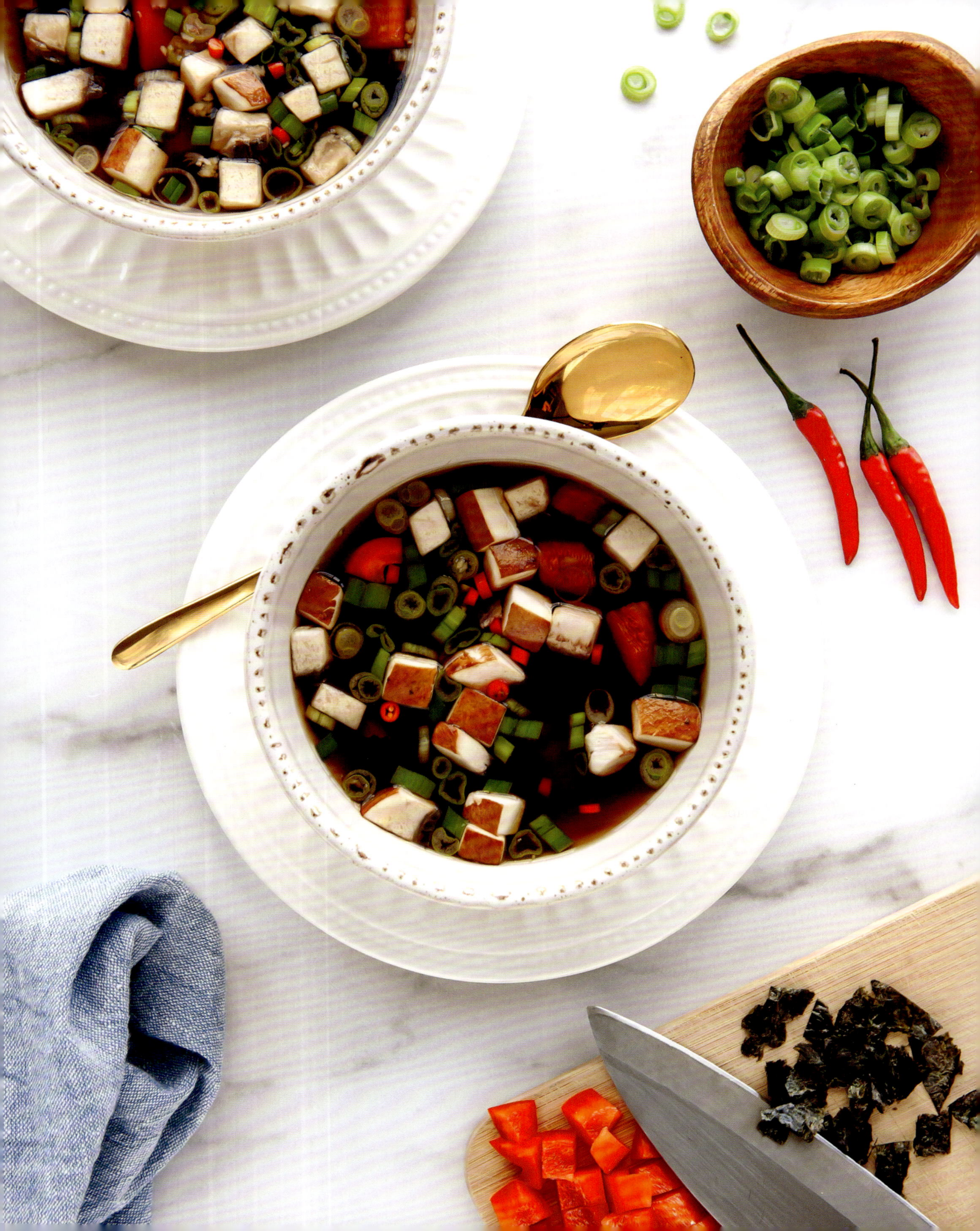

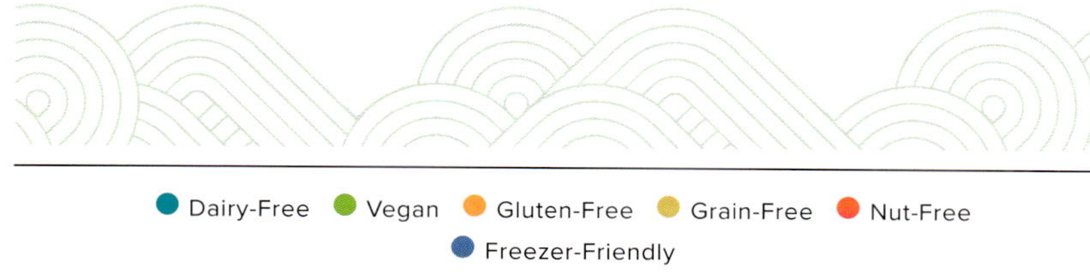

Dairy-Free · Vegan · Gluten-Free · Grain-Free · Nut-Free · Freezer-Friendly

Miso Mineral Soup

Sea vegetables such as nori, kelp, wakame, and kombu are among the most mineral-rich foods in the world. Seaweed is an especially potent source of the mineral iodine, which is essential for infant brain development. This recipe calls for nori because it is the most widely available, but feel free to use whatever sea vegetable you like.

Spice it up! If you like a spicy soup or are looking to clear up some congestion from a cold, finely chop a few slices of red chili pepper and add to your bowl.

10 MINUTES PREPPING • 20 MINUTES COOKING • MAKES 2 TO 3 SERVINGS

WHAT YOU NEED:

- 1 ½ tbsp (22 mL) olive oil
- 1 ½ cups (375 mL) portobello mushrooms, chopped
- 2 carrots, chopped
- ½ red bell pepper, chopped
- 2 small cloves garlic, minced
- 1 tbsp (15 mL) fresh ginger, minced
- 4 cups (1 L) water
- 1 sheet of nori, crumbled
- 2 stalks green onion, sliced
- 2 to 3 tbsp (30 to 45 mL) miso paste
- 2 tbsp (30 mL) hot water
- 1 tbsp (15 mL) tamari (substitute soy sauce for non-GF)

HOW TO MAKE IT:

1. Heat olive oil in medium/large pot set to medium heat. Add the mushrooms, carrots, red pepper, garlic, and ginger, and sauté 2 to 3 minutes.
2. Add the 4 cups (1 L) of water to the pot, top with the lid, bring to a boil, and let simmer, about 10 minutes.
3. Add the nori and green onions and simmer 5 more minutes. Meanwhile, in a small dish, whisk together the miso paste, hot water, and tamari.
4. Pour the miso mixture into the soup, stir, turn off the heat, and enjoy.

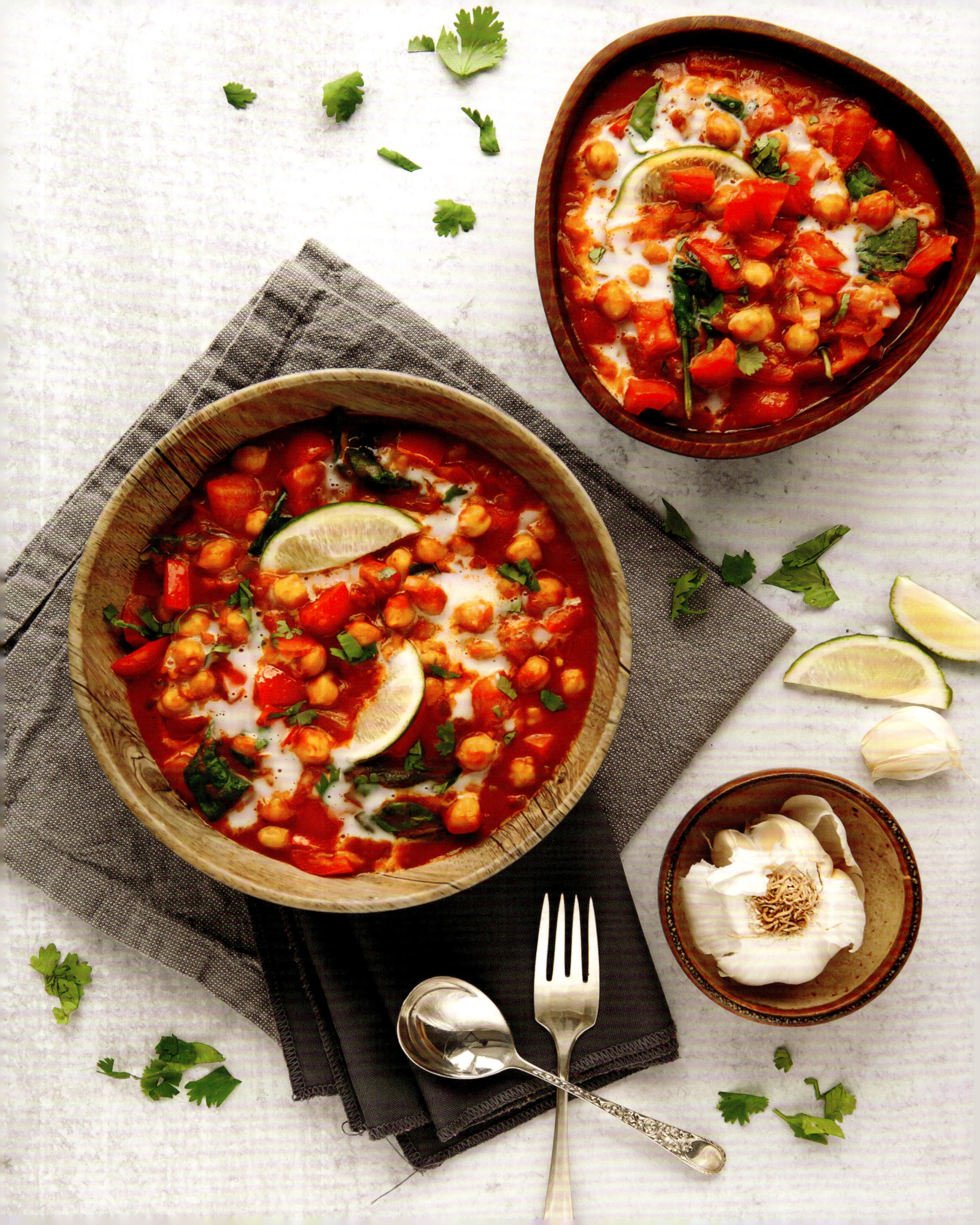

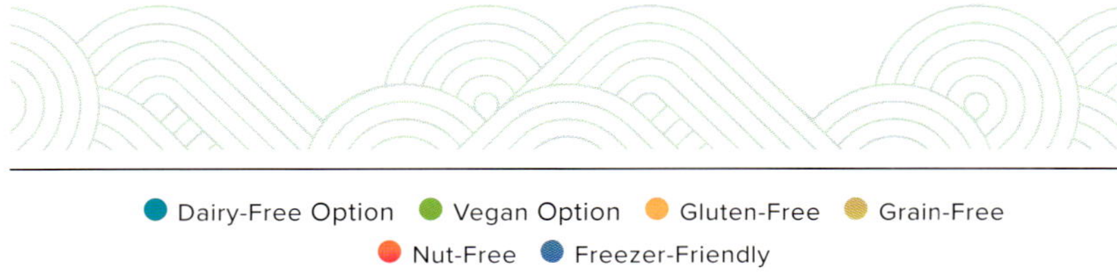

Dairy-Free Option · Vegan Option · Gluten-Free · Grain-Free · Nut-Free · Freezer-Friendly

Heal in a Curry

This is a quick curry, full of warming spices. It's easy to double, easy to freeze, and can be made with whatever vegetables or greens you have on hand. The fat in the coconut milk helps keep you full and ensures that the vitamins in the veggies get absorbed into your system.

15 MINUTES PREPPING • 20 MINUTES COOKING • MAKES 4 TO 6 SERVINGS

WHAT YOU NEED:

- 1 tbsp (15 mL) ghee or avocado oil
- ½ large onion (about 1 cup/250 mL), finely chopped
- 3 cloves garlic, minced
- 1 tsp (5 mL) ginger, minced
- 1 tbsp (15 mL) tomato paste
- 2 tsp (10 mL) cumin
- 1 tsp (5 mL) turmeric
- 1 tsp (5 mL) coriander
- 1 tsp (5 mL) paprika
- ½ tsp (2.5 mL) sea salt
- 1 cup (250 mL) strained tomatoes/passata
- 1 can (19 oz/540 mL) chickpeas, drained and rinsed
- 2 cups (500 mL) red bell pepper, chopped (or veggies of choice)
- 1 can (13.5 oz/400 mL) coconut milk, full fat
- 1 to 2 large handfuls of spinach (or greens of choice)

HOW TO MAKE IT:

1. Heat ghee/oil in a large pan over medium heat, and add the onion, garlic, and ginger. Sauté for 2 minutes.
2. Add the tomato paste and spices, and stir for 1 minute or until fragrant.
3. Add remaining ingredients (except spinach), bring to a simmer, and cook, 15 to 20 minutes, stirring occasionally. Stir in spinach, remove pan from heat, and serve over rice or quinoa.

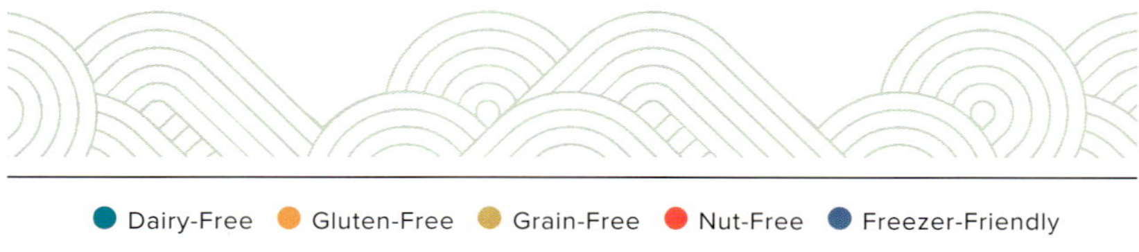

Dairy-Free • Gluten-Free • Grain-Free • Nut-Free • Freezer-Friendly

Simplest Roast Chicken

Simplified down to a basic but full-flavour recipe, you can get the chicken in the oven in under 5 minutes. This roast chicken recipe ensures you have protein on hand for the week to go with bowls, sandwiches, tacos, or salads. What's left can be repurposed into the healing Everyday Bone Broth, page 181.

5 MINUTES PREPPING • 45 TO 60 MINUTES COOKING • MAKES 1 CHICKEN

WHAT YOU NEED:

- 1 organic whole chicken
- 1 tbsp (15 mL) smoked paprika
- 2 tsp (10 mL) dried rosemary
- 1 tsp (5 mL) garlic powder
- 1 tsp (5 mL) sea salt

HOW TO MAKE IT:

1. Preheat oven to 425°F (220°C).
2. Rub spices all over chicken, then place chicken right-side up on a roasting tray, baking dish, or cast-iron pan.
3. Roast chicken in oven for 45 to 60 minutes, or until a meat thermometer placed in the thickest part of the thigh reads 165°F (74°C). Depending on the size of your chicken, you may want to cover with tinfoil for the last 10 to 20 minutes to prevent skin from burning.

Link-up

Consider roasting two chickens at a time, and save the extra meat to make the **Rosemary Chicken Noodle Soup** (page 213) or **Chicken + Spinach Enchiladas** (page 218).

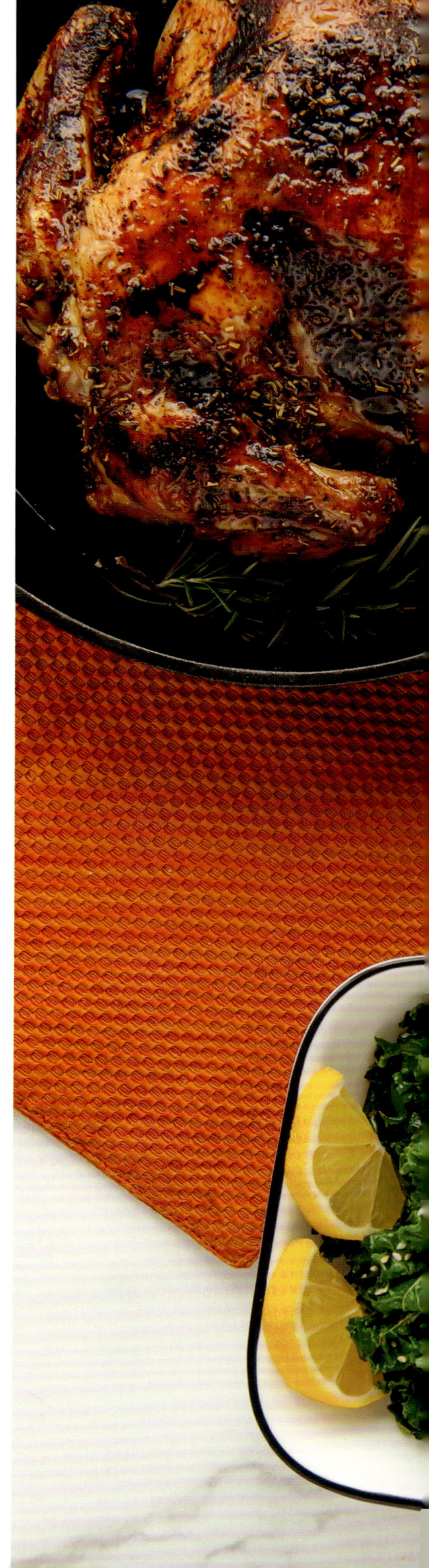

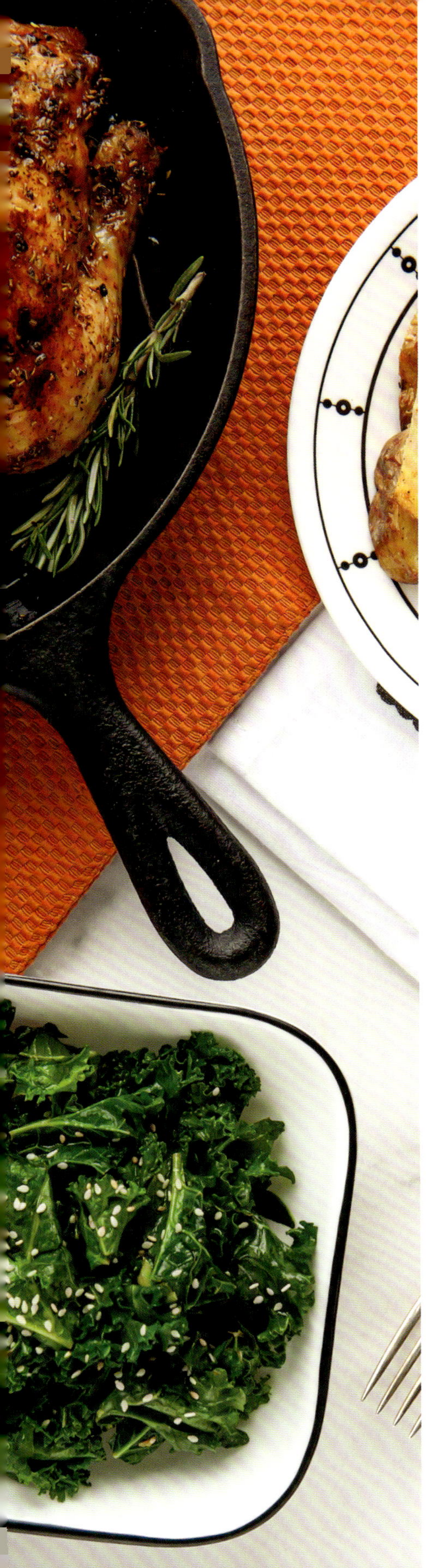

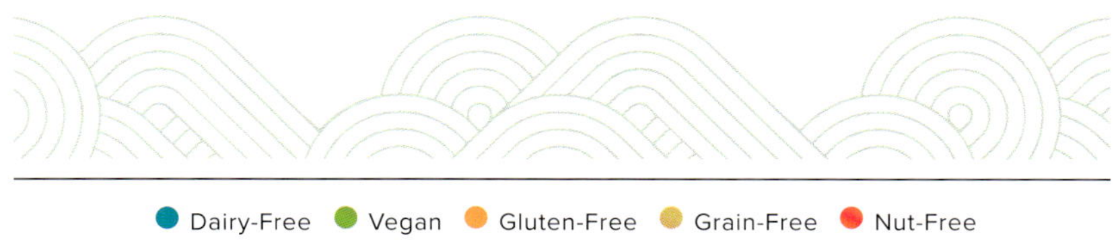

Dairy-Free · Vegan · Gluten-Free · Grain-Free · Nut-Free

Garlic Sesame Kale

In the fall or winter months when raw greens or green smoothies might not be your jam, this super-fast sautéed kale is as delicious as it is perfect for postpartum. Both sesame seeds and kale top the list of calcium superfoods, a mineral that's often low in new moms whose calcium stores did double duty building baby's teeth and bones.

10 MINUTES PREPPING • 5 MINUTES COOKING • MAKES 3 SERVINGS

WHAT YOU NEED:

1 bunch kale, washed, destemmed, and roughly chopped

1 tbsp (15 mL) lemon juice

2 tbsp (30 mL) olive oil, divided

1 pinch sea salt

4 cloves of garlic, minced

1 tbsp (15 mL) sesame seeds

Drizzle of sesame oil (optional)

HOW TO MAKE IT:

1. In a large bowl, top kale with lemon juice, 1 tbsp (15 mL) of the olive oil, and salt. Massage kale for 3 to 5 minutes until kale is noticeably darker and softer (and has reduced in size).
2. In a large pan set to medium heat, add remaining tbsp (15 mL) olive oil. Add garlic and cook, 2 minutes, stirring frequently.
3. Add kale to pan and cook, stirring frequently, 2 to 3 minutes, until kale is bright green and hot throughout but not wilted. Move pan away from heat, sprinkle kale with sesame seeds and sesame oil (if using), and serve immediately.

Link-up

Use leftovers in the **7-Minute Ultimate Breakfast Bowl** (page 39) and enjoy.

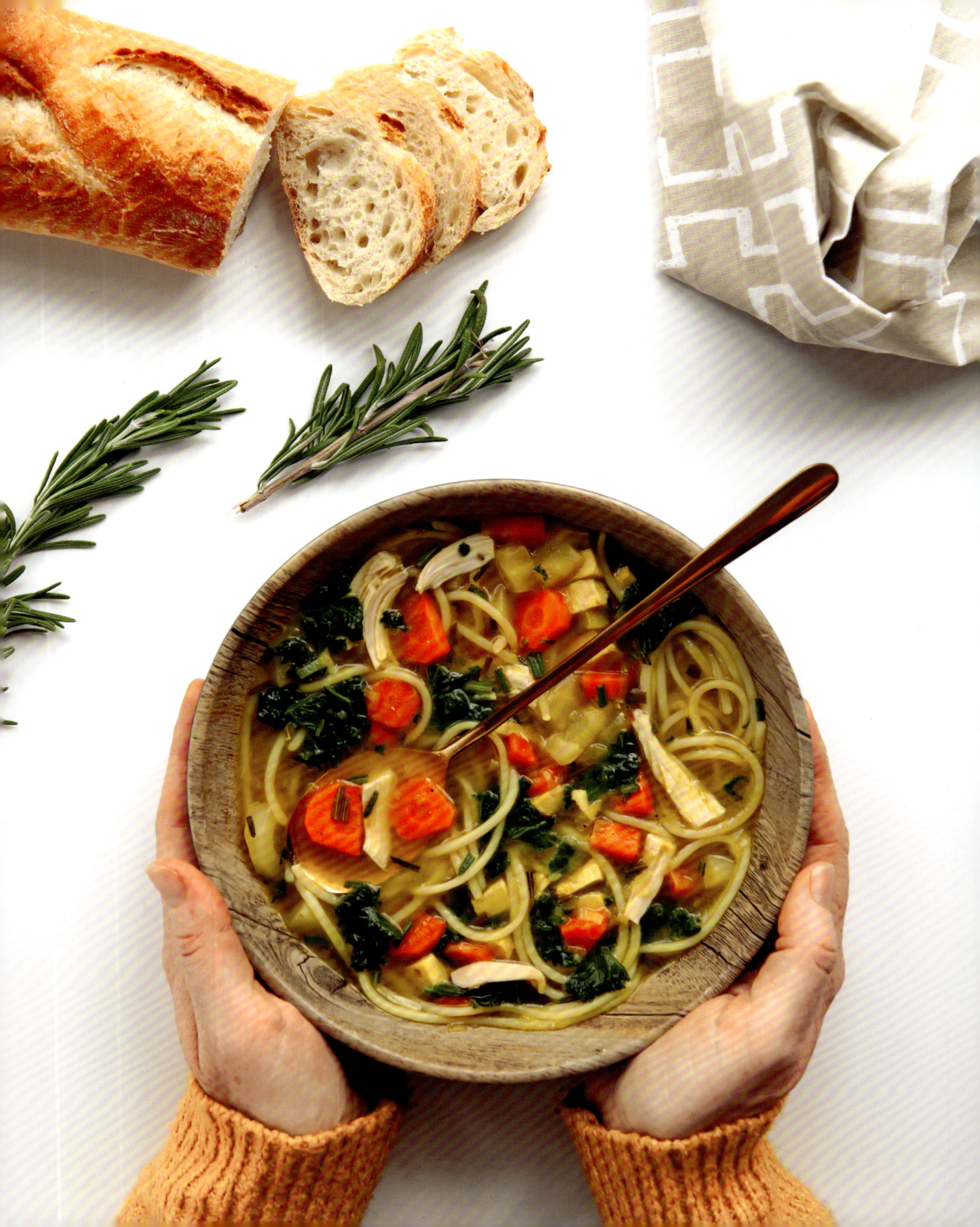

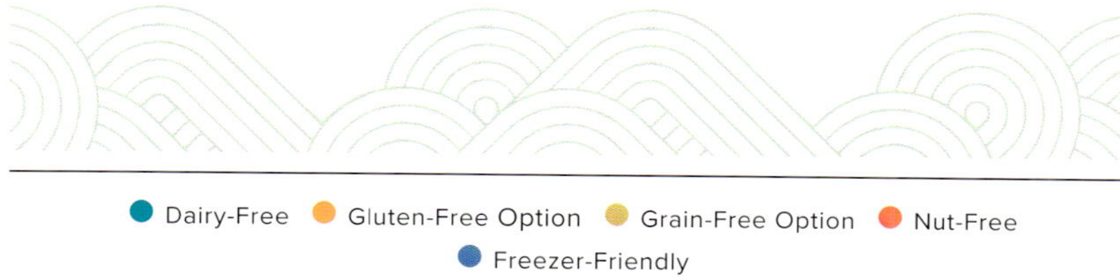

Dairy-Free · Gluten-Free Option · Grain-Free Option · Nut-Free · Freezer-Friendly

Rosemary Chicken Noodle Soup

I've been making this soup for years and it always goes over well. It's exactly what chicken noodle soup should be: nurturing, comforting, warming, and, most of all, delicious. Post-holidays, I make this soup using leftover turkey and it's just as amazing. If you have extra herbs on hand such as thyme or parsley, go ahead and sprinkle some into your bowl.

15 MINUTES PREPPING • 40 MINUTES COOKING • MAKES 4 TO 6 SERVINGS

WHAT YOU NEED:

- 1 tbsp (15 mL) olive oil
- 2 shallots, finely chopped
- 5 carrots (about 1 ⅔ cups/400 mL), sliced into rounds
- 9 cups (2.25 L) Everyday Bone Broth (page 181) or store-bought chicken broth
- 3 cups (750 mL) cooked chicken, roughly diced
- 1 ½ tsp (7.5 mL) fresh rosemary, finely chopped
- ¾ tsp (4 mL) sea salt, divided
- ½ tsp (2 mL) pepper
- 2 cups (500 mL) kale, destemmed and roughly chopped
- 100 g pasta of choice (I use half a box of quinoa noodles)

HOW TO MAKE IT:

1. In a large pot, heat oil over medium heat, then add shallots and ¼ tsp (1 mL) of sea salt, and stir, 2 to 3 minutes.
2. Add carrots and cook, 5 more minutes, stirring often.
3. Add the broth, chicken, rosemary, remaining ½ tsp (2 mL) of sea salt, and pepper to the pot, reserving the kale and pasta. Turn heat to high, bring to a boil, then lower heat to a simmer for 15 to 20 minutes.
4. Add pasta of choice (make sure to check cook time for your particular pasta), and cook until it's done to your liking, stirring occasionally. Add kale in the last 5 minutes of cook time, then turn off heat and serve.

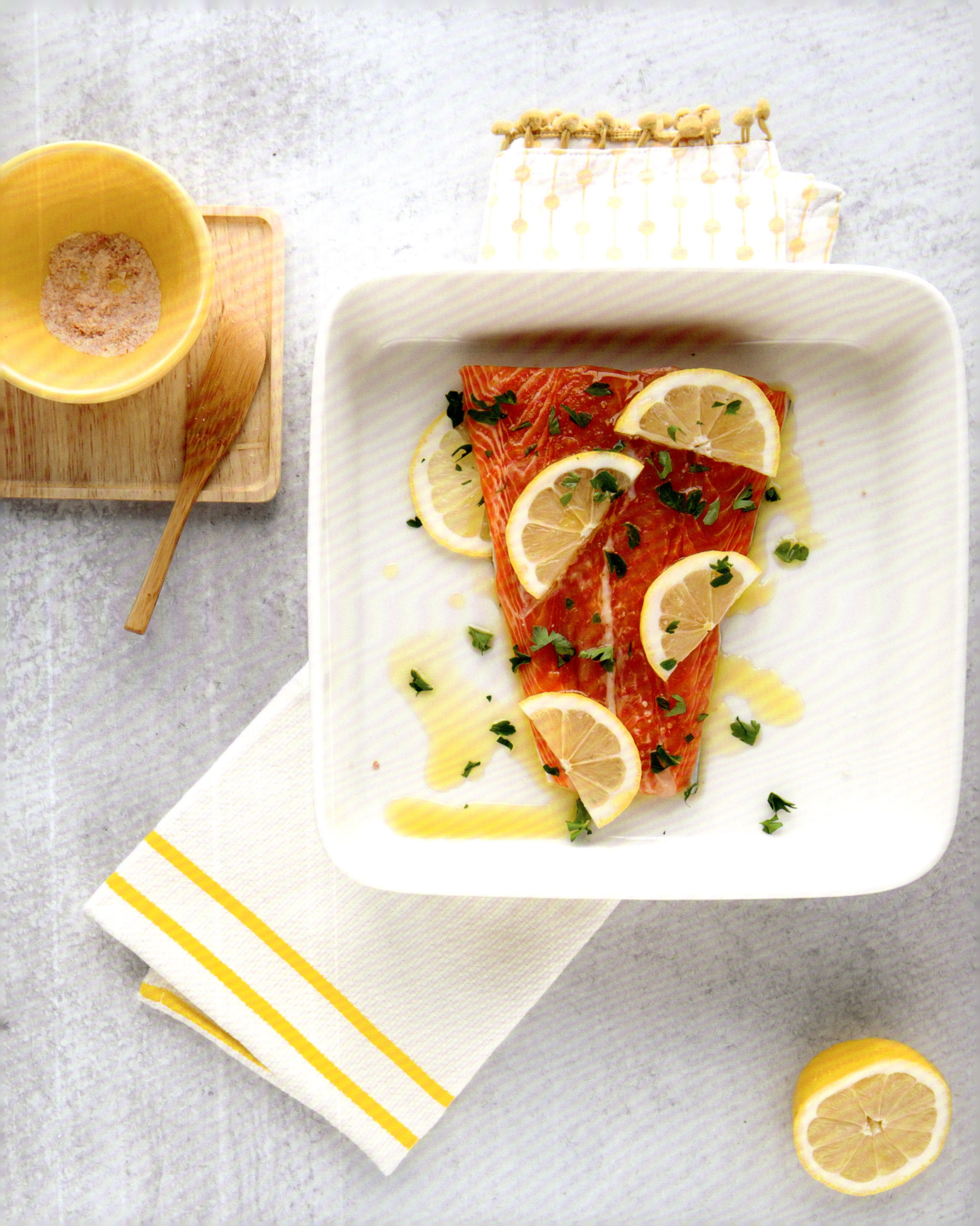

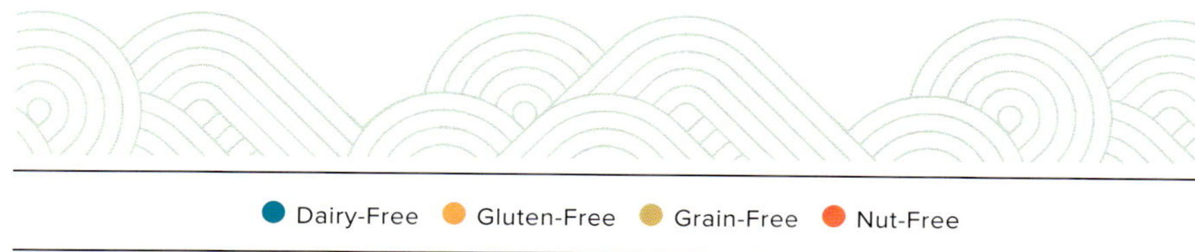

Dairy-Free • Gluten-Free • Grain-Free • Nut-Free

Simple Salted Lemon Salmon

Admittedly, I've had to learn to like salmon. This recipe has made it possible for me to add salmon to my diet — it's just so fast and easy. Plus, not much beats the nutritional profile of salmon, namely the dose of omega-3 fatty acid DHA, which is a super nutrient for mom and baby.

5 MINUTES PREPPING • 20 MINUTES COOKING • MAKES 4 TO 6 SERVINGS

WHAT YOU NEED:

1 large salmon filet (about 2 lb/900 g)

2 tbsp (30 mL) olive oil

1 lemon, half sliced, half left whole

¼ tsp (1 mL) fine sea salt

¼ tsp (1 mL) pepper

1 tbsp (15 mL) fresh parsley, chopped (optional)

Link-up

Leftover parsley? Consider making **Hidden Greens Meatballs**, page 113, or **Warm Golden Cauliflower + Carrot Salad with Cinnamon Maple Dressing**, page 205.

HOW TO MAKE IT:

1. Heat oven to 350°F (180°C) and get out a baking dish or pan that will fit your salmon (if using a baking pan, line it with parchment paper).
2. Brush both sides of the salmon with olive oil, laying the fish skin-side down in your baking dish.
3. Sprinkle salmon with salt and pepper, then arrange lemon slices around the salmon. Squeeze some lemon juice from the half lemon onto the fish, and place the fish in the oven.
4. Salmon is done after about 15 to 20 minutes, or when fish flakes when pierced with a fork.
5. Serve salmon with fresh parsley, if using, and an additional squeeze of lemon juice. Enjoy over salad or with rice and a side of Garlic Sesame Kale (page 211).

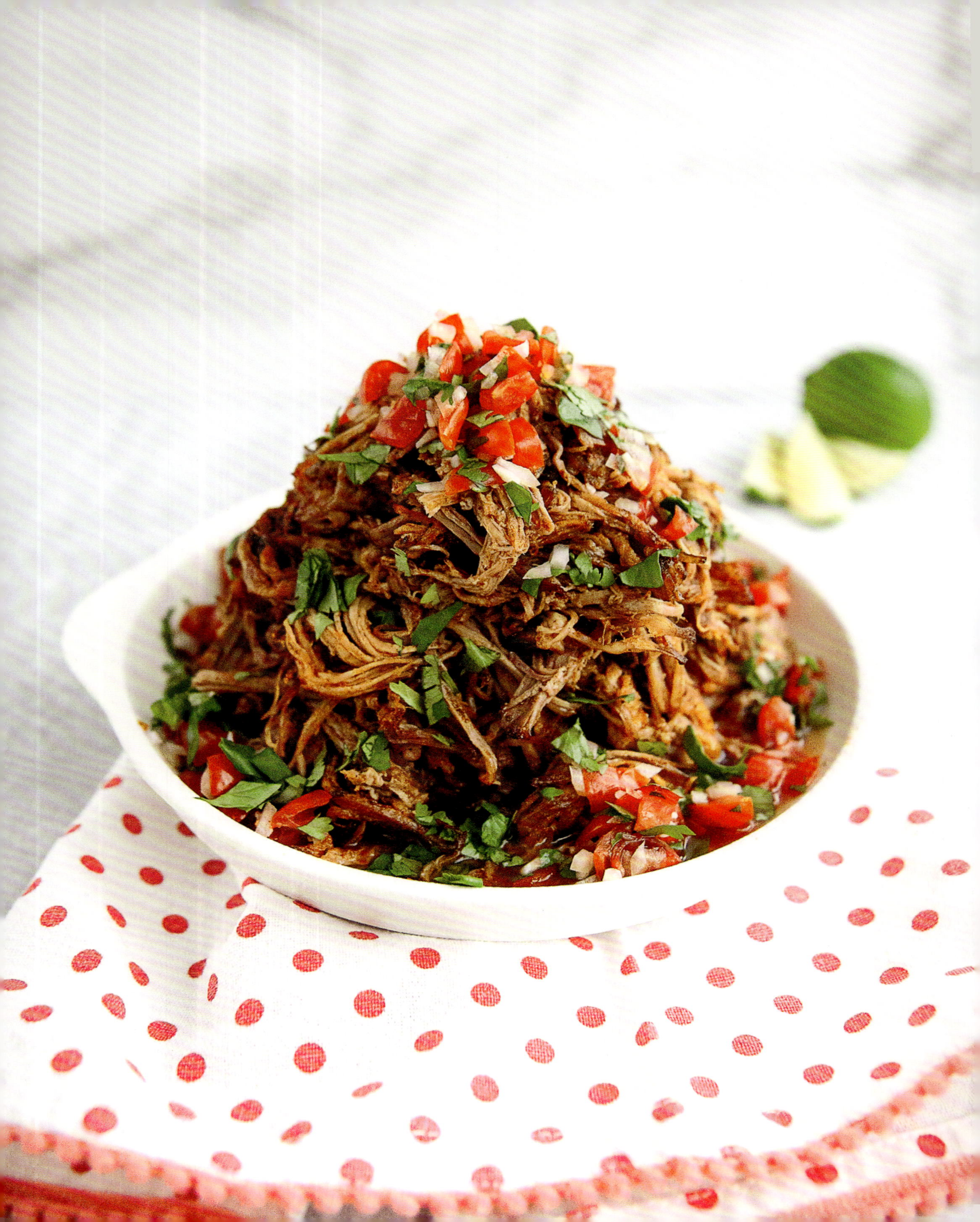

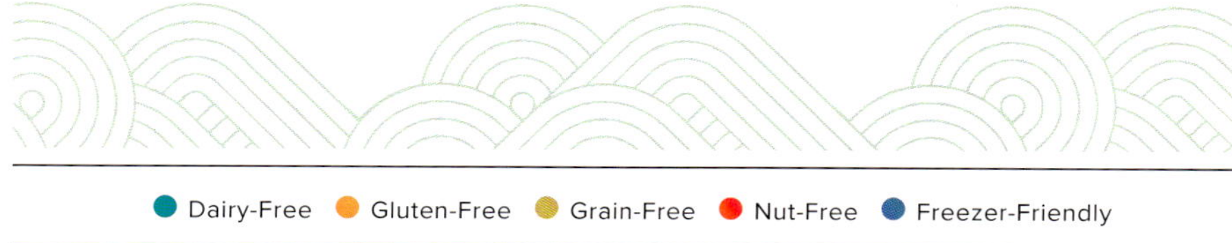

● Dairy-Free ● Gluten-Free ● Grain-Free ● Nut-Free ● Freezer-Friendly

Paprika + Cinnamon Pulled Pork

This dish is so tasty you're not going to want to stop eating it. Full of protein and collagen-building amino acids, pulled pork fits into the category of postpartum healing foods right along with soups and stews. It's a hands-off recipe in the slow cooker, so let it hang out and slow cook all day. I make this recipe to enjoy carnitas for days, but there's no wrong way to eat this amazing pulled pork.

10 MINUTES PREPPING • 8 HOURS COOKING • MAKES 6 TO 8 SERVINGS

WHAT YOU NEED:

- 3 ½ to 4 lb (1.5 to 1.8 kg) pork shoulder (bone in or out)
- 2 tbsp (30 mL) smoked paprika
- 2 tsp (10 mL) sea salt
- 2 tsp (10 mL) cinnamon
- 1 tsp (5 mL) pepper
- 1 cup (250 mL) Everyday Bone Broth, page 181, or store-bought
- ½ cup (125 mL) freshly squeezed orange juice

HOW TO MAKE IT:

1. Add broth and orange juice to slow cooker and set to low setting.
2. Combine spices in a small bowl, then rub all over the pork, using up all of the spices (it seems like a lot, but it's worth it!).
3. Add pork to slow cooker, cover with lid, and let cook for 8 hours.
4. After 8 hours, remove pork from slow cooker and shred with two forks. Store in large glass container, with the juices, until ready to eat.
5. (optional, but highly recommended) When ready to eat, set oven to broil, and line a baking sheet with parchment paper. Add the shredded pork and juices to the prepared sheet and broil for 5 minutes. Remove from oven and, using tongs, flip shredded pork over. Broil for 5 more minutes until nice and crispy, then enjoy on tacos, in a bowl, or on its own!

Link-up

Try pulled pork in the **Fajita Bump Bowl**, page 101. So good!

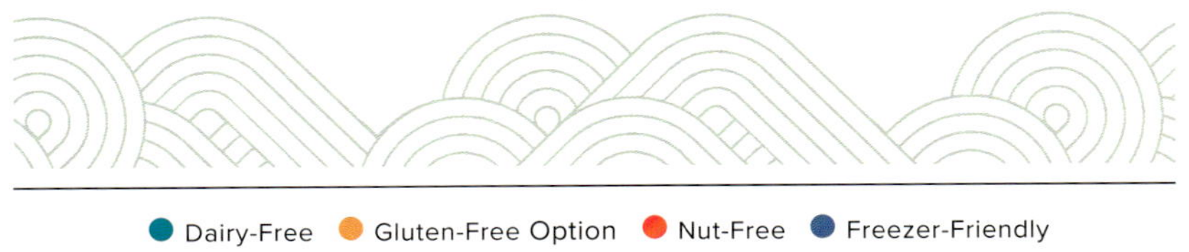

Dairy-Free • Gluten-Free Option • Nut-Free • Freezer-Friendly

Chicken + Spinach Enchiladas

Everyone needs a delicious enchilada recipe in their meal rotation! It's friendly for food prep (you can make both the veggie and chicken mixture and the enchilada sauce in advance, keeping them in the fridge or freezer until you're ready to make your enchiladas). This recipe can easily keep your family happy and well fed for several days.

15 MINUTES PREPPING • 40 MINUTES COOKING • MAKES 8 SERVINGS

WHAT YOU NEED:

1 ½ tbsp (22 mL) olive oil

½ large sweet onion, diced (1 cup/250 mL)

2 ½ bell peppers, diced (3 cups/750 mL)

2 to 2 ½ cups (500 to 625 mL) cooked chicken, diced

2 cups (500 mL) baby spinach, roughly chopped

1 tbsp (15 mL) fajita spice mix (page 71)

1 batch/about 2 cups (500 mL) Lazy Enchilada Sauce (or store bought)

8 tortillas of choice

Optional toppings: pico de gallo, avocado, sliced green onions, cilantro, cheese, or hot sauce

HOW TO MAKE IT:

1. Preheat oven to 375°F (190°C) and grease a 9 × 13-inch casserole dish with avocado oil or butter/ghee.
2. Add the olive oil to a large pan set to medium heat and add the onion and bell peppers. Sauté for 5 minutes, until onion appears softened.
3. Add the cooked chicken, spinach, fajita spice mix, and ½ cup (125 mL) of enchilada sauce to the pan and cook, 3 minutes more, until spinach has wilted and everything is heated through.
4. Spoon ½ to ¾ cup (125 to 175 mL) enchilada sauce into your greased casserole dish to coat lightly.
5. Assemble your enchiladas. Into each tortilla, scoop ½ cup (125 mL) of the chicken and veggie mixture and, folding in the sides, roll into an enchilada and place seam-side down on your casserole dish. Continue until all 8 tortillas have been filled.
6. Top enchiladas with sauce until coated to your liking and bake uncovered, about 20 to 25 minutes, until edges have just started to look golden.
7. Let enchiladas stand for about 5 minutes before serving with desired toppings.

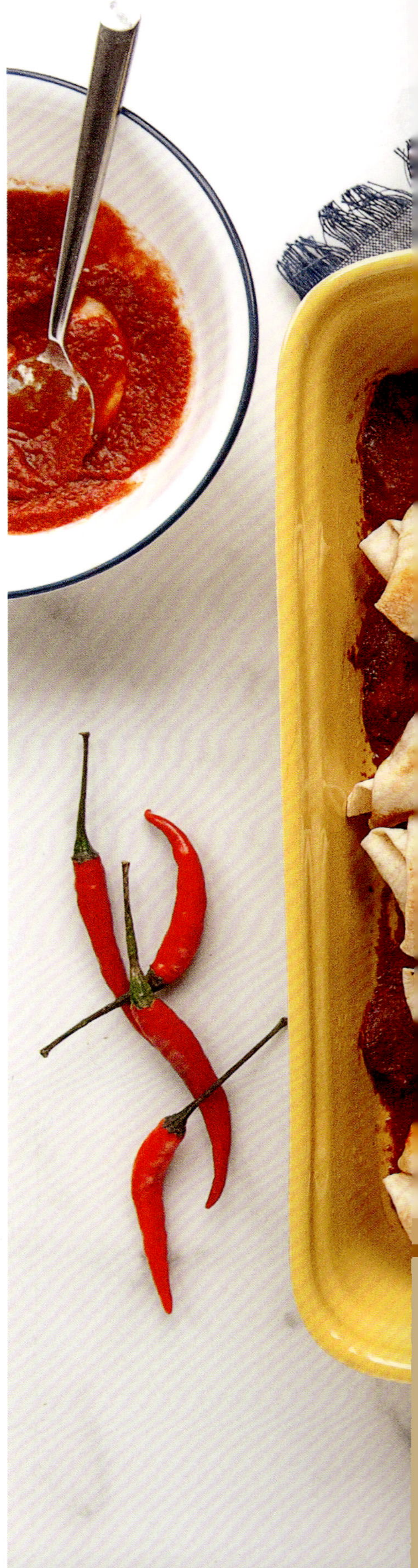

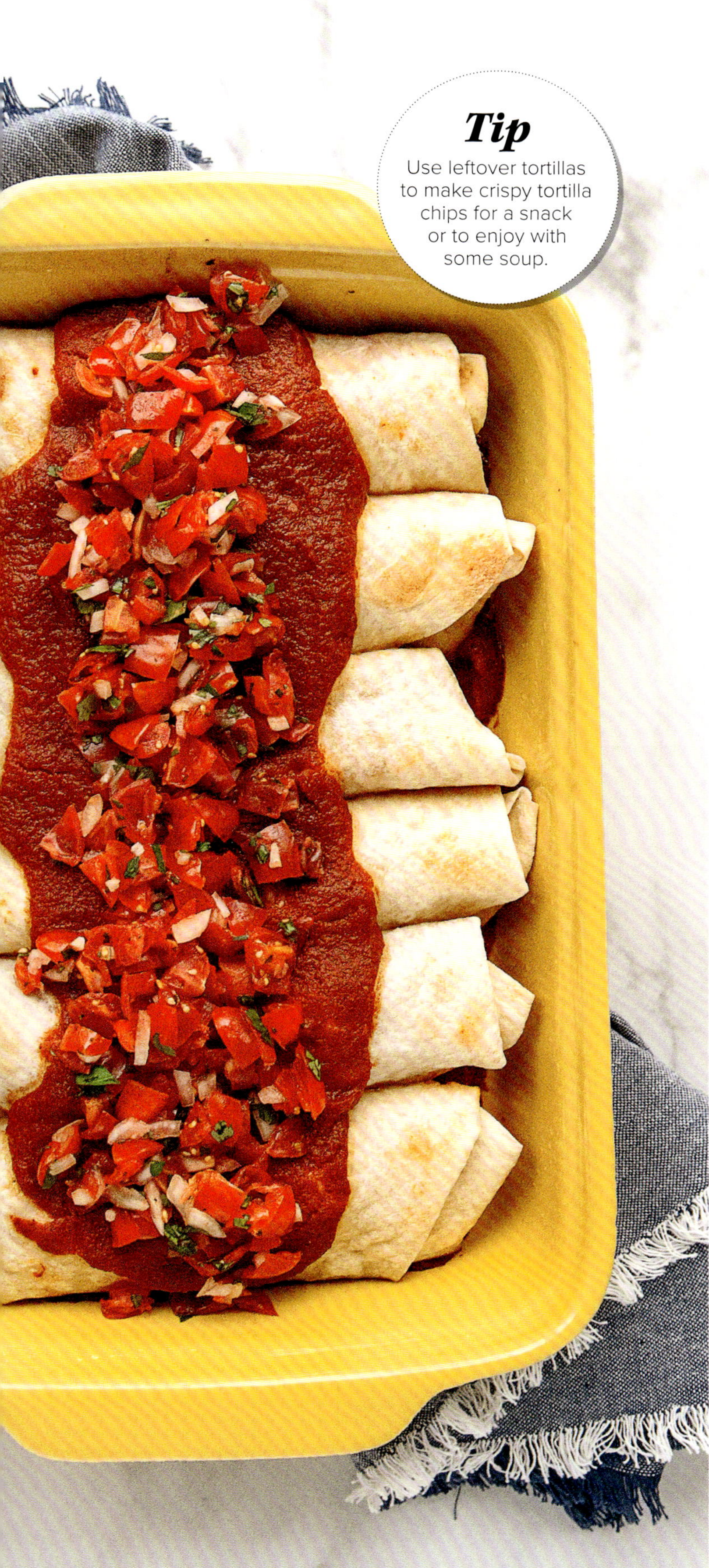

Tip

Use leftover tortillas to make crispy tortilla chips for a snack or to enjoy with some soup.

LAZY ENCHILADA SAUCE

WHAT YOU NEED:

1 jar (23 oz/680 mL) passata/strained tomatoes

1 ½ tbsp (22 mL) chili powder

1 tbsp (15 mL) onion powder

½ tsp (2 mL) garlic powder

¼ tsp (1 mL) fine sea salt

HOW TO MAKE IT:

1. Add all ingredients to a medium pot set over medium-high heat and bring to a boil. Reduce heat to low and simmer for about 5 minutes.
2. Freeze cooled leftover sauce in a glass jar for up to 3 months.

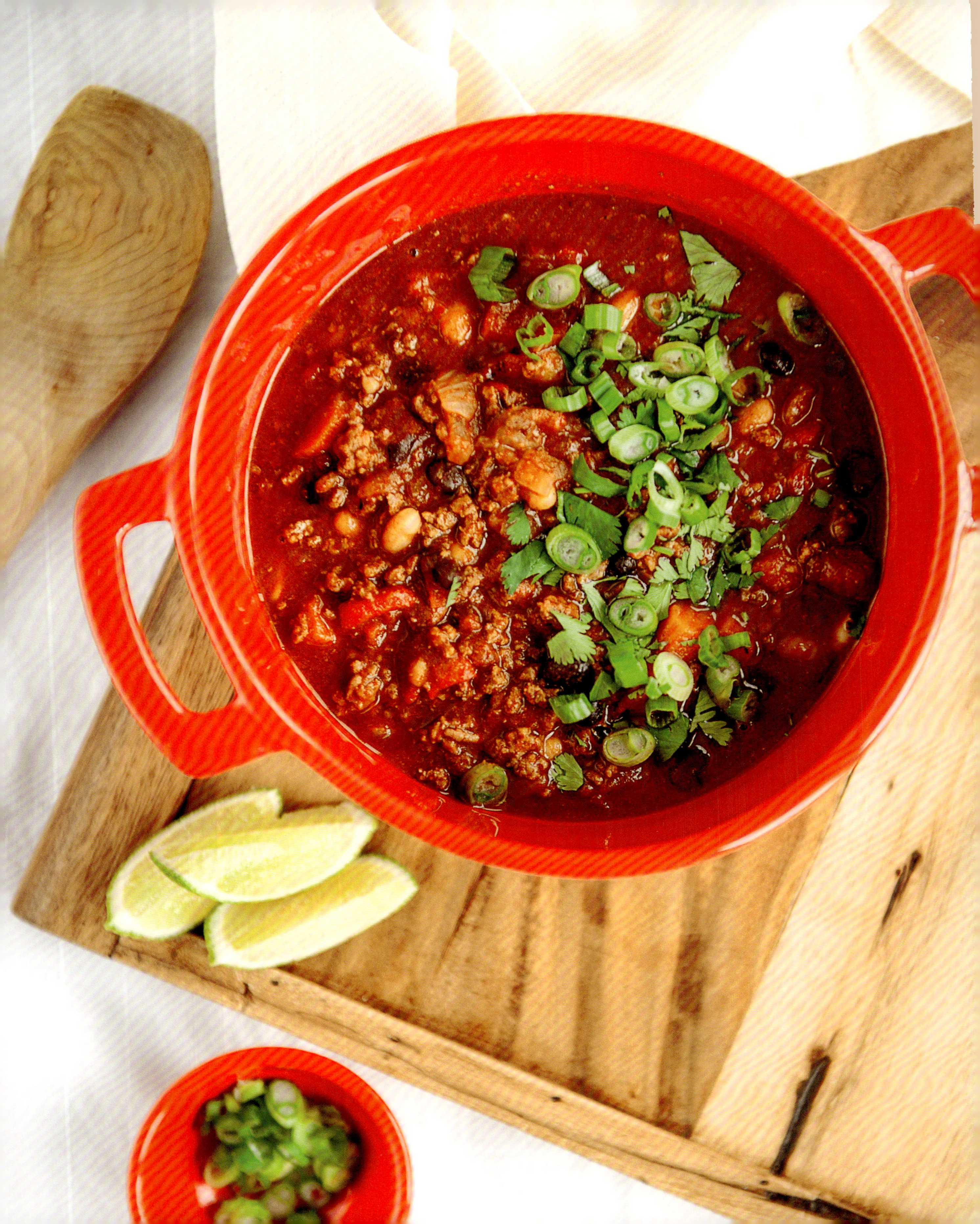

Gluten-Free Option • Grain-Free • Nut-Free • Freezer-Friendly

Stout + Chocolate Chili

My sister's partner, Tom, a great cook and family friend, once made me the best chili I've ever tasted. When finalizing the chili for this book, I had Tom in the kitchen to show me his secrets. I love the addition of stout, a traditional breastfeeding choice thanks to the barley and hops, and chocolate, which really is never a wrong choice.

15 MINUTES PREPPING • 45 MINUTES COOKING • MAKES 6 SERVINGS

WHAT YOU NEED:

- 2 tbsp (30 mL) olive oil
- 1 medium/large onion, finely chopped (2 cups/500 mL)
- 2 to 3 carrots, chopped into small pieces (1 ½ cups/375 mL)
- 2 roasted red peppers, from a jar*
- 2 ½ lb (1.1 kg) lean ground beef
- 1 tsp (5 mL) fine sea salt, divided
- 2 ½ tbsp (37 mL) chili powder
- 2 tbsp (30 mL) cumin
- 2 tsp (10 mL) garlic powder
- 1 ½ tsp (7.5 mL) cinnamon
- 1 ½ tsp (7.5 mL) smoked paprika
- 1 can (19 oz/540 mL) tomatoes, crushed or strained
- 1 can (19 oz/540 mL) tomatoes, diced
- 2 cans (19 oz/540 mL) beans of choice
- 1 cup (250 mL) stout beer**
- 2 to 3 oz (56 to 84 g) semi-sweet, high-quality chocolate, finely grated

HOW TO MAKE IT:

1. Heat olive oil in large pot set to low-medium heat. Add chopped onion and carrots and sauté with ¼ tsp (1 mL) sea salt until onions are translucent, about 5 to 7 minutes.
2. Add ground beef and remaining salt and spices, and sauté until the meat is browned and fully cooked.
3. Add roasted red peppers, both cans of tomatoes, beans, and beer and bring to a simmer. Grate in the chocolate, stir, and let chili simmer, 20 to 30 minutes minimum. Taste the chili, and add additional salt or spices to taste.

NOTE

*Use fresh bell peppers as a substitute for the roasted red peppers, adding them to the pot in step 1 with the carrots and onions.

**Use bone broth (homemade or store-bought) as a gluten-free and alcohol-free substitute for the beer.

Link-up

Use up the rest of the jar of roasted red peppers in the **Red Pepper Basil Egg Cups** recipe, page 185.

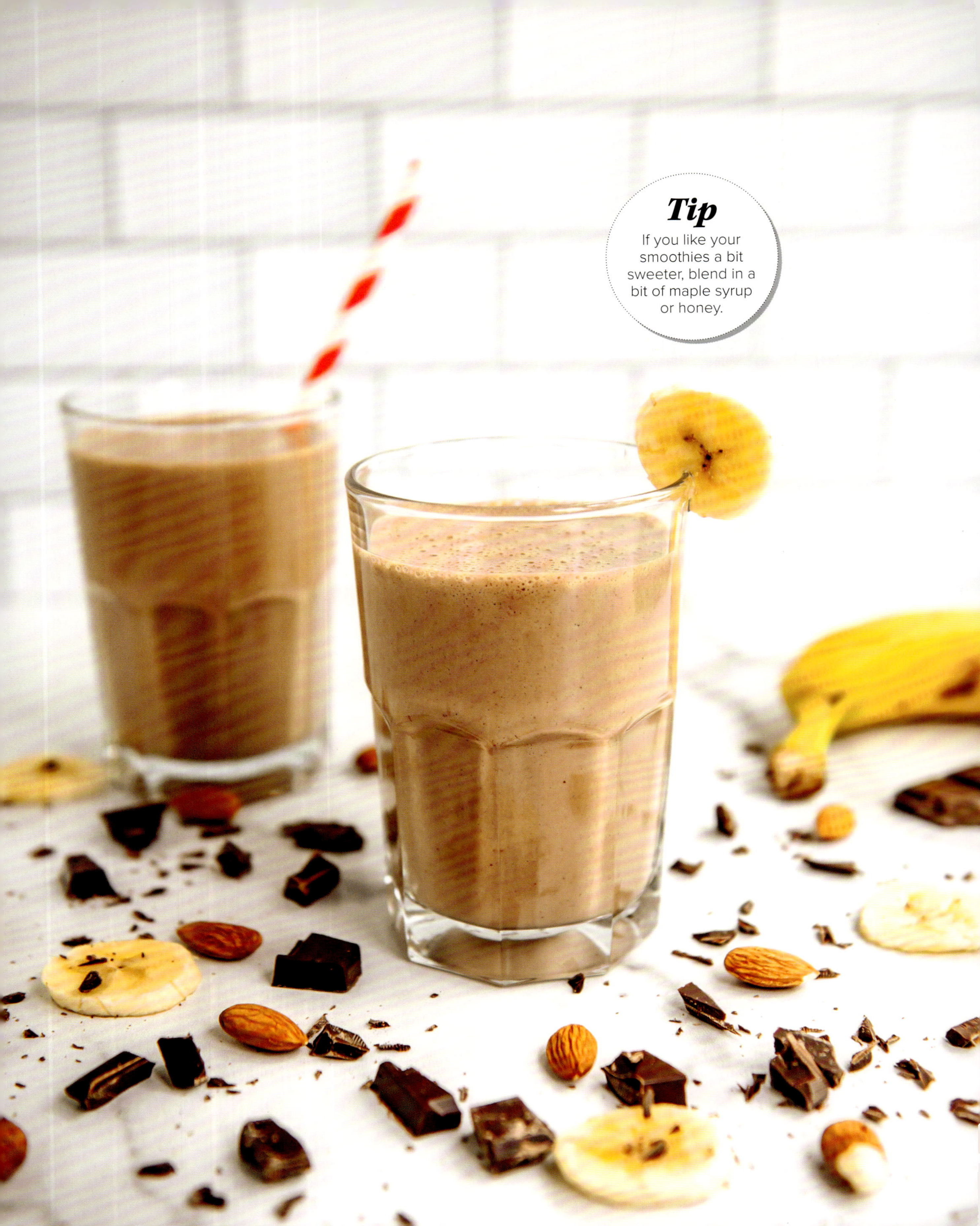
Tip
If you like your smoothies a bit sweeter, blend in a bit of maple syrup or honey.

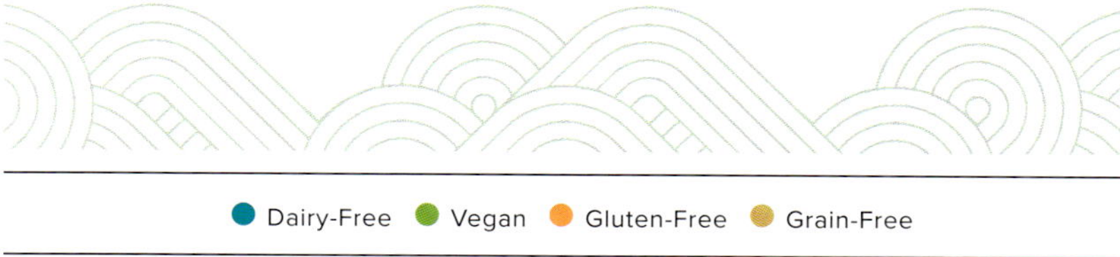

Dairy-Free • Vegan • Gluten-Free • Grain-Free

Sip to Sleep Chocolate Smoothie

AKA the nighttime smoothie. This makes a great protein-and-fat powered before-bed or middle-of-the-night snack when you're up feeding baby. Simply make the smoothie before bed, keep it in the refrigerator, and drink it when needed during the night. For an extra-cold smoothie, add a few ice cubes when blending.

5 MINUTES PREPPING • 1 MINUTE BLENDING • MAKES 1 LARGE OR 2 SMALL SERVINGS

WHAT YOU NEED:	HOW TO MAKE IT:
1 ½ cups (375 mL) Cashew Hemp Milk (page 189) or milk of choice	1. Add all ingredients in a high-powered blender and blend for about 1 minute, or until smoothly combined.
1 to 2 tbsp (15 to 30 mL) ground flaxseed	
1 tbsp (15 mL) almond butter, or nut/seed butter of choice	
½ tbsp (7 mL) cacao powder	
½ a frozen banana	
¼ tsp (1 mL) cinnamon	

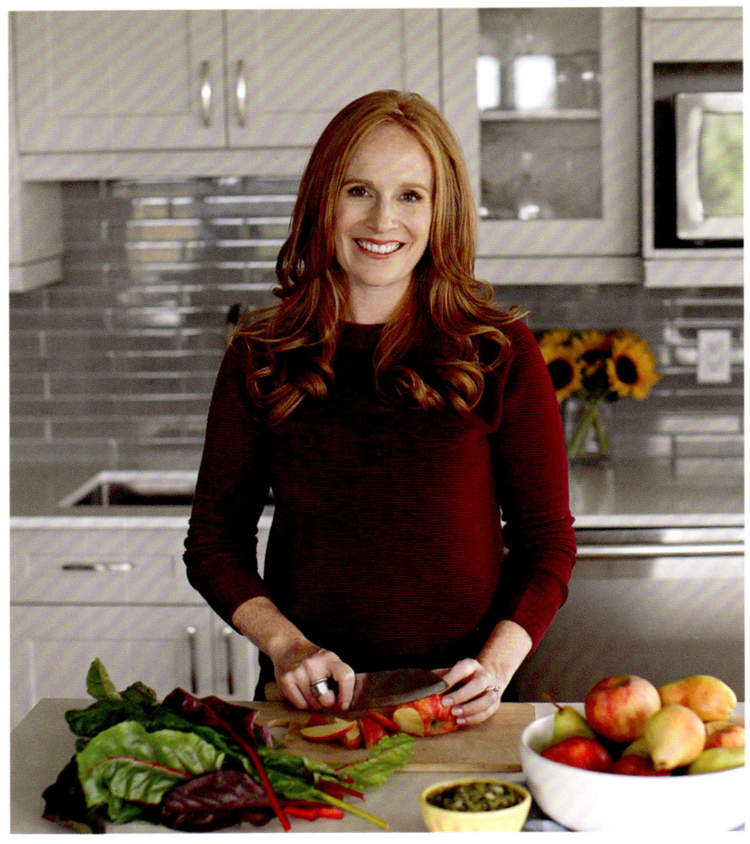

LINDSAY TAYLOR loves food, and promotes real-food nutrition for health and wellness. She believes strongly that eating healthy can be fun, easy, enjoyable, and rewarding for everyone.

As a mom, certified culinary nutrition expert, and doula with a background in public health and academic research, Lindsay understands the impact of pregnancy and motherhood on women's lives. She knows the importance of eating wholesome, nourishing food to optimize the well-being of both moms and their babies — hence this book.

Lindsay delights in sharing what she knows about how to cope with the ups and downs of pregnancy and new-mom life, and the benefits of real-food choices. She creates easy-to-follow recipes for cooking up nutritious meals, and includes practical tips and tricks to enhance the prepping and cooking experience. For Lindsay, writing *The Food Doula Cookbook* has been a commitment — and a labour of love.

ACKNOWLEDGEMENTS

COOKING IS VERY RARELY an innate skill, but learned through family, community, and, let's face it, necessity. I couldn't put together more than grilled cheese and salads for most of my life, despite my lifelong interest in nutrition. That's the thing about nutrition — it can exist in facts without ever being translated to the plate. Cooking is a practice, so thank you for being willing to do just that — practise with a new recipe, a new ingredient, and this book. I'm so grateful for you!

A huge thank you to Maggie Goh, President and Publisher of Rubicon Publishing and Plumleaf Press, for believing in this project. You gave me an opportunity that I had only dreamed of. To my editor Kim Koh, the hardest- and fastest-working person I know, thank you for making my vision a reality. To Terri, Jennifer, Robin, Christine, and the whole team at Rubicon for their dedication to and excitement for this book.

I am so thankful to all of these (mostly) women and mothers who were so giving of their time (during a pandemic) and who tested, retested, and made every recipe better than I could have done on my own. Thank you to Kristin Olive, Ainsley Harpur, Laura Cornacchione, Laura Guglick, Deb Schnarr, Kim and Ali Schnarr, Jennifer Ryder, Lisa Williamson, Jen Schnarr, Brooke Taylor (who made the pumpkin pancakes at least five times with twin newborns and a two-year-old at home to ensure it was fit to be a new-mom staple!), Erin Hollingsworth, Sarah Rawski, Laura Mack, Monique Aucoin, Pamela Ritchie, Jaklyn Andrews, Victoria Hull, Denise Taylor, Katie Compton, Heather Travis, Andria Hinton, Jacqueline Szwedo, Jess Taylor, Tom Duff, Philippa Taylor, Christina Gianonne, Mary Kutarna, Sacha Taylor, Mary Bracken, Erin Romeo, Jillian Stewart, Scott Taylor, Cheryl and Penny Stubbs. I am so glad I asked for help.

To Meghan Telpner and the Academy of Culinary Nutrition for *getting it*. For teaching comfort in the kitchen and know-how with real food, and for giving me the confidence that what I had to say and offer with this book was valuable.

To my sisters, both biological and chosen, who are my sounding board and have been instrumental in seeing and pushing me toward the dreams that they knew were there all along. Christina, Katie, Alex, Jess and Jill — these women are strong, talented, giving, and kind. So beyond thankful for you.

To Tom, Scott and Maria, for brightening up my life with your infectious energy and positivity, for being family, for loving food, and for happily collaborating with me on the world's best chili (just waiting for that certification).

I am so grateful for my parents. My four-year-old likes my dad better than me; doesn't that say a lot? My mom — my biggest cheerleader, whose love and positivity radiate always. Some people have food stylists, prop stylists, photographers, and assistants to make recipes look great — I had my mom. She ironed linens, helped me chop veggies, and parented so that I could get it done. She's the best!

Mike, you are the reason this book is here. The reason I was able to put these words on the page, tear apart our kitchen testing recipes, and somehow manage to be my own food photographer. Your love, support, patience, and partnership are unwavering, and I am so lucky to be doing life with you.

Finally, thank you to the families who have let me into their homes, relied on me to help them thrive, and trusted me to share recipes that were doable and could be part of their family mealtime memories. It is a privilege to be part of your life.

REFERENCES

Calcium

Cullers, A., King, J. C., Van Loan, M., Gildengorin, G., & Fung, E. B. (2019). Effect of prenatal calcium supplementation on bone during pregnancy and 1 y postpartum. *The Americal Journal of Clinical Nutrition*, 109(1), 197–206.

Hacker, A. N., Fung, E. B., & King, J. C. (2012). Role of calcium during pregnancy: Maternal and fetal needs. *Nutrient Reviews*, 70(7), 397–409.

Hofmeyr, G. J., Lawrie, T. A., Atallah, A. N., & Torloni, M. R. (2018). Calcium supplementation during pregnancy for preventing hypertensive disorders and related problems. *Cochrane Database of Systematic Reviews*, 10(10).

Schoenaker, D. A., Soedamah-Muthu, S. S., & Mishra, G. D. (2014). The association between dietary factors and gestational hypertension and pre-eclampsia: A systematic review and meta-analysis of observational studies. *BMC Medicine*, 12(157).

Choline

Beluska-Turkan, K., Korczak, R., Hartell, B., Moskal, K., Maukonen, J., Alexander, D. E., Salem, N., Harkness, L., Ayad, W., Szaro, J., Zhang, K., & Siriwardhana, N. (2019). Nutritional gaps and supplementation in the first 1000 days. *Nutrients*, 11 (12), 2891.

Masih, S. P., Plumptre, L., Ly, A., Berger, H., Lausman, A. Y., Croxford, R., Kim, Y., & O'Connor, D. L. (2015). Pregnant Canadian women achieve recommended intakes of one-carbon nutrients through prenatal supplementation but the supplement composition, including choline, requires reconsideration. *The Journal of Nutrition*, 145 (8), 1824–1834.

Zeisel, S. H. (2008). Choline: Critical role during fetal development and dietary requirements in adults. *Annual Review of Nutrition*, 26, 229–250.

Zeisel, S. H. (2013). Nutrition in pregnancy: The argument for including a source of choline. *International Journal of Women's Health*, 5, 193–199.

Dates

Al-Kuran, O., Al-Mehaisen, L., Bawadi, H., Beitawi, S., & Amarin, Z. (2011). The effect of late pregnancy consumption of date fruit on labour and delivery. *Journal of Obstetrics and Gynaecolgy*, 31(1), 29–31.

Khadem, N., Sharaphy, A., Latifnejad, R., Hammond, N., & Ibrahimzadeh, S. (2007). Comparing the efficacy of dates and oxytocin in the management of postpartum hemorrhage. *Shiraz E-Medical Journal*, 8(2).

Razali, N., Mohd Nahwari, S. H., Sulaiman, S., & Hassan, J. (2017). Date fruit consumption at term: Effect on length of gestation, labour and delivery. *Journal of Obstetrics and Gynaecology*, 37(5), 595–600.

Eating During Labour

Ciardulli, A., Saccone, G., Anastasio, H., & Berghella, V. (2017). Less-Restrictive Food Intake During Labour in Low-Risk Singleton Pregnancies: A Systematic Review and Meta-Analysis. *Obstetrics and Gynecology*, 129 (3); 473–480.

Moola, S., Baxter, H., Di Lallo, S., Handa, M., Hanvey, L., Jefferies, A., & Watts, N. (2018). Public Health Agency of Canada: Family-Centred Maternity and Newborn Care: National Guidelines. Retrieved from: https://www.canada.ca/en/public-health/services/publications/healthy-living/maternity-newborn-care-guidelines-chapter-4.html#a7.

Public Health Agency of Canada (2012). Canadian Hospitals Maternity Policies and Practises Survey (Ottawa). Retrieved from: http://www.mncyn.ca/wp-content/uploads/2016/03/2011_CHMPPS-report.pdf.

Singata, M., Tranmer, J., & Gyte, G. M. (2013). Restricting oral fluid and food intake during labour. *Cochrane Database of Systematic Review*, 2013(8).

Ginger

Lete, I. & Allué, J. (2016). The Effectiveness of Ginger in the Prevention of Nausea and Vomiting during Pregnancy and Chemotherapy. *Integrated Medicine Insights*, 11, 11–17.

Greens

Shahrook, S., Ota, E., Hanada, N., Sawada, K., & Mori, R. (2018). Vitamin K Supplementation during pregnancy for improving outcomes: a systematic review and meta-analysis. *Nature Scientific Reports*, 8, 11459.

Iron

Allen, L. H. (2000). Anemia and iron deficiency: Effects on pregnancy outcome. *The American Journal of Clinical Nutrition*, 71(5), 1280S–1284S.

Alwan, N. A. & Hamamy, H. (2015). Maternal iron status in pregnancy and long-term health outcomes in the offspring. *Journal of Pediatric Genetics*, 4(2), 111–123.

Georgieff, M. K. (2011). Long-term brain and behavioural consequences of early iron deficiency. *Nutrition Reviews*, 69(1), S43–S48.

Juul, S. E., Derman, R. J., & Auerbach, M. (2019). Perinatal iron deficiency: Implications for mothers and infants. *Neonatology*, 115, 269–274.

Wiegersma, A. M., Dalman, C., & Lee, B. K. (2019). Association of prenatal maternal anemia with neurodevelopmental disorders. *JAMA Psychiatry*, 76(12), 1294–1304.

Lemon

Yavari Kia, P., Safajou, F., Shahnazi, M., & Nazemiyeh, H. (2014). The Effect of Lemon Inhalation Aromatherapy on Nausea and Vomiting of Pregnancy: A Double-Blinded, Randomized, Controlled Clinical Trial. *Iranian Red Crescent Medical Journal*, 16(3), 14360.

Maternal Nutrition

Abu-Saad, K. & Fraser, D. (2010). Maternal Nutrition and Birth Outcomes. *Epidemiologic Reviews*, 32(1), 5–25.

Gallo, L. A., Tran, M., Moritz, K. M., & Wlodek, M. E. (2013). Developmental programming: Variations in early growth and adult disease. *Clinical and Experimental Pharmacology and Physiology*, 40; 795–802.

Gresham E., Collins, C. E., Mishra, G. D., Byles, J. E., & Hure, A. J. (2016). Diet quality before or during pregnancy and the relationship with pregnancy and birth outcomes: the Australian Longitudinal Study on Women's Health. *Public Health Nutrition*, 19(16), 2975–2983.

Han, Z., Mulla, S., Beyene, J., Liao, G., & McDonald, S. D. (2011). Maternal underweight and the risk of preterm birth and low birthweight: A systematic review and meta analyses. *International Journal of Epidemiology*, 40(1), 65–101.

Igwebuike, U. M. (2010). Impact of maternal nutrition on ovine foetoplacental development: A review of the role of insulin-like growth factors. *Animal Reproduction Science*; 121 (3–4), 189–196.

Koletzko, B., Godfrey, K. M., Poston, L., Szajewska, H., van Goudoever, J. B., de Waard, M., Brands, B., Grivell, R. M., Deussen, A. R., Dodd, J. M., Patro-Golab, B., & Zalewski, B. M. (2019). Nutrition During Pregnancy, Lactation, and Early Childhood and its Implications for Maternal and Long-Term Child Health: The Early Nutrition Project Recommendations. *Annals of Nutrition and Metabolism*, 74, 93–106.

Meher, A., Sundrani, D., & Joshi, S. (2015). Maternal nutrition influences angiogenesis in the placenta through peroxisome proliferator activated receptors: A hypothesis. *Molecular Reproduction and Development*, 82(10); 726–734.

Milk Composition

Brenna, J. T., Varamini, B., Jensen, R. G., Diersen-Schade, D. A., Boettcher, J. A., & Arterburn, L. M. (2007). Docosahexaenoic and arachidonic acid concentrations in human breast milk worldwide. *The American Journal of Clinical Nutrition*, 85(6), 1457–1464.

Dror, D. K. & Allen L. H. (2018). Vitamin B-12 in Human Milk: A Systematic Review. *Advances in Nutrition*, 9(1), 358S–366S.

Hahn-Holbrook, J., Fish, A., & Glynn, L. M. (2019). Human milk omega-3 fatty acid composition is associated with infant temperament. *Nutrients*, 11(12), 2964.

Hay, G., Clausen, T., Whitelaw, A., Trygg, K., Johnston, C., Henriksen, T., & Refsum, H. (2010). Maternal folate and cobalamin status predicts vitamin status in newborns and 6-month-old infants. *The Journal of Nutrition*, 140(3), 557–564.

Pawlak, R., Vos, P., Shahab-Ferdows, S., Hampel, D., Allen, L. H., & Perrin, M. T. (2018). Vitamin B-12 content in breast milk of vegan, vegetarian, and nonvegetarian lactating women in the United States. *American Journal of Clinical Nutrition*, 109(1), 525–531.

Milk Supply

Bazzano, A. N., Hofer, R., Thibeau, S., Gillispie, V., Jacobs, M., & Theall, K. P. (2016). A review of herbal and pharmaceutical galactagogues for breast-feeding. *The Ochsner Journal*, 16(4), 511–524.

Kominiarek, M. A. & Rajan, P. (2016). Nutritional recommendations in pregnancy and lactation. *The Medical Clinics of North America*, 100(6), 1199–1215.

Morning Sickness

Campbell, K., Rowe, H., Azzam, H., & Lane, C. (2016). The Management of Nausea and Vomiting of Pregnancy. *Journal of Obstetrics and Gynecology Canada*, 38(12), 1127–1137.

Crozier, S., Inskip, H. M., Godfrey, K. M., Cooper, C., & Robinson S. M. (2017). Nausea and vomiting in early pregnancy: Effects on food intake and diet quality. *Maternal and Child Nutrition*, 13(4), e12389.

Deuchar, N. (2000). The psychological and social aspects of nausea and vomiting of pregnancy. *Nausea and Vomiting of Pregnancy: State of the Art 2000, Vol 1.* Toronto: Motherrisk, 10–14.

Nutrient Status of a New Mom

Centres for Disease Control and Prevention (2020). Breastfeeding: Maternal Diet. Retrieved from: https://www.cdc.gov/breastfeeding/breastfeeding-special-circumstances/diet-and-micronutrients/maternal-diet.html

Kominiarek, M. A. & Rajan, P. (2016). Nutrition recommendations in pregnancy and lactation. *The Medical Clinics of North America*, 100(6), 1199–1215.

Prado, E. L. & Dewey, K. G. (2014). Nutrition and brain development in early life. *Nutrition Reviews*, 72(4), 267–284.

Omega-3 Fatty Acids

Braarud, H. C., Markhus, M. W., Skotheim, S., Stormark, K. M., Frøyland, L., Graff, I. E., & Kjellevold, M. (2018). Maternal DHA Status during Pregnancy Has a Positive Impact on Infant Problem Solving: A Norwegian Prospective Observation Study. *Nutrients*, 10(5), 529.

Koletzko, B., Boey, C. C., Campoy, C., Carlson, S. E., Chang, N., Guillermo-Tuazon, M. A., Joshi, S., Prell, C., Quak, S. H., Sjarif, D. R., Su, Y., Supapannachart, S., Yamashiro, Y., & Osendarp, S. J. (2014). Current information and Asian perspectives on long-chain polyunsaturated fatty acids in pregnancy, lactation, and infancy: systematic review and practice recommendations from an Early Nutrition Academy workshop. *Annals of Nutrition and Metabolism*, 65(1), 49–80.

Lauritzen, L., Brambilla, P., Mazzocchi, A., Harsløf, L. B., Ciappolino, V., & Agostoni, C. (2016). DHA Effects in Brain Development and Function. *Nutrients*, 8(1), 6.

Massari, M., Novielli, C., Mandò, C., Di Franceesco, S., Della Porta, M., Cazzola, R., Panteghini, M., Savasi, V., Maggini, S., Schaefer, E., & Cetin, I. (2020). Multiple Micronutrients and Docosahexaenoic Acid Supplementation during Pregnancy: A Randomized Controlled Study. *Nutrients*, 12(8), 2432.

Middleton, P., Gomersall, J. C., Gould, J. F., Shepherd, E., Olsen, S. F., & Makrides, M. (2018). Omega-3 fatty acid addition during pregnancy. Cochrane Database of Systematic Reviews, 11.

Weiser, M. J., Butt, C. M., & Mohajeri, M. H. (2016). Docosahexaenoic Acid and Cognition throughout the Lifespan. *Nutrients*, 8(2), 99.

Overall Dietary Patterns

Chia, A. R., Chen, L. W., Lai, J. S., Wong, C. H., Neelakantan, N., van Dam, R. M., & Chong, M. F. F. (2019). Maternal dietary patterns and birth outcomes: A systematic review and meta-analysis. *Advances in Nutrition*, 10(4), 685–695.

Kibret, K. T., Chojenta, C., Gresham, E., Tegegne, T. K., & Loxton, D. (2018). Maternal dietary patterns and risk of adverse pregnancy (hypertensive disorders of pregnancy and gestational diabetes mellitus) and birth (preterm birth and low birth weight) outcomes: A systematic review and meta-analysis. *Public Health Nutrition*, 22(3), 506–520.

Perinatal Mood

Brandenbarg, J., Vrijkotte, T. G., Goedhart, G., & van Eijsden, M. (2012). Maternal early-pregnancy vitamin D status is associated with maternal depressive symptoms in the Amsterdam Born Children and Their Development cohort. *Psychosomatic Medicine*, 74(7), 751–757.

Chatzi, L., Melaki, V., Sarri, K., Apostolaki, I., Roumeliotaki, T., Georgiou, V., Vassilaki, M., Koutis, A., Bitsios, P., & Kogevinas, M. (2011). Dietary patterns during pregnancy and the risk of postpartum depression: the mother-child 'Rhea' cohort in Crete, Greece. *Public Health Nutrition*, 14(9), 1663–1670.

Chong, M. F., Wong, J. X., Colega, M., Chen, L. W., van Dam, R. M., Tan, C. S., Lim, A. L., Cai, S., Broekman, B. F., Lee, Y. S., Saw, S. M., Kwek, K., Godfrey, K. M., Chong, Y. S., Gluckman, P., Meaney, M. J., Chen, H., & GUSTO study group (2014). Relationships of maternal folate and vitamin B12 status during pregnancy with perinatal depression: The GUSTO study. *Journal of Psychiatric Research*, 55, 110–116.

Gould, J. F., Best, K., & Makrides, M. (2017). Perinatal nutrition interventions and post-partum depressive symptoms. *Journal of Affective Disorders*, 224, 2–9.

Miyake, Y., Tanaka, K., Okubo, H., Sasaki, S., & Arakawa, M. (2015a) Intake of dairy products and calcium and prevalence of depressive symptoms during pregnancy in Japan: a cross-sectional study. *BJOG: An International Journal of Obstetrics & Gynaecology*, 122(3), 336–343.

Mokhber, N., Namjoo, M., Tara, F., Boskabadi, H., Rayman, M. P., Ghayour-Mobarhan, M., Sahebkar, A., Majdi, M. R., Tavallaie, S., Azimi-Nezhad, M., Shakeri, M. T., Nematy, M., Oladi, M., Mohammadi, M., & Ferns, G. (2011). Effect of supplementation with selenium on postpartum depression: a randomized double-blind placebo-controlled trial. *The Journal of Maternal-Fetal & Neonatal Medicine,* 24(1), 104–108.

Nielsen, N. O., Strøm, M., Boyd, H. A., Andersen, E. W., Wohlfahrt, J., Lundqvist, M., Cohen, A., Hougaard, D. M., & Melbye, M. (2013). Vitamin D status during pregnancy and the risk of subsequent postpartum depression: a case-control study. *PloS one*, 8(11), e80686.

Rees, A. M., Austin, M.-P., Owen, C., & Parker, G. (2009). Omega-3 deficiency associated with perinatal depression: case control study. *Psychiatry Research*, 166(2–3), 254–259.

Roy, A., Evers, S. E., Avison, W. R., & Campbell, M. K. (2010). Higher zinc intake buffers the impact of stress on depressive symptoms in pregnancy. *Nutrition Research*, 30(10), 695–704.

Sparling, T. M., Henschke, N., Nesbitt, R. C., & Gabrysch, S. (2017). The role of diet and nutritional supplementation in perinatal depression: A systematic review. *Maternal & Child Nutrition*, 13(1).

Sparling, T. M., Nesbitt, R. C., Henschke, N., & Gabrysch, S. (2017). Nutrients and perinatal depression: A systematic review. *Journal of Nutritional Science*, 6(61).

Strøm, M., Mortensen, E. L., Halldorsson, T. I., Thorsdottir, I., & Olsen, S. F. (2009). Fish and long-chain n-3 polyunsaturated fatty acid intakes during pregnancy and risk of postpartum depression: A prospective study based on a large national birth cohort. *The American Journal of Clinical Nutrition*, 90(1), 149–155.

Preconception

Bao, W., Bowers, K., Tobias, D., Olsen, S. F., Chavarro, J., Vaag, A., Kiely, M., & Zhang, C. (2014) Prepregnancy low-carbohydrate dietary pattern and risk of gestational diabetes mellitus: a prospective cohort study. *American Journal of Obstetrics and Gynecology*, 99(6), 1378–84.

Bhutta, Z. A., Das, J. K., Rizvi, A., Gaffey, M. F., Walker, N., Horton, S., Webb, P., Lartey, A., & Black, R. E. (2013). Evidence-based interventions for improvement of maternal and child nutrition: What can be done and at what cost? *The Lancet*, 382 (9890), 452–77.

Gardiner, P., Nelson, L., Shellhaas, C. S., Dunlop, A. L., Long, R., Andrist, S., & Jack, B. W. (2008). The clinical content of preconception care: nutrition and dietary supplements. *American Journal of Obstetrics and Gynecology*, 199(6), S345–56.

Grieger, J. A., Grzeskowiak, L. E., & Clifton, V. L. (2014). Preconception dietary patterns in human pregnancies are associated with preterm delivery. *The Journal of Nutrition*, 144(7), 1075–80.

Maconochie, N., Doyle, P., Prior S., & Simmons R. (2007). Risk factors for first trimester miscarriage — results from a UK-population-based case-control study. *BJOG: An International Journal of Obstetrics & Gynaecology*, 114(2), 170–86.

McMillen, I. C., MacLaughlin, S. M., Muhlhausler, B. S., Gentili, S., Duffield, J. L., & Morrison, J. L. (2008). Developmental origins of adult health and disease: the role of periconceptional and foetal nutrition. *Basic & Clinical Pharmacology & Toxicology*, 102(2), 82–89.

Schoenaker, D. A., Soedamah-Muthu, S. S., Callaway, L. K., & Mishra, G. D. (2015). Prepregnancy dietary patterns and risk of developing hypertensive disorders of pregnancy: results from the Australian Longitudinal Study on Women's Health. *American Journal of Clinical Nutrition*, 102(1), 94–101.

Tobias, D. K., Zhang, C., Chavarro, J., Bowers, K., Rich-Edwards, J., Rosner, B., Mozaffarian, D., & Hu, F. B. (2012). Prepregnancy adherence to dietary patterns and lower risk of gestational diabetes mellitus. *American Journal of Clinical Nutrition*, 96(2), 289–95.

Protein

Elango, R. & Ball, R. O. (2016) Protein and Amino Acid Requirements during Pregnancy. *Advances in Nutrition*, 7(4), 839(S)–844(S).

Red Raspberry Leaf Tea

Parsons, M., Simpson, M., & Ponton, T. (1999). Raspberry leaf and Its effect on labour: Safety and efficacy. *Australian College of Midwives Incorporated Journal,* 12(3), 20–25.

Simpson, M., Parsons, M., Greenwood, J., & Wade, K. (2001). Raspberry leaf in pregnancy: Its Safety and efficacy in labor. *J Midwifery Women's Health*, 46(2), 51–59.

Soft Cheeses

Desai, R. W. & Smith, M. A. (2017). Pregnancy-related listeriosis. *Birth Defects Research*, 109(5), 324–335.

Jackson, K. A., Gould, L. H., Hunter, J. C., Kucerova, Z., & Jackson, B. (2018). Listeriosis Outbreaks associated with soft cheeses, United States, 1998–2014. *Emerging Infectious Diseases*, 24(6), 1116–1118.

Moran, L. J., Verwiel, Y., Khomami, M. B., Roseboom, T. J., & Painter, R. C. (2018). Nutrition and listeriosis during pregnancy: a systematic review. *Journal of Nutritional Science*, 7(25).

Staying Healthy

Rondanelli, M., Miccono, A., Lamburghini, S., Avanzato, I., Riva, A., Allegrini, P., Faliva, M. A., Perioni, G., Nichetti, M., & Perna, S. (2018). Self Care for Common Colds: The Pivotal Role of Vitamin D, Vitamin C, Zinc, and Echinacea in Three Main Immune Interactive Clusters (Physical Barriers, Innate and Adaptive Immunity) Involved during an Episode of Common Colds – Practical Advice on Dosages and on the Time to Take These Nutrients/Botanicals in order to Prevent or Treat Common Colds. *Evidence Based Complementary and Alternative Medicine.*

Vitamin A

Azais-Braesco, V. & Pascal, G. (2000). Vitamin A in pregnancy: requirements and safety limits. *The American Journal of Clinical Nutrition*, 71(5), 1325S–1333S.

Vitamin B6

Ebrahimi, N., Maltepe, C., & Einarson, A. (2010). Optimal management of nausea and vomiting of pregnancy. *International Journal of Women's Health*, 2, 241–248.

Water

American Pregnancy Association. Premature & Preterm Labour. Retrieved from: https://americanpregnancy.org/labor-and-birth/premature-labor/

Zhang, N., Zhang, F., Chen, S., Han, F., Lin, G., Zhai, Y., He, H., Zhang, J., & Ma, G. (2020). Associations between hydration state and pregnancy complications, maternal-infant outcomes: protocol of a prospective observational cohort study. *BMC Pregnancy and Childbirth*, 20 (1), 82.

IMAGE CREDITS

[cover: border–Magnia; endpaper–sorninai; 4: pomegranates–Studio PhotoDFlorez; 11: food–Natalia Lisovskaya; 13: oatmeal–Foxys Forest Manufacture; 14: almond flour–M. Unal Ozmen; ghee–Robyn Mackenzie; heart note–Peter Hermes Furian; honey–New Africa; olive oil–baibaz; organic flour–New Africa; syrup–PhenomenalPhoto; 15: broccoli–Nataly Studio; chocolate–rvlsoft; eggs–Olexandr Panchenko; flax–xpixel; lentils–pukao; raspberries–mayakova; salmo–Smit; 15: spinach–New Africa] Shutterstock.com; 17: pregnancy test–LumiNola/iStock.com; [18: toast–Rimma Bondarenko; 19: blueberries–Zeeking; peanut butter–bigacis; 20: peas–domnitsky; quinoa–Nataly Studio; seeds–Aitormmfoto; 21: jello–SunnyToys; nuts–Fascinadora; 22: ginger–Nataly Studio; ginger–Nataly Studio; lemons–Nataly Studio; marble–nattha99; 23: mangold–StudioPhotoDFlorez; pineapple–Nataly Studio; spinach–Fascinadora; sunflower seeds–milart; 24: avocados–baibaz; bananas–mayakova; olives–Spalnic; pickled–Chamille White; sauerkraut–BW Folsom; 25: fork–nevodka; napkin–Duplass; 26: clocks–Stephanie Frey; 28: berries–MaraZe; egg avocado–Elena Shashkina; kitchen–Didecs; 29: edamame–SOMMAI; waffles–Air Kanlaya; 31: grey table–KREUS; note card–Brumarina; spinach–Smit; 32: ginger tea–K.Decor] Shutterstock.com; 75: pregnant belly–PeopleImages/iStock.com; [76: chickpeas–timquo; garlic–Tim UR; ginger–Lotus Images; honey–Jr images; inhaling steam–goodbishop; orange–Tim UR; tea–Aleksey Patsyuk; 77: chips–Indigo Photo Club; food background–VICUSCHKA; ice cream–MaraZe; pickle–domnitsky; 78: smoothies–Olga Pink; 79: woman pouring smoothie–wavebreakmedia; 80: vegetables–casanisa; 82: burrito–vitals; quiche–RESTOCK images; salad–Magdanatka; 83: sack cloth–Maryia_K; texture pattern–StevanZZ; tomatoes–Svetlana Serebryakova] Shutterstock.com; 121: pregnant woman_iS-damircudic/iStock.com; [122: pregnant woman–Syda Productions; 123: blackberry smoothie–baibaz; soup–Julija Lavrinaite; tea–isak55; water wave–Olga Nikonova; water–Palo_ok; 124: eggs–Bozena Fulawka; herring–Angorius; olive oil–Valentyn Volkov; steak–YARUNIV Studio; sunflower seeds–Katerina Voevodskaya] Shutterstock.com; 125: chopping–hobo/iStock.com; [126: cookware–New Africa; 128: packing–Onjira Leibe; 129: napkin–MaraZe; table–Artur Sipachov] Shutterstock.com; 167: mother–Nastasic/iStock.com; [168: woman napping–Syda Productions; 169: broth–Anna Hoychuk; iced coffee–baibaz; pizza–bestv; strawberries–Nataly Studio; sushi–Evikka; 171: crying–paulaphoto; 173: broth–Fattyplace; 174: beef–nadianb; olives–nadianb; 175: water–Joshua Resnick; 176: food rainbow–Denise I Johnson; 177: salmon–New Africa; 178: containers–New Africa; 179: table–primopiano] Shutterstock.com.

INDEX

RECIPES FOR SPECIAL DIETARY NEEDS

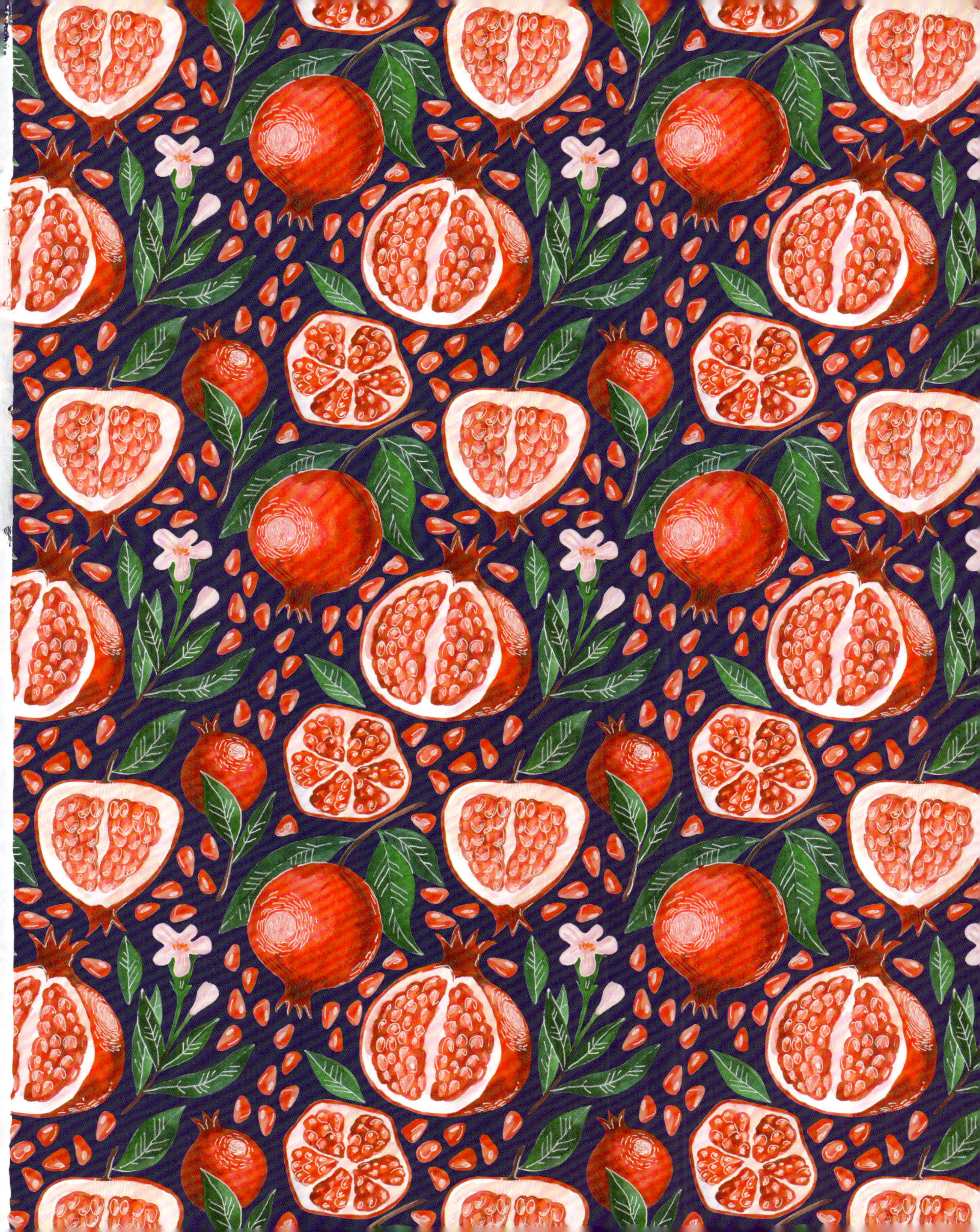

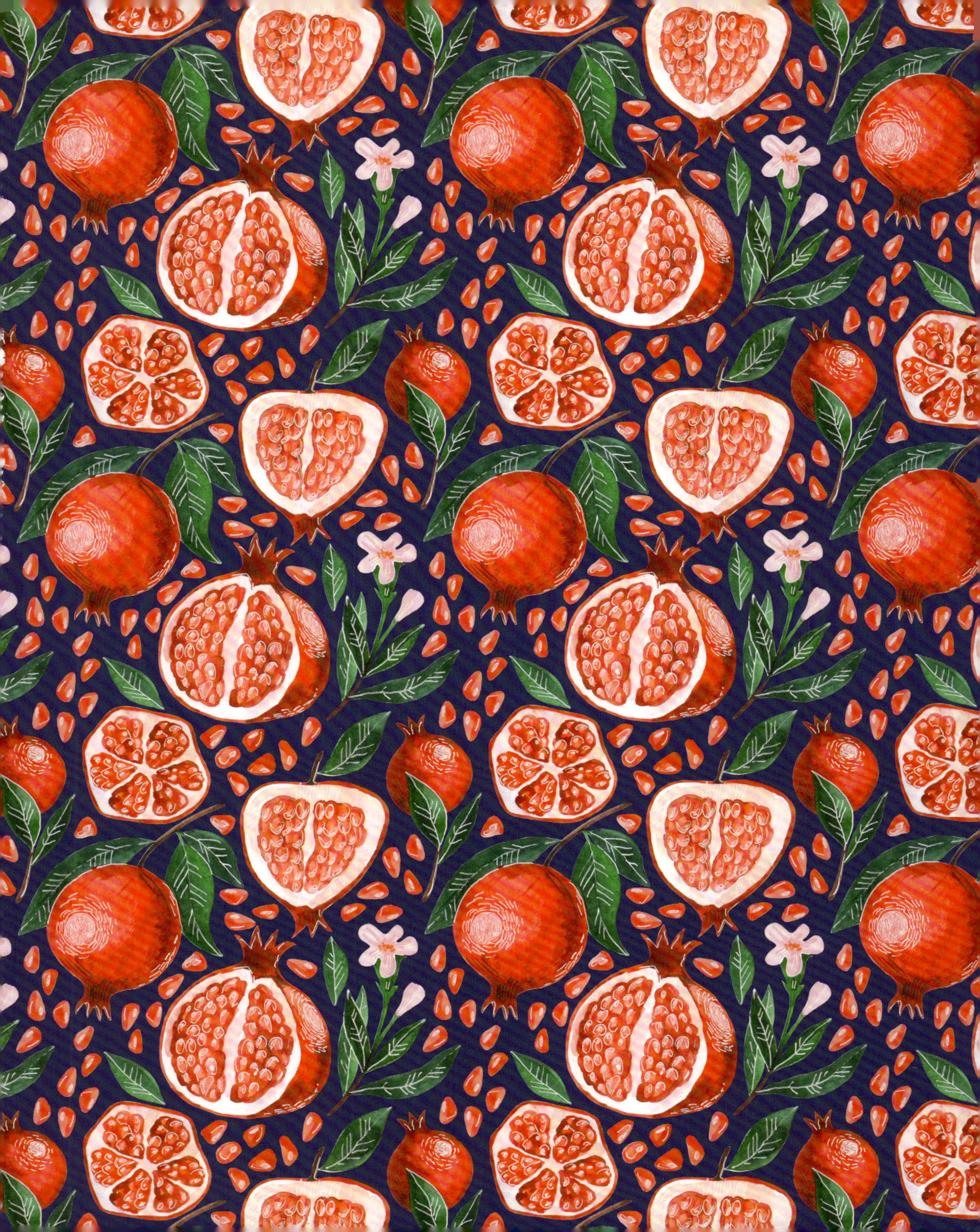